Amyotrophic Lateral Sclerosis

A Comprehensive Guide to Management

Amyotrophic Lateral Sclerosis

A Comprehensive Guide to Management

EDITED BY

Hiroshi Mitsumoto, M.D.

ALS Center and Neuromuscular Program
Department of Neurology
Cleveland Clinic Foundation
Cleveland, Ohio

and

Forbes H. Norris, M.D.

ALS Research Foundation
San Francisco, California

Demos Publications, 386 Park Avenue South, New York, New York 10016

Library of Congress Cataloging-in-Publication Data

Amyotrophic lateral sclerosis : a comprehensive guide to management /
  edited by Hiroshi Mitsumoto and Forbes H. Norris.
    p.   cm.
  Includes index.
  ISBN 0-939957-58-2 (pbk.) : $39.95
  1. Amyotrophic lateral sclerosis. I. Mitsumoto, Hiroshi.
II. Norris, Forbes H. (Forbes Holten), 1928—
  [DNLM: 1. Amyotrophic Lateral Sclerosis—congresses. WE 550
A5306 1994]
RC406.A24A478 1994
616.8′3—dc20
DNLM/DLC
for Library of Congress   94-13438
                                     CIP

Made in the United States of America

Preface

The science of amyotrophic lateral sclerosis (ALS) has been heightened as never before. In addition to increased media coverage of the disease and those afflicted with it, each year local, national, and international conferences are being held to study advances in the search for a cause and possible cure.

Although it is obvious that the science of ALS, as well as related diseases, is going through a period of awareness and progress, unfortunately this had not yet led to an effective treatment. For most patients, the prognosis is dim. We take refuge in the long survivals of some and perhaps the erroneous diagnosis of others, but on the whole, clinical diagnosis is usually reliable, and for the vast number of those so diagnosed, the ultimate result is fatal.

The question before us, then, is can ALS be managed and managed successfully? The answer is definitely yes. There is a great deal that can be done to treat the symptoms of ALS, to improve the quality of life of a patient, and to help caregivers and the family cope with the disease.

Where can physicians, patients, caregivers, and family members look to get this information? Where do they go for guidance, for comprehensive and practical advice? We have both been confronted with this problem in the past, and this book is the result.

We have assembled materials from a group of leading professionals who have worked with ALS. What you will find is each aspect of the management of ALS covered in detail, with the best possible approach to measures that will be most helpful to all—to physicians, other health care professionals, patients, caregivers, and family members.

Each chapter is complete in its in-depth analysis of the issues involving the management of amyotrophic lateral sclerosis. From the physician's viewpoint, we look at the classification and clinical features of ALS, its diagnosis, care of patients, therapeutic trials, and unorthodox treatments. There is a probing study of speech problems and physical therapy. Nutrition and environmental adaptations are also very important to the well-being of the patient. For caregivers, family members, and other health care professionals, we investigate ventilatory care in the hospital and at home, nursing care, long-term care, financial resources, and the role played by support groups. There is much more to the intricate portrait of ALS, with an all-encompassing look at hospital care, life support systems, legal, ethical, psychosocial, and spiritual overviews. We close with the role of the national voluntary health agency—so important in all aspects of dealing with the puzzle of ALS.

Some may call our efforts a stopgap medical approach, but without hope there would be no life. And we are talking here about more time. We are talking about tomorrow. Someone once said, "Tomorrow is the most important thing in life. It comes into us at midnight very clean. It's perfect when it arrives and puts itself in our hands. It hopes we've learned something from yesterday."

H. M.
F. H. N.

Acknowledgments

It has been a true privilege and a delight to co-edit this book with Dr. Forbes H. Norris, who was undoubtedly the foremost authority on ALS patient care. Only with his tireless and masterful help have I managed to co-edit this book. The theme of this entire book is *care*. This echoes the teaching of my own mentors, Dr. Joseph M. Foley and Dr. Walter G. Bradley, who always maintained that *care* comes before anything else for the desperately ill.

The ALS symposium on which this book is based was held in Cleveland in June 1991 and was initiated by the ALS Association. Lynn M. Klein, Vice President of the Association, has been instrumental in making possible the publication of this book. We also express our special gratitude to Dr. Lewis P. Rowland for his support of the symposium. We very much appreciate Dr. Diana M. Schneider, President of Demos Publications, for her strong encouragement and continuous support throughout the project.

We are especially grateful to each chapter author, all of whom made excellent contributions despite tight time constraints. We are indebted to Mrs. Mary Kay Schoepf and Ms. Teri Mohar for their secretarial help. We also greatly appreciate Joan Wolk of Demos Publications for her patience and help in the production of the book. Lastly, I personally thank my family for their support.

Hiroshi Mitsumoto

Dedication

This book is dedicated to Forbes H. Norris, Jr. (May 1, 1928–June 18, 1993), a steadfast warrior who took up the charge against ALS and made a difference in the lives of many.

"It is surmounting difficulties that makes heroes."

Louis Kossuth

Contents

Contributors

Helen Ann Bower, M.S.W., L.C.S.W., Director, Psychosocial Services, Kimberly Quality Care Hospice, 10789 Santa Monica Boulevard, Suite 395, Los Angeles, California 90025-4732

Walter G. Bradley, D.M., F.R.C.P., Department of Neurology, University of Miami, P.O. Box 016960, Miami, Florida 33101

Mark B. Bromberg, M.D., Ph.D., Motor Neuron Disease Clinic, Department of Neurology, University of Michigan Medical Center, 1500 East Medical Center Drive, Ann Arbor, Michigan 48109-0316

Eileen Carr-Davis, R.D., L.D., Cleveland Clinic Foundation, 9500 Euclid Avenue, Cleveland, Ohio 44195

Hideaki Hayashi, M.D., Department of Neurology, Tokyo Metropolitan Neurological Hospital, 3-18-22, Honkomagome, Bunkyo-Ku, Tokyo, Japan

Patricia Heidkamp Casey, M.S., O.T.R/L, ALSA Center, University of Chicago, Les Turner Foundation, MDA Clinics, Chicago, Illinois

Marlene A. Ciechoscki, M.S., R.N., 314 Park Lane, Wilmington, Delaware 19804-2353

Ann Kuckelman Cobb, Ph.D., R.N., School of Nursing, University of Kansas Medical Center, 39th and Rainbow Boulevard, Kansas City, Kansas 66103

Karen L. Fernengel, R.N., M.N., St. Mary College, 4100 S. Fourth Street Trafficway, Leavenworth, Kansas 66048

Brian Gould, M.D., United HealthCare Corporation, 9900 Bren Road East, P.O. Box 1459, Minneapolis, Minnesota 55440

Mark R. Glasberg, M.D., Marcus J. Lawrence Medical Center, 202 South Willard Road, Cottonwood, Arizona 86326

Catherine M. Howell, M.S., P.T., 574 North Trigo Lane, Paso Robles, California 93446

Sany T. Khabbaz, M.D., Department of Neurology, University of Chicago, 5841 South Maryland Avenue, Chicago, Illinois 60637

Lynn M. Klein, Vice President for Patient Services, the ALS Association, 21021 Ventura Boulevard, Suite 321, Woodland Hills, California 91364

Barbara T. Beal Libby, R.N., M.N., P.H.N., 5973 Coit Avenue N.E., Grand Rapids, Michigan 49505-1147

James M. Mancinelli, M.S., CCC-SL P/L, Department of Orthopedic Surgery and Rehabilitation, and the ALS Clinic, Hahnemann University Hospital, Broad and Vine Streets, Philadelphia, Pennsylvania 19102

Evelyn R. McDonald, M.S., The New Road Map Foundation, P.O. Box 15981, Seattle, Washington 98115

Kristen O'Donovan, L.S.W., Department of Social Work, Cleveland Clinic Foundation, 9500 Euclid Avenue, Cleveland, Ohio 44195

Hiroshi Mitsumoto, M.D., ALS Center and Neuromuscular Program, Department of Neurology, Cleveland Clinic Foundation, 9500 Euclid Avenue, Cleveland, Ohio 44195-5226

N. Michael Murphy, M.D., St. Peter's Hospice, 315 South Manning Boulevard, Albany, New York, 12208

Forbes H. Norris, M.D., ALS Research Foundation, 2351 Clay Street, San Francisco, California 94115 (deceased)

Edward Anthony Oppenheimer, M.D., Pulmonary and Critical Care Medicine, Southern California Permanente Group, 4950 Sunset Boulevard, Los Angeles, California 90027-5822

Mary Beth Parks, R.N., Gulf Coast Medical Personnel, P.O. Box 5965, Kingwood, Texas 77325-5965

JoAnn B. Reckling, R.N., M.N., M.A., University of Kansas School of Nursing, 39th and Rainbow Boulevard, Kansas City, Kansas 66103

Raymond P. Roos, M.D., Department of Neurology, University of Chicago, 5841 South Maryland Avenue, Chicago, Illinois 60637

Lewis P. Rowland, M.D., Department of Neurology, Columbia University College of Physicians and Surgeons, 710 West 168th Street, New York, New York 10032

Barbara Thompson, O.T.R., ALS Regional Center, St. Peter's Hospital, 315 South Manning Boulevard, Albany, New York 12208

1

Classification and Clinical Features of Amyotrophic Lateral Sclerosis

Hiroshi Mitsumoto, M.D.

Charcot (1) published the first full account of the clinical and pathological features of amyotrophic lateral sclerosis (ALS) in 1874. His description of the clinical and histopathologic aspects of the disease is thorough and valid. Although we have accumulated an incredible amount of new information about this disease in the past 120 years, ALS remains enigmatic.

The terms *amyotrophic lateral sclerosis* and *motor neuron disease* (MND) are often used interchangeably, but MND usually refers to a broad, heterogeneous group of clinical syndromes that include ALS (2). Motor neuron disease thus encompasses disorders of motor neurons in the spinal cord, brainstem, and cerebral motor cortex that are manifested by muscular weakness, atrophy, and corticospinal tract signs in varying combinations. ALS is the most common MND syndrome among adults and refers specifically to a relentlessly progressive, generalized, and fatal wasting disease of skeletal muscle that in the sporadic, classical form has a focal onset and is accompanied by fasciculations and spasticity (3,4). In addition to these clinical signs, the syndrome includes the corresponding characteristic pathological changes of lower and upper motor neuron degeneration (5).

The clinical signs and outcome of the disease are generally consistent, and the diagnosis of ALS is made with impressive uniformity in the clinical practice (6). However, it is also true that misdiagnosis in patients with ALS is not at all rare, particularly in its early stages or when it presents with atypical features (7,8). In fact, the true clinical limits of ALS still remain unclear (6). Given the increasing research activities and clinical trials on patients with ALS in recent years, it is imperative that we use uniform diagnostic criteria for ALS (9). Otherwise we cannot fully interpret the information and data on ALS, not only in patient care but also in research in general. This chapter describes the classification of ALS, its clinical signs and symptoms, its diagnostic criteria, and its prognosis.

Classification of ALS

The classification of MNDs presented by the World Federation of Neurology is based on heredity and presumed causes (10). This classification provides a long and complete list of MNDs, in which "sporadic" ALS is classified in the category of undetermined cause. In this chapter we use a more clinical classification of ALS (Table 1-1). These syndromes are described below.

Amyotrophic Lateral Sclerosis

Amyotrophic lateral sclerosis (ALS) was distinguished by Charcot in the 1860s from the condition known heretofore as progressive muscular atrophy, which had been described earlier by Aran in 1850 (11) and Duchenne in 1855 (12). Charcot subsequently established ALS as a separate entity (1,13).

The average age of onset is the mid-fifties but varies considerably and ranges from the late teens to the eighties. The incidence of age-specific mortality rates increases to ages seventy to seventy-four and then declines (6,14). Although a

Table 1-1. Classification of Amyotrophic Lateral Sclerosis

1. Sporadic ALS
    A. Classical ALS
    B. Progressive bulbar palsy (PBP)
    C. Progressive muscular atrophy (PMA)
    D. Primary lateral sclerosis (PLS)
2. Familial ALS
3. Western Pacific ALS/Parkinson's Disease/Dementia Complex
4. Juvenile ALS with Intracytoplasmic Inclusions
5. ALS-Like Motor Neuron Diseases with Definable Causes
    Polyradiculopathy/myelopathy
    Post-polio syndrome
    Motor neuropathy with anti-GM_1 antibody
    MND and gammopathy/paraproteinemia
    Heavy metal intoxication
    Hexosaminidase-A deficiency
    Paraneoplastic motor neuronopathy syndrome
    Syringomyelia/syringobulbia

study done in Rochester, Minnesota, suggested that the incidence of ALS increases with age (15), this trend has not been found in other epidemiological studies (16,17).

Men are somewhat more frequently affected with ALS than women, the ratio ranging from 1.2:1 to 1.6:1. The annual incidence rate of classical ALS is 0.4 to 2.4 per 100,000 population and is remarkably uniform throughout the world (14). Data compiled by Kurtzke (14) suggest an increased incidence worldwide since the early 1970s. This increase does not seem to be explained by increased recognition of the disease or improvement in diagnosis. A few reports of "clusters" of a small number of ALS cases in unusual settings have been reported and at times have been highly publicized. However, the epidemiological significance of such small clusters is still unknown.

ALS without family history is called sporadic ALS. ALS may be subclassified in the following forms (18,19):

Classical ALS is the ALS that was originally described by Charcot (1), and thus it is often called Charcot's disease in Europe. Classical ALS is a distinct syndrome characterized by a combination of upper motor neuron and lower motor neuron involvement. Table 1-2 describes the diagnostic criteria for classical ALS proposed by the World Federation of Neurology (9). In approximately two-thirds of patients with ALS, the disease takes this classical form.

Progressive bulbar palsy (PBP) was originally described by Duchenne in 1860 (20). In approximately 25 percent of patients with ALS, the initial symptoms begin in muscles innervated by the lower brainstem cranial nerves in or near the medulla that control articulation, mastication, and deglutition. Sometimes the disease remains in this form for years, but usually it progresses to generalized muscle weakness, that is, to ALS. When the disease is strictly

Table 1-2. Diagnostic Criteria of ALS (World Federation of Neurology El Escorial Criteria*)

A. The diagnosis of ALS *requires* the *presence* of
  1. Signs of lower motor neuron (LMN) degeneration by clinical, electrophysiological, or neuropathological examination;
  2. Signs of upper motor neuron (UMN) degeneration by clinical examination; and
  3. Progressive spread of signs within a region or to other regions.
B. Together with the *absence* of
  1. Electrophysiological evidence of other disease processes that might explain the signs of LMN and/or UMN degeneration; and
  2. Neuroimaging evidence of other disease processes that might explain the observed clinical and electrophysiological signs.

---

* The criteria are discussed in Brooks et al. (9).

limited to the bulbar muscles clinically and electrodiagnostically, it is PBP, not classical ALS.

Patients with *progressive muscular atrophy* (PMA) constitute roughly 8 percent to 10 percent of patients with sporadic ALS. PMA is sometimes called Aran-Duchenne type of MND (11,12). The initial symptoms are manifestations of lower motor neuron involvement of the spinal cord and, in a later stage, of the lower brainstem. If upper motor neuron disease does not develop within two years, the disease is likely to remain PMA.

Primary lateral sclerosis (PLS) was first described by Erb in 1875 (21). The clinical signs of PLS consist only of upper motor neuron signs. It is the rarest of all the forms of ALS, and in fact there are very few autopsy-proven cases (22,23). It is said that the disease will stay in this form if no lower motor neuron signs have developed within two years after onset. However, we have seen clinically "typical" PLS progress to ALS after eight years. To establish the diagnosis of PLS, all other causes of myelopathy must be excluded.

Whether the above forms of sporadic ALS represent a spectrum of the same disease or whether they are in fact distinct is not yet known (6). However, autopsy studies often find both upper and lower motor neuron involvement in cases where clinical examination showed one but not the other (24). Thus, the diagnosis and classification of these forms based solely on neurological examination may not be definitive.

Familial Amyotrophic Lateral Sclerosis

Familial ALS cases comprise 5–10 percent of all cases of ALS (25). Familial ALS is inherited as an autosomal dominant trait with high penetrance in most cases. Recent molecular genetic studies located the abnormal gene to be in Cu/Zn superoxide dismutase gene on the long arm of chromosome 21 (26). Autopsy studies show that familial ALS involves the posterior columns, Clarke's columns, and the spinocerebellar tracts more frequently than sporadic ALS, indicating that sporadic and familial ALS are different (5). However, there are no differences between familial and sporadic ALS on neurological examination: the identification of another family member with ALS is the sole distinguishing factor (25).

Western Pacific Amyotropic Lateral Sclerosis

A fifty- to one hundred-fold increase in ALS among the Chamorro people on the island of Guam was observed in the 1950s (27). A similar cluster has been noted in the Kii Peninsula of Japan and in two isolated groups who live on New Guinea. The ALS patients on Guam have the same clinical characteristics seen in sporadic ALS. The most unique feature of this form of ALS, however, is the presence of neurofibrillary tangles in the central nervous system (CNS) (5).

On Guam, another CNS disease called Parkinson's disease-dementia complex (PD-complex) is also characterized histologically by the widespread presence of CNS neurofibrillary tangles (5). PD-complex occurs concurrently with ALS, not only in the same Chamorro family, but even in the same patient. The incidence of this form of ALS, however, has drastically fallen in recent years (28). The unique mineral composition of soil and water and exposure to the neurotoxin cycasin in food substances have been implicated as potential causes (28,29). Rare cases of ALS that clinically and neuropathologically resemble Western Pacific ALS/PD-complex have been reported in the rest of the world, suggesting that this specific ALS form may not be restricted to the Western Pacific (5,30).

Juvenile Amyotropic Lateral Sclerosis

Exceedingly rare cases of adolescent MND that are clinically and neuropathologically indistinguishable from ALS except for basophilic intracytoplasmic inclusions in upper and lower motor neurons have been reported. Onset is between ages twelve and sixteen (31). Although ALS perhaps can occur at such young ages, these cases are probably different from sporadic ALS.

ALS-Like Motor Neuron Diseases with Definable Causes

When we deal with the potential diagnosis of ALS, which has a dismal prognosis, it is essential to exclude treatable diseases and other less severe diseases, although they are very rare (32) (see Chapters 2 and 3).

A combination of *chronic cervical and lumbosacral polyradiculopathy and spondylitic myelopathy* can cause a variety of upper and lower motor neuron signs without sensory symptoms and can closely resemble ALS. Particularly when bulbar signs are absent in patients with ALS, this polyradiculopathy myelopathy is the most frequent condition to be distinguished from ALS. Neuroimaging tests, such as MRI, of the appropriate portion of the spinal cord and electrodiagnostic tests are crucial to the diagnosis.

Post-poliomyelitic muscular atrophy is characterized by progressive muscle atrophy and weakness that develops at least fifteen years after recovery from acute poliomyelitis (33). It usually affects the muscles previously affected by polio. In general it does not cause upper motor neuron signs and remains focal and asymmetric. Nevertheless, unsuspected spondylitic cervical myelopathy can cause misleading upper motor neuron signs in patients who have otherwise typical post-poliomyelitic muscular atrophy. Wear and tear in surviving motor neurons years after polio infection is believed to be the main process of this condition. However, recently an aberrant immunological process has been implicated in post-poliomyelitis (34).

Motor neuropathy with high anti-ganglioside (anti-GM$_1$ and anti-asialo GM$_1$)

antibodies is manifested as predominantly lower motor neuron disease with multifocal conduction block on electrodiagnostic studies (35). This condition is potentially treatable, particularly with cyclophosphamide (Cytoxan) (35) and perhaps with intravenous immunoglobulin. However, anti-ganglioside antibodies themselves are found in other conditions, including demyelinating polyneuropathy, connective tissue disease, and ALS (36,37,38). We have seen a patient with "classical" ALS who had high anti-asialo GM_1 antibodies. His muscle strength improved over several months with long-term intravenous immunoglobulin therapy. It is possible that ALS with high titers of anti-GM_1 antibody may differ from classical ALS.

Monoclonal gammopathy is more frequently found in patients with ALS than in the general population of similar age groups (39). *IgM paraproteinemia* also is reported in rare cases of MND of predominantly lower motor neuron involvement. Aggressive immunotherapy may improve these MNDs. Evidence that some patients with ALS have monoclonal gammopathy, positive anti-GM_1 antibody, or both, led to a hypothesis that ALS is an unconventional autoimmune disease (40).

Lead intoxication may cause pure demyelinating motor neuropathy, whereas *chronic mercury intoxication* is reported to produce upper and lower motor neuron signs along with other CNS manifestations (32). We screen for heavy metals only when patients with ALS report potential exposure in the past or when the disease is sufficiently atypical.

Adult hexosaminidase-A deficiency is associated with protean CNS manifestations. It causes pure lower motor neuron disease, which mimics spinal muscular atrophy, but the disease can resemble ALS when both upper and lower motor neurons are involved (41). In this rare condition, there are almost always other neurological manifestations, such as ataxia, dementia, or peripheral neuropathy, suggesting that the disease is a multisystem degeneration. The screening test should be done when ALS has atypical features; that is, young age of onset and signs suggesting multisystem involvement (41).

ALS is rarely associated with cancer. However, subacute paraneoplastic MND definitely exists. We have seen two patients with small-cell lung cancer and positive antineuronal antibodies in whom rapidly progressive generalized upper and lower motor neuron signs developed (42,43). At autopsy the gray matter of the spinal cord revealed unusually prominent reactive gliosis and neuronal degeneration, along with the features of limbic encephalopathy. Hodgkin's lymphoma and other lymphomas or leukemias are also associated with predominantly lower motor neuron disease (44). Some cases show definite upper motor neuron signs. The clinical course in most cases appears to be benign.

Several other conditions cause various motor syndromes, including *hyperthyroid* and *hyperparathyroid diseases* and *diabetes mellitus*. *Syringomyelia* and *syringobulbia* can cause a combination of upper and lower motor neuron signs.

A detailed discussion of the differential diagnoses is included in Chapters 2 and 3.

Clinical Signs and Symptoms of ALS

Table 1-3 lists the common signs and symptoms of ALS.

Upper Motor Neuron Signs

Upper motor neurons reside predominantly in the precentral motor cortex. Giant Betz motor neurons are among the largest neurons. They control direct volitional muscle contraction and constitute less than 5 percent of all nerve fibers

Table 1-3. Clinical Signs and Symptoms of ALS

Upper Motor Neuron Signs
  Spasticity
  Hyperreflexia
  Pathological reflexes (Babinski's sign)
Lower Motor Neuron Signs
  Muscle weakness
  Truncal muscle weakness
  Muscle atrophy
  Fasciculations
  Hyporeflexia
  Hypotonicity or flaccidity
  Muscle cramps
Bulbar Signs
  Dysarthria
  Dysphagia
  Sialorrhea (drooling)
  Pseudobulbar signs
Respiratory Signs
Other Signs
  Fatigue
  Weight loss and ALS cachexia
  Tendon shortening
  Joint contracture
Uncommon Manifestations
  Dementia
  Sensory impairment
  Ocular palsy
  Bladder and bowel dysfunction
  Decubiti

arising from the motor cortex. Disease or functional impairment in these neurons, their nerve fibers [corticopontine, corticobulbar, and corticospinal (pyramidal) tracts], or both, causes upper motor neuron symptoms and signs.

Spasticity

Spasticity is a state of sustained increase in tension of a muscle when it is lengthened. For example, in spasticity, if one contracts a muscle, the antagonist muscle suddenly increases in tension instead of relaxing, preventing the normal uniform muscle contraction. Spasticity is associated with the loss of or release from the normal inhibiting action of the pyramidal system on the anterior horn cells (45). It is difficult to evaluate muscle strength in a muscle with significant spasticity.

Hyperreflexia

Muscle stretch reflexes are easily elicited in healthy persons. When the pyramidal system is affected, these reflexes are exaggerated. In hyperreflexia, only a slight or distant stimulus is needed to elicit a reflex response. For example, tendon-tapping (muscle-stretch) causes reflexes in neighboring muscles (spreading), and stretching muscle tendons induces sustained clonus (repeated rhythmic muscle contractions). If these responses are elicited, the muscle-stretch reflexes are abnormal (45). In ALS, one finds a unique situation: severely wasted, nearly paralyzed muscles have markedly brisk reflexes. A variety of cutaneous reflexes, such as the superficial abdominal reflexes and cremasteric reflexes, are intact in ALS

Extensor Plantar Reflex

When this reflex is elicited, the pyramidal tract on the same side is affected. This pathological reflex (Babinski's sign, a spontaneous extension of the great toe often accompanied by fanning of the other toes) is elicited by stroking the outer edge of the sole upwards from the heel with a fairly sharp (but not needle-sharp) object. In normal people, the great toe flexes by the same stimulation. It is intriguing to note that we often encounter patients with ALS who have generalized pathological hyperreflexia but normal plantar reflexes (3).

Lower Motor Neuron Signs

Lower motor neurons are contained in the motor cranial nerve nuclei in the brainstem and spinal cord anterior horns. Disease or functional impairment in these motor neurons or their nerve fibers that reach the innervated muscles causes lower motor neuron signs and symptoms.

Muscle Weakness

This is the cardinal sign and symptom in ALS. It is manifested not only by loss of strength, but also by fatigability, variation in strength, and diminished range of motion. Muscle weakness is also recognized by diminished rate of movement, loss of coordination, clumsiness, and lack of ability to carry out skilled acts, some of which are clearly the result of upper motor neuron impairment (45). One should remember that both upper and lower motor neuron disease causes muscle weakness.

Truncal Muscle Weakness

Whereas cervical flexor muscle weakness is seen in many muscle diseases, including muscular dystrophy and polymyositis, truncal muscle weakness involving the cervical extensor muscles is rare. When such weakness occurs, it is seen almost exclusively in myasthenia gravis and ALS. The weakness in neck extensor muscles causes heaviness of the head, and patients often hold their head with one hand so as not to let the head fall forward. In a more advanced stage of the disease, the head is completely flexed, and patients become unable to look more than a few feet away, resulting in serious impairment with feeding and breathing. A compensatory lordosis may occur as patients attempt to maintain their posture while walking. Muscle pains from overstretched neck extensor muscles are not uncommon. Electrophysiological analyses reveal evidence of active denervation in the truncal paraspinal muscles in patients with ALS (46).

Muscle Atrophy

When the impulse from motor axons no longer reaches the muscle for whatever reason, the muscle lies flaccid and no longer contracts voluntarily or reflexively. All the affected muscle fibers lose their volume and decrease in size, and as a result there is wasting of the entire muscle mass (45). Almost all ALS patients have muscle atrophy in affected muscles. A unique combination of severe muscle atrophy and pathological hyperreflexia occurs in ALS because upper and lower motor neurons are simultaneously affected. Atrophy is most frequently observed in the intrinsic hand muscles, particularly the first dorsal interosseous muscles.

Fasciculations

Fasciculations are fine, rapid, flickering, vermicular twitching movements that appear with spontaneous contraction of a bundle of muscle fibers belonging to a single motor unit. The impulse for the fasciculation appears to be generated along the entire motor axon from the cell body. However, the pathogenesis of fasciculation remains unknown. In general, the larger the muscle, the larger the size of the fasciculation. In the tongue muscles, fasciculations are small vermicular movements on the surface of the tongue.

Fasciculations are found in nearly all ALS patients but rarely are they the

Table 1-4. Presenting Symptoms and Signs of ALS*

Symptoms or Signs		Frequency (%)
Weakness		63.2%
One arm	10.7%	
One leg	11.9%	
Both arms	8.5%	
Paraparesis	19.8%	
Hemiparesis	3.8%	
Generalized	8.5%	
Atrophy		9.7%
Fasciculation		3.5%
Spasticity		1.3%
Bulbar signs		22.0%
Pain and cramps		8.8%
Paresthesia		3.5%
Weight loss		2.2%
Data not available		4.1%

* Based on 318 patients with ALS from Gubbay et al. (55), modified by permission.

presenting symptom (Table 1-4). When we cannot confirm the presence of fasciculation by clinical examination or by electromyography, we are cautious to conclude that the diagnosis is ALS. It is important to remember that fasciculations are common phenomena in many healthy persons. Thus, fasciculations without abnormal neurological findings have no clinical significance (benign fasciculations).

Hyporeflexia

If the disease involves lower motor neurons alone, the muscle stretch reflexes are sluggish or absent. When muscles become totally paralyzed or atrophied, any hyperreflexia noted earlier may disappear.

Hypotonicity or Flaccidity

Hypotonicity is a decrease or loss of normal muscle tone. The muscle lies inert, flaccid, flabby, and soft to palpation, in contrast to the spasticity seen in upper motor neuron involvement.

Muscle Cramps

In a true cramp, the abrupt, involuntary, and painful shortening of muscle is attended by visible or palpable knotting of the muscle, often with an abnormal posture of the affected joint that is relieved by stretching or massage. It is useful to adopt a practical definition when discussing this with patients: a muscle cramp is a charley horse; a sudden, involuntary, sustained muscle contraction with severe pain that interrupts activity. Nocturnal muscle cramps interrupt sleep. Like muscle fasciculations, the pathogenesis of the muscle cramp is not well understood, although it is believed to be caused by irritability of lower motor neurons. Again, it is a common phenomenon in healthy people, particularly in the calves. In ALS it occurs not only in these muscles but also in the hands, abdomen, neck, jaw, or even tongue. Muscle cramp is one of the most common symptoms in ALS, and when patients do not report having muscle cramps, one may need to be cautious about the diagnosis.

Bulbar Signs and Symptoms

Muscles controlling articulation, mastication, and deglutition are innervated by the cranial nerves VII (facial), IX (glossopharyngeal), X (vagus), and XII (hypoglossal), whose nuclei are anatomically located in the bulb (medulla). Cranial nerve V (trigeminal) is usually also included because it controls jaw movement (45). When these brainstem motor neurons are primarily affected, the condition is called "paretic" or "flaccid bulbar palsy," whereas when upper motor neurons and their descending tracts, the corticobulbar tracts, are affected, "spastic bulbar palsy" develops. In ALS, a mixed bulbar palsy, consisting of a varying mixture of spastic and paretic components, is usual. In the pure paretic form, facial muscles are flaccid; the tongue is atrophied and fasciculating, and the gag reflex and jaw reflex are absent. Contrary to the paretic form, in spastic bulbar palsy (or pseudobulbar palsy), facial atrophy and weakness are absent; the tongue is not wasted and fasciculating; and the gag reflex and jaw reflex are pathologically brisk.

Dysarthria

Impaired articulation is called dysarthria, which again can be spastic, flaccid, or mixed. Initial complaints include the inability to yell or sing, a weakening voice, and slurring of speech. When the vocal cords become paretic, the voice sounds hoarse or weak. When the velopharyngeal port is incompetent, air leaks into the nose and the voice sounds nasal. On the other hand, in spastic dysarthria the voice sounds as if it is produced by effort through a narrowed upper airway. Repetitive movements of the lips, tongue, and pharynx become especially difficult. Eventually enunciation becomes more difficult, and in a more advanced stage speech becomes impossible (anarthria) (see Chapter 6).

Dysphagia

Impaired mastication and deglutition is called dysphagia. It usually follows dysarthria in ALS patients. Handling food inside the mouth becomes difficult.

Food may pool between gum and cheek, and patients may be unable to move food into the throat and may experience weak or uncoordinated movements of swallowing. Liquid is generally more difficult to swallow than solid food. Liquid may regurgitate into the nose through an incompetent velopharyngeal port. Small, dry, crumbling food is more difficult to consume than soft, smooth, consistent food. Eventually, swallowing may trigger coughing, which warns of serious dysphagia. Patients require more time to finish a meal at this stage, and eating itself becomes a major chore. When the cough reflex is weakened by flaccid paralysis of pharyngolaryngeal and respiratory muscles, the risk of aspiration of food and saliva into the airway becomes imminent (Chapter 6).

Sialorrhea (Drooling)

Patients with ALS frequently complain of drooling that is often severely disabling and embarrassing. The drooling results from the lack of spontaneous automatic swallowing to clear excessive saliva in the mouth and may result in insidious aspiration of saliva into the airway.

Pseudobulbar Palsy

The difficulties with articulation, mastication, and deglutition here are similar to those of progressive flaccid bulbar palsy, but the underlying mechanism is different. Pseudobulbar palsy is caused by bilateral lesions that interrupt the pathways of the suprasegmental fibers (corticobulbar tracts from upper motor neurons) to the bulbar nuclei (spastic bulbar palsy). Frequently, emotional control appears to be deficient, resulting in spontaneous or unmotivated crying and laughing. Some people call this symptom "emotional incontinence," but that is not a proper term because the phenomenon is not due to lack of continence. It is thought to be caused by disinhibition of the bulbar and respiratory muscles for crying or laughing.

Respiratory Symptoms

Exertional dyspnea is one of the early respiratory symptoms of ALS. Later, at rest, patients may experience excessive yawning or frequent sighing. Examination sometimes shows use of accessory respiratory muscles. The diaphragm may be particularly vulnerable in some ALS patients. They report profound dyspnea only when supine. Paradoxical respiration (the abdomen depresses instead of elevates with inspiration when supine) is found on examination in these patients. We routinely measure forced vital capacity both sitting and supine to detect the early diaphragmatic weakness in ALS patients.

On rare occasions, patients present with impending respiratory failure. As the first manifestation of ALS, this symptom is associated with a very poor prognosis. These patients often need immediate respiratory care in the intensive care unit, resulting in some delay in reaching a correct diagnosis of ALS. Rarely, sleep apnea is reported to occur when respiratory regulation in the brainstem is impaired.

Other Signs and Symptoms

Fatigue

Fatigue is a common complaint in neuromuscular diseases. In ALS, however, a fatigue identical to that which occurs in myasthenia gravis may be superimposed. The neuromuscular junctions in the muscles undergoing denervation and reinnervation are electrophysiologically unstable. Furthermore, motor axon sprouting to reinnervate denervated muscle fibers is equally unstable. Such a circumstance causes fatigue on repetitive muscle contractions (6).

Weight Loss

Progressive depletion of muscle mass and reduced caloric intake secondary either to progressive dysphagia or to loss of appetite can cause progressive weight loss in ALS patients. However, on occasion weight loss is far more profound than expected in those who have little or mild muscle wasting. This unusual weight loss is called *ALS cachexia* (3) and primarily involves the loss of body fat, ranging from 30—50 percent of body weight. ALS cachexia is a grave prognostic sign.

Tendon Shortening

The Achilles tendon can shorten in patients who have a relatively slow course of the disease because the anterior compartment muscles weaken more than the posterior compartment muscles.

Joint Contracture

Contractures develop relatively quickly in immobile fixed joints as a result of muscle paralysis. Joint contracture can cause severe pain and discomfort on voluntary action and passive movement.

Uncomon Manifestations of ALS

Dementia

Dementia is diagnosed in a few patients with otherwise classical ALS (3.5 percent). In our experience, when dementia is superimposed, the form of ALS is likely to involve bulbar muscles. Progressive dementia in ALS appears to differ from Creutzfeldt-Jakob disease (47) and Alzheimer's disease (48). It is not clear whether ALS with dementia represents a variation in expression of ALS—a point along a spectrum of the disease—or a different disease (49).

Sensory Impairment

There have been extensive investigations on the sensory system in ALS (32). Detailed morphological studies of cutaneous sensory nerves by biopsy and dorsal root ganglia by autopsy, quantitative sensory testing, and electrophysiological (somatosensory evoked potentials) analyses have all shown that the sensory system is indeed affected in ALS. We have seen a few patients with otherwise classical ALS who showed markedly abnormal sensory nerve action potentials on electrodiagnostic tests (50). Nevertheless, it is important to remember that in clinical practice ALS is a pure motor syndrome.

Ocular Palsy

Abnormalities of extraocular muscles in ALS can be detected by sophisticated ocular motility testing (32). In fact, ocular palsy develops in a surprisingly high proportion of patients with ALS who are sustained by mechanical ventilation, suggesting that ocular nuclei, which are ontogenetically older motor neurons, appear to be preserved until the late stage of this disease (51).

Bladder and Bowel Dysfunction

Special sacral motor neurons, lying in Onuf's nucleus and controlling vesicourethral sphincter muscles and the muscles of the pelvic floor, are spared in ALS (52). However, detailed analysis of bladder function reveals subtle dysfunction in patients with ALS (53).

Decubiti

When Charcot (1) described ALS in 1874, he pointed out that decubiti were not seen despite long-term bed rest. Intact sensory perception and normal cutaneous autonomic function may prevent decubiti in ALS patients. Recent studies suggest that cutaneous collagen fibrils in ALS patients differ from those of healthy people (54).

Presenting Symptoms

Gubbay et al. (55) summarized the frequency of presenting symptoms of ALS (Table 1-4). The most frequent presenting symptom is weakness, which occurs in nearly two-thirds of all patients with ALS. In the majority, the clinical presentation is typical: weakness that is focal in onset spreads rapidly to other myotomes. When the disease involves only one side of the body, however, it is called Mills' variant (hemiparetic form), which results in diagnostic difficulty (8). We have seen several patients who had upper and lower motor neuron signs in one extremity almost exclusively for a year or more before typical widespread muscle involvement ensued in the course of disease. Muscle atrophy or wasting only occurs in fewer than 10 percent of patients as the presenting symptom. Atrophy noted by patients is usually localized in intrinsic hand muscles, but sometimes generalized muscle atrophy is reported.

The second most common initial complaint is for bulbar symptoms, which occur in 22 percent of patients. Fewer than 10 percent of patients present with pains and muscle cramps but, as discussed earlier, cramps are one of the most frequent symptoms during the course of the disease. Pains and other ill-defined sensory symptoms, such as numbness and tingling, are not at all rare in ALS (6), despite the fact that the sensory system is largely spared.

Prognosis

Approximately 50 percent of ALS patients die in three to four years after the onset of symptoms; 20 percent live for five years. About 10 percent live for ten years, and a few can live for as long as twenty years (6). We believe that patients with ALS now live longer. Life expectancy is obviously low shortly after the diagnosis is established, but it gets significantly better forty-six months after onset (56). Generally speaking, life expectancy is shorter when the initial symptoms involve respiratory muscles or bulbar muscles (in paretic form) and when the patients are older. Patients who have low compound motor action potentials on electrodiagnostic studies are likely to have severe functional impairment and a poor prognosis (57). In contrast, the younger the patient, the longer the life expectancy. When the disease involves exclusively upper motor neurons, as in PLS, the prognosis is much better than in classical ALS. Prognosis is also better in the case of pure lower motor neuron disease (PMA). When bulbar symptoms are caused by pure upper motor neuron involvement (pseudobulbar palsy), the prognosis is again better. The variation of prognosis is much too great to generalize to any individual patient with ALS. It is important to remember that there are rare patients who spontaneously improve or stabilize from disease thought to be ALS (58,59).

Concluding Remarks

In the first chapter of this book, we review the fundamental aspects of ALS, namely, the classification, clinical features, diagnostic criteria, and prognosis of the disease. More detailed discussion on specific topics is available in several recently published, excellent monographs (60,61,62).

Despite the fact that we have accumulated enormous knowledge about ALS, the cause remains undetermined and, thus, a definitive classification is not available. In this chapter we have recommended a practical classification of ALS. Although such a classification is useful, it is frustrating to realize that we still do not know if conditions such as PMA and PLS are really different expressions of the same disease or truly different diseases. Daily interaction with patients with ALS fosters a sense of urgency to do something more. As a diagnostician, I believe it is important to remember that clinical acumen is the best tool for sorting out the diagnosis and classification of ALS at present. It has been said from time to time that clinical observation has little more to offer neurology; yet clinical observations continue to discover new syndromes and to reinterpret old symptoms. Careful clinical observations and analysis, therefore, continue to be crucial for both patient care in our personal experience and the study of the disease in our professional experience.

Acknowledgments

I am grateful to all the health professionals at our ALS Clinic at the Cleveland Clinic Foundation for their excellent service, dedicated care for patients, and hard work. I also express my gratitude to many patients and their families who came to see us. Tom Lang and Hershel Goren, M.D., gave helpful criticism of the manuscript.

References

1. Charcot JM. De la sclérose latérale amyotrophique. *Prog Med* 1874, 2:325–327, 341–342, and 453–455.
2. Rowland LP. Diverse forms of motor neuron disease. *Adv Neurol* 1982, 36:1–14.
3. Norris FH, Denys EH, Ü KS. Old and new clinical problems in amyotrophic lateral sclerosis. In: Tsubaki T, Toyokura Y, eds. *Amyotrophic Lateral Sclerosis*. Baltimore: University Park Press, 1979.
4. Tandan R, Bradley WG. Amyotrophic lateral sclerosis: I. Clinical features, pathology and ethical issues in management. *Ann Neurol* 1985, 18:271–280.
5. Hirano A, Hirano M, Dembitzer HM. Pathological variation and extent of the disease process in amyotrophic lateral sclerosis. In: Hudson AJ, ed. *Amyotrophic Lateral Sclerosis: Concepts in Pathogenesis and Etiology*. Toronto: Univ Toronto Press, 1990.
6. Mulder DW. Clinical limits of amyotrophic lateral sclerosis. *Adv Neurol* 1982, 36: 15–22.
7. Belsh JM, Schiffman PL. Misdiagnosis in patients with amyotrophic lateral sclerosis. *Arch Intern Med* 1990, 150:2301–2305.
8. O'Reilly DF, Brazis P, Rubino FA. The misdiagnosis of unilateral presentation of amyotrophic lateral sclerosis. *Muscle Nerve* 1982, 5:724–726.
9. Brooks BR, Sufit RL, DePaul R, Tan Y, Sanjak M, Robbins J. Design of clinical therapeutic trials in amyotrophic lateral sclerosis. *Adv Neurol* 1991, 56:521–546.
10. DeJong JMBV. The world federation of neurology classification of spinal muscular atrophies and other disorders of motor neurons. In: Vinken PJ, Bruyn GW, Klawans HL, eds. *Handbook of Clinical Neurology: Diseases of the Motor System*, Amsterdam: Elsevier, 1991.

11. Aran FA. Recherches sur une maladie non encore décrite du système musculaire (atrophie musculaire progressive). *Arch Gen Med* 1850, 24:5–35, 172–214.
12. Duchenne (de Bologne), Guillaume BA. De l'atrophie musculaire avec transformation graisseuse, *De L'électrisation Localisée.* Paris: Baillière, 1855.
13. Goldblatt D. Motor neuron disease: hitorical introduction. In: Norris FH, Kurland LT, eds. *Motor Neuron Disease: Research on Amyotrophic Lateral Sclerosis and Related Disorders.* New York, Grune and Stratton, 1969, 2–11.
14. Kurtzke JF. Risk factors in amyotrophic lateral sclerosis. *Adv Neurol* 1991, 56: 245–270.
15. Juergens SM, Kurland LT, Okazaki H, Mulder DW. ALS in Rochester, Minnesota, 1925–1977. *Neurology* 1980, 30:463–470.
16. Norris FH. Amyotrophic lateral sclerosis. In: Smith RA. *Handbook of Amyotrophic Lateral Sclerosis.* New York: Marcel Dekker, 1992, 1–38.
17. Annegers JF, Appel SH, Perkins P, Lee JR-J, Perkins P. Incidence and prevalence of amyotrophic lateral sclerosis in Harris County, Texas, 1985–1988. *Arch Neurol* 1991, 48: 589–593.
18. Rowland LP. Motor neuron diseases: the clinical syndrome. In: Mulder DW, ed. *The Diagnosis and Treatment of Amyotrophic Lateral Sclerosis,* Boston: Houghton Mifflin, 1980, 7–27.
19. Hudson AJ. Amyotrophic lateral sclerosis: clinical evidence for differences in pathogenesis and etiology. In: Hudson AJ, ed. *Amyotrophic Lateral Sclerosis: Concepts in Pathogenesis and Etiology,* Toronto: Univ Toronto Press, 1990, 108–143.
20. Duchenne (de Bologne), Guillaume BA. Paralysie musculaire progressive de la langue de voile de palais et des lèvres. *Arch Gen Med* 1860, 16:283–296,431–445.
21. Erb WA. Über einen wenig bekannten spinalen Symptomen-Complex. *Klin Woch* 1875, 12:357–359.
22. Beal MF, Richardson EP Jr. Primary lateral sclerosis. *Arch Neurol* 1981,38:630–633.
23. Younger DS, Chou S, Hays AP, et al. Primary lateral sclerosis: a clinical diagnosis reemerges. *Arch Neurol* 1988, 45:1304–1307.
24. Brownell B, Oppenheimer DR, Hughes JY. The central nervous system in motor neuron disease. *J Neurol Neurosurg Psychiat* 1970, 33:338–357.
25. Mulder DW, Kurland LT, Offord KP, Beard CM. Familial adult motor neuron disease: amyotrophic lateral sclerosis. *Neurology* 1986, 36:511–517.
26. Rosen DR, Siddique T, Patterson D, et al. Mutations in Cu/Zn superoxide dismutase gene are associated with familial amyotrophic lateral sclerosis. *Nature* 1993, 362: 59–62.
27. Yanagihara RT, Garruto RM, Gajdusek DC. Epidemiological surveillance of amyotrophic lateral sclerosis and parkinsonism-dementia in the commonwealth of the northern Mariana Islands. *Ann Neurol* 1983, 13:79–86.
28. Lavine L, Steele JC, Wolfe N. Amyotrophic lateral sclerosis/parkinsonism-dementia complex in Southern Guam: is it disappearing? *Adv Neurol* 1991, 56:271–286.
29. Yase Y. The pathogenetic role of metals in motor neuron disease—the participation of aluminum. *Adv Exp Med Biol* 1987, 209:89–96.
30. Meyers KR, Dorencamp DG, Suzuki K. Amyotrophic lateral sclerosis with diffuse neurofibrillary changes. *Arch Neurol* 1974, 30:84–89.
31. Oda M, Akagawa N, Tabuchi Y, Tanabe H. A sporadic juvenile case of amyotrophic

lateral sclerosis with neuronal intracytoplasmic inclusions. *Acta Neuropathol* 1978, 44:211–216.
32. Mitsumoto H, Hanson MR, Chad DA. Amyotrophic lateral sclerosis: recent advances in pathogenesis and therapeutic trials. *Arch Neurol* 1988, 40:189–202.
33. Dalakas MC, Elder G, Hallett, et al. A long-term follow-up study of patients with post-poliomyelitis neuromuscular symptoms. *N Engl J Med* 1896, 314:959–963.
34. Cwick VA, Mitsumoto H. Postpoliomyelitis syndrome. In: Smith RA. *Handbook of Amyotrophic Lateral Sclerosis.* New York: Marcel Dekker, 1992, 77–91.
35. Pestronk A, Cornblath DR, Ilyas AA, et al. A treatable mutifocal motor neuropathy with antibodies to GM_1 ganglioside. *Ann Neurol* 1988, 24:73–78.
36. Lange DJ, Trojaborg E, Latov N, et al. Multifocal motor neuropathy with conduction block: is it a distinct clinical entity? *Neurology* 1992, 42:497–505.
37. Sadiq SA, Thomas FP, Kilidireas K, et al. The spectrum of neurologic disease associated with anti-GM_1 antibodies. *Neurology* 1990, 40:1067–1072.
38. Pestronk A, Adams RN, Cornblath D, et al. Patterns of serum IgM antibodies to GM_1 and GD_{1a} gangliosides in amyotrophic lateral sclerosis. *Ann Neurol* 1989, 25:98–102.
39. Shy ME, Rowland LP, Smith T, et al. Motor neuron disease and plasma cell dyscrasia. *Neurology* 1986, 36:1429–1436
40. Drachman DB, Kuncl RW. Amyotrophic lateral sclerosis: an unconventional autoimmune disease? *Ann Neurol* 1989, 26:269–274.
41. Mitsumoto H, Sliman RJ, Schafer IA, et al. Motor neuron disease and adult hexosaminidase A deficiency in two families: evidence for multisystem degeneration. *Ann Neurol* 1985, 17:378–385.
42. Dalmau J, Furneaux HM, Rosenblum MK, et al. Detection of the anti-Hu antibody in specific regions of the nervous system and tumor from patients with paraneoplastic encephalomyelitis/sensory neuronopathy. *Neurology* 1991, 41:1757–1764.
43. Wong MCW, Salange VD, Chou S, Mitsumoto H, Kozachuk W. Immune-associated paraneoplastic motor neuron disease and limbic encephalopathy. *Muscle Nerve* 1987, 10:661–662.
44. Younger DS, Rowland LP, Latov N, et al. Lymphoma, motor neuron diseases, and amyotrophic lateral sclerosis. *Ann Neurol* 1991, 29:78–86.
45. DeJong RN. *The Neurological Examination. 3rd Ed.* New York: Harper and Row, 1970.
46. Kuncl RW, Cornblath DR and Griffin JW. Assessment of thoracic paraspinal muscles in the diagnosis of ALS. *Muscle Nerve* 1988, 11:484–492.
47. Salazar AM, Masters CL, Gadjusek C, Gibbs CJ. Syndromes of amyotrophic lateral sclerosis and dementia: relation to transmissible Creutzfeldt-Jakob disease. *Ann Neurol* 1983, 14:17–26.
48. Mitsuyama Y. Presenile dementia with motor neuron disease in Japan: clinico-pathologicval review of 26 cases. *J Neurol Neurosurg Psychiat* 1984, 47:953–959.
49. Hudson AJ. Amyotrophic lateral sclerosis and its association with dementia, parkinsonism, and other neurological disorders: a review. *Brain* 1981, 104:217–247.
50. Mitsumoto H. Wilbourn AJ, Hanson MR, Phillips RC, Schwartzman MJ. Spectrum of sensory abnormalities in adult motor neuron disease. *Neurology* 1989, 39 (suppl 1):111.
51. Hayashi H, Kata S, Kawada, Tsubaki T. Amyotrophic lateral sclerosis: oculomotor function in patients in respirators. *Neurology* 1987, 37:1431–1432.

52. Mannen T, Iwata M, Toyokura Y, Nagashima K. Preservation of a certain motoneuron group of the sacral cord in amyotrophic lateral sclerosis. *J Neurol Neurosurg Psychiat* 1982, 58:464–469.
53. Hattori T. Negative symptoms and signs of amyotrophic lateral sclerosis: Disturbance of micturition. *Rinsho Sinkeigaku* 1984, 24:1254–1256.
54. Ono S, Mechanic GL, Yamauchi M. Cross-linking of skin collagen in patients with amyotrophic lateral sclerosis. *Ann Neurol* 1991, 30:254.
55. Gubbay SS, Kahana E, Zilber N, Cooper G, Pintov S, Leibowitz Y. Amyotrophic lateral sclerosis. A study of its presentation and prognosis. *J Neurol* 1985, 232: 295–300.
56. Kondo K, Hemmi I. Clinical statistics in 515 fatal cases of motor neuron disease. *Neuroepidemiology* 1984, 3:129–148.
57. Mitsumoto H, Schwartzman M, Levin KH, Schields RW, Wilbourn AJ. Electromyographic (EMG) changes and disease progression in ALS. *Neurology* (Suppl 1) 1990.
58. Mulder DW, Howard FM. Patient resistance and prognosis in amyotrophic lateral Sclerosis. *Mayo Clin Proc* 1976, 51:537–541.
59. Tucker T, Layzer RB, Miller RG, Chad D. Subacute reversible motor neuron disease. *Neurology* 1991, 41:1541–1544.
60. Rowland LP, ed. *Adv Neurol vol 56. Amyotrophic Lateral Sclerosis and Other Motor Neuron Diseases*, New York: Raven Press, 1991.
61. Hudson AJ, ed. *Amyotrophic Lateral Sclerosis: Concepts in Pathogenesis and Etiology*, Toronto: Univ Toronto Press, 1990.
62. Smith RA, ed. *Handbook of Amyotrophic Lateral Sclerosis*. New York: Marcel Dekker, 1992.

2

Amyotrophic Lateral Sclerosis: The Diagnostic Process

Walter G. Bradley, D.M., F.R.C.P.

A few years ago, I reviewed the management of patients with ALS and Duchenne muscular dystrophy from diagnosis to death and beyond and doctor-patient relationships during the course of these diseases (1). The present chapter provides the opportunity to consider ALS and its diagnosis in greater depth. It is important to consider the clinical, scientific, and psychological aspects at each stage, and also to consider not only the patient but also the family and the doctor.

Clinical Features of ALS That Are Relevant to the Diagnosis

The clinical features of ALS are well known. The disease usually affects adults, particularly those in the latter half of life. The symptoms and signs are those of a relatively slowly progressive condition advancing over months or years to produce weakness, cramps, fasciculations in the muscles, dysarthria, dysphagia, and dyspnea. Examination reveals both upper and lower motor neuron damage without significant involvement of the autonomic and sensory nervous systems, the cerebellum, basal ganglia, or cortical function. An interesting feature is the pleomorphic presentation of the disease. It can begin with difficulty in speech and swallowing, lower motor neuron weakness and wasting of the muscles of an arm or a leg, progressive spastic paraplegia, or isolated respiratory failure.

The "typical" presentation is easy to diagnose. The more unusual cases cause many practitioners great difficulty. Paresthesias, which are seen in about 25 per-

21

cent of patients, can lead an unsuspecting practitioner away from the diagnosis. Asymmetric involvement at presentation is the rule rather than the exception. A clinical sign of considerable help in pointing to the diagnosis is the presence of increased tendon reflexes in muscles already considerably atrophied due to lower motor neuron denervation. Few diseases other than motor system degeneration cause this picture.

In the bulbar territory, it is often difficult to define whether the problem lies in the upper or lower motor neuron. Since spontaneous movements of the tongue are so frequent in normal individuals, I do not diagnose lower motor neuron damage in the tongue unless there is significant atrophy. Tongue movements may be slow, with weak protrusion. Speech is often strained and monotonous or slurred. The jaw jerk and facial reflexes may be increased or normal.

All of these features should be sought in the history and physical examination, but it must be recognized that the absence of any one of them does not rule out the diagnosis of ALS.

Diagnostic Definition of the Disease

The clinical features need to be fitted into a template of requirements for the diagnosis of ALS. The reason for such diagnostic criteria is that there is no laboratory test that can prove the presence of ALS. A working clinical definition of the disease is the following: a syndrome of upper and lower motor neuron dysfunction of the arms, legs, bulbar, and/or respiratory motor systems, slowly progressing over months or years in adults, without involvement of any other part of the nervous system or the presence of any specific cause.

A number of caveats need to be expressed in relation to this definition. In the early stages of the disease, only one part of the motor system, such as the upper or the lower motor neuron, may be involved. Similarly in the early stage, only one limb or only the bulbar territory may be involved. At the end stage of the disease, extensive lower motor neuron degeneration and paralysis may erase previously evident upper motor neuron signs. Yet another caveat relates to the involvement of other parts of the nervous system. Pathologically, and sometimes with refined *in vivo* investigations, it is possible to demonstrate minor involvement of other parts of the nervous system, such as the sensory system. This does not rule out the diagnosis of ALS. A final caveat is that there are rare cases in which an identical syndrome is associated with, and perhaps even caused by, a different underlying disease. The importance of this last caveat is that many of these diseases are treatable, which will halt or even cure the progressive motor neuron syndrome. Regrettably, such curable instances of ''symptomatic ALS'' are rare.

Investigations of Relevance to the Diagnosis of ALS

The first point to make is that in many countries ALS is a purely clinical diagnosis. In these countries, no investigation is usually undertaken other than the "investigation of time," that is, to watch the typical and inexorable progression of the disease and confirm its progressive nature and distribution. This approach is particularly striking to the U.S. neurologist who may expend $10,000 or $20,000 investigating a patient presenting with ALS to rule out disorders of thyroid and parathyroid glands, disorders of nutrition including vitamin B_{12} deficiency, immunological disorders including multiple sclerosis, chronic inflammatory demyelinating polyneuropathy, chronic granulomatous diseases, vasculitis, specific antibody disorders such as anti-GM_1 ganglioside antibodies, chronic infections such as the retroviruses, Lyme disease, and syphilis, specific enzyme deficiencies such as hexosaminidase A deficiency, heavy metal intoxication such as lead poisoning, paraneoplastic conditions associated with asymptomatic cancer, lymphoma, or bone marrow dyscrasia, gammopathies, or focal lesions of the neuraxis. The tests can include such expensive items as magnetic resonance imaging, electrophysiological studies, and muscle, nerve, and bone marrow biopsies.

Personally, I feel that many such tests are unnecessary in a typical case. For instance, why should we do an MRI scan of the cervical region when the clinical examination clearly shows bulbar involvement and lower motor neuron changes in the legs? Why should we perform bone marrow biopsy when the patient has no demonstrable gammopathy? Since "symptomatic ALS" is so rare, we should ask whether such tests are cost-effective in view of the spiraling costs of health care.

In many cases, some abnormality of these tests is detected. By definition, "abnormal" in most laboratory studies is a value exceeding ±3 standard deviations of the mean. Hence, one or two patients in every one hundred normal subjects will have an "abnormal" result in every test. Such "abnormal" results often lead to a secondary cascade of investigations, including repeated and yet more complex studies to validate or refute the previously "abnormal" result.

Some of the investigations help document the presence of disease which is not recognizable clinically. This is generally a search for lower motor neuron signs by needle EMG of several muscles in two or more limbs.

These investigations play an important role in assuaging the concerns of the doctor that nothing has been missed and that the diagnosis must be ALS. They also play the same role for the patient, who in the United States usually feels that a "death sentence" like the diagnosis of ALS cannot be made without many expensive tests.

It is unfortunate that the diagnostic pathway often appears to be so difficult for physicians and patients. Physicians often have difficulty seeing the forest for the trees and lack the clarity of diagnostic skills to conclude that the patient has ALS. They sometimes get wrapped up in the "abnormal" test results and keep the patient unaware of the diagnosis even after many tests and many return visits. The patient often becomes aware that the condition is serious, that it is progressively deteriorating, and that the doctor is concerned since all of these tests are being done. If the patient is not told anything, he or she may lose confidence in the doctor at this stage, and seek another or several other opinions. On the other side, it is not infrequent for the doctor to lack the confidence or perhaps the moral courage to tell the patient the likely diagnosis. Such a doctor will refer the patient without sharing the diagnosis. All of us who specialize in ALS have seen many patients arrive confused, with no idea of the diagnosis, but with reports of a $20,000 workup and copies of letters from the original doctor going back several months saying that this is probably a motor neuron disorder.

I believe it should be the duty of the initial neurologist to at least share the possibility of this diagnosis with the patient at an earlier stage, and this is my standard procedure. At the first consultation, unless there is real clinical uncertainty, I share in overall terms the possibility of conditions entering into the differential diagnosis. I explain what tests have to be done and why. Often patients have some suspicion of the presence of ALS or of an equally terrifying disease like cancer when they come to see the doctor. If the patient wants more information, I prefer to put off a detailed discussion until the follow-up visit after the planned tests have been completed. However, if the patient clearly exhibits a considerable fear that this is ALS, I point out that that condition is often more benign than many people believe. With this approach, the patient leaves with no greater fears about the condition than were brought into the office at the beginning of the consultation. The patient feels that the doctor understands the disease and has things under control with regard to the investigations.

Follow-Up Visit

I usually schedule a follow-up visit one to three weeks after the initial consultation, as soon as the necessary test results are available. Those results are important, but the patient must not be left uncertain of the outcome for too long. The patient and a close family member should be present at the time of this follow-up visit. The reason is that the spouse or other relative is going to be heavily involved in the future problems of the disease. Of even more importance is the fact that two sets of ears and two memories are better than one. On leaving a doctor's office after an interview such as this, patients usually retain less than one-third of what the doctor said.

I usually begin this follow-up interview by reviewing the initial impression that I obtained from the clinical examination at the first visit. I discuss the confirmatory nature of the tests and what they mean. I interpret any abnormal results and confirm the initial impression that the patient has ALS, if that is the case.

Unless there is some special reason not to, I deal frankly but optimistically with the details of this disease. It is generally helpful for the patient to receive an outline of the salient features of what is happening with regard to motor neuron degeneration and what it produces. It is reassuring to know that, although the muscles of the body are likely to be affected, many other parts of the nervous system such as sensation, mentation, bowel, bladder, sexual function, vision, and hearing are spared. Since patients often have contact with others suffering from the same disease, it is helpful if they realize that the condition is very pleomorphic and can affect different parts of the body at variable rates.

I share with the patient what they usually already know, that individuals with ALS often die within a few years of diagnosis of the condition. However, I emphasize that 50 percent live five years, 10 percent live more than ten years, and perhaps 5 percent live more than twenty years with the disease. I emphasize that we now realize that this disease is considerably more benign than was originally thought. I point out that the condition can "burn itself out" or arrest at a certain stage. I tell them about the three patients that I have seen and the several other cases in the literature (2), who clearly had a syndrome of ALS but who spontaneously went into remission.

With this basis, it is necessary to discuss next what we know about the cause of ALS. As a preface, it is essential to say that we do not know the cause or the cure of the disease. I outline the major theories of the cause of motor neuron degeneration in ALS and how research is progressing to investigate those theories. It is helpful to the patients to see how each of these theories has already, or may in the future, spawn attempted treatments. Research is often an enigmatic process for the lay person, but patients soon come to realize the significance of research with regard to their own disease. I give patients the names, addresses, and phone numbers of the ALS Association, the Muscular Dystrophy Association, and local chapters or support groups for ALS. I encourage patients and their families to contact these organizations and to be placed on the mailing list for the receipt of updated information about research and patient care.

It is important that we plant the idea that although the disease may not be curable, it is most certainly treatable. Perhaps of greater importance is to plant this concept in the minds of neurologists throughout the country. In fact, a patient with ALS needs to be seen frequently to help circumvent as far as possible each of the manifestations of the disease.

Toward the end of the follow-up interview, I usually discuss the research and therapeutic trials in which the patient can become involved. The patient and the next of kin usually have many questions at this stage. It is important to allow them to have all of these questions answered and to point out that they are welcome to bring many more questions on every occasion. Typically, patients want to know how they got the disease, what caused it, and whether anything that they were exposed to in the past might have been relevant. They want to know if someone close can catch it. They particularly want to know if it is inherited and if their children might suffer from it. They find it impossible to believe that the disease is untreatable. They want to know how it may be slowed down and what treatment should be taken. Should they take vitamins, acupuncture, or other modalities of treatment? At this stage, and at each crucial point of deterioration in the future, I believe it is important to offer the patient a referral for a second opinion.

At the end of the follow-up visit, I draft a letter to the referring physician and, unless there is some specific contraindication, send the patient a copy of the letter of my first consultation, together with a copy of this follow-up letter. Then at least the patient has all of that information available to review and can come back on the next occasion with more informed questions. I urge patients to obtain pamphlets and manuals from the ALS Association and the Muscular Dystrophy Association so that they have some independent information about the condition prior to the next visit.

The Confirmatory Second Opinion

For many readers of this chapter, a patient will have presented with symptoms awaiting diagnosis. For many specialists in ALS, the patient usually has an established diagnosis but seeks a second opinion. Even in this circumstance, there is sometimes reason to offer yet a further confirmatory consultation to the patient. It is important to make clear to the patient and the family what is to be achieved by this second opinion. The patient should be told about the skills and experience of the person from whom the second opinion is to be sought. The availability of the second opinion helps the patient and the family feel that the door is always left open, and that the initial physician's mind is not closed to other possibilities. ''A grief shared is a grief halved'' might be a good motto. This further opinion may be obtained from a center with a special research program that may be of value to the patient. I always say that I hope the patient will come back to see me for continuing care after the second opinion, and that perhaps this can be undertaken in collaboration with the secondary referral center.

It is important to know what should not be asked of a second opinion. The referring neurologist should not ask that the person giving the second opinion take on the task of disclosing the diagnosis of ALS when this is already obvious. The referring doctor should not say what has been said to so many patients in the past: ''This is ALS, and you are going to die within two to three years. Go home and put your affairs in order. There is no point in coming to see me again, since there is nothing further that I can do.'' Not only is this untrue, but it is also a gross abrogation of the physician's responsibility to the patient, albeit often resulting from the difficulty that the doctor has in dealing with an incurable disorder.

Psychological Reactions in the Doctor, Patient, and Family at the Time of Diagnosis of ALS

I have previously outlined the psychological reactions in the patient and the doctor throughout the course of ALS and Duchenne muscular dystrophy (1). I will expand here on the situation with regard to ALS at the time of diagnosis. The education of physicians in the current era emphasizes the scientific knowledge of disease and the many conditions that can be treated or cured by modern science. We have relatively little training in the care of patients with incurable disease. In this day and age, especially for the relatively younger doctor, an incurable disease like ALS is a psychological blow to the prowess of the physician. This may be one reason why so many doctors are unwilling to make a diagnosis of ALS despite having all of the necessary skills, knowledge, and information.

As a neurologist becomes a little longer in the tooth, with fewer or grayer hairs, and particularly if he or she specializes in neuromuscular diseases, there are other reactions to making the diagnosis of ALS. Too many patients have gone before who have presented in an initially healthy independent state but have been followed through the severely dependent stage to death in only a few years. Many physicians become "burnt out" by the emotional strain of looking after ALS patients. All of us are aware of the sinking feeling in our spirits when we first make the diagnosis that a patient has ALS.

It is important to remember, however, that if *our* feelings are dragged down by the diagnosis, those of the patient and family are even more disastrously affected. In a frail eighty-year-old, the diagnosis of ALS is not such a burden to the doctor, but in the all-too-frequent patient in the twenties or thirties with a young family and so much life before him or her, ALS is a tragedy.

The patient's reactions over the course of the disease range through the classical stages of shock, denial, anger, bargaining, depression, and eventual acceptance, in a very similar fashion to those seen in cancer patients (3), and are beyond the scope of this particular chapter. It is worth noting, however, that these reactions are often not in the neat order given here, and that often a mixture of such reactions can be seen in the patient and the family at the time of the first or second interview.

Conclusions

The diagnosis is simply the initial part of the management of the patient with ALS. In clinical terms, the diagnosis of ALS is easy in most cases, even for the neurologist with relatively limited experience. It is important to make a professional and personal commitment to the ongoing care of that patient at the time of diagnosis and to make clear this commitment to the patient and the family. It is important to recognize the very serious psychological aspects of the initial consultation and follow-up interviews, both for the patient and for the doctor. Involvement in research, particularly therapeutic trials, is a very significant aspect of the care of patients with ALS. Such trials are of great psychological benefit, not only to the patients but also to the doctors, though they have problems of their own. Such problems include the difficulty of dealing with patients who are not eligible, the difficulty of convincing patients and their families of the need for a placebo group, and ways to maintain compliance when it is clear that the trial drug is not a "wonder cure." Nevertheless, such trials, or research studies in general, provide the psychological and sometimes the material underpinnings of ALS clinics around the world. Discussion about such res⸺ ˙ is an important part of the diagnostic pathw⸺ ⸺ ˙ throughout the course of A

1. Bradley W⸺   lystrophy: the
   diseases and   ', Wolf SG, et
   al., eds. *Rea*   Philadelphia:
   Charles Pres
2. Tucker T, L⸺   iron disease.
   Neurology 1⸺
3. Kubler-Ross ⸺

3

Care of the Amyotrophic Lateral Sclerosis Patient

Forbes H. Norris, M.D.

Giving the Diagnosis

The care of the ALS patient begins with the diagnosis, which must be very carefully considered in light of other possible diagnoses and of the fact that we have no positive diagnostic test for ALS, even after so many years of clinical and laboratory research. The diagnosis remains one of "exclusion," as Dr. Bradley discussed in the preceding chapter. A patient with the typical picture of ALS should receive that diagnosis only after the disorders that might mimic such a clinical state have been carefully excluded. A very careful and deliberate exclusion process also serves to aid the physician in becoming better acquainted with the patient and the family, so that when the diagnosis of ALS does seem unavoidable, it can be given with maximum consideration of their reactions and after they have developed some confidence in the physicians.

In many university clinics, the preliminary diagnostic work is done by house staff or junior attending physicians, who are often unable or too pressed for time to explain adequately to the patient and the family just what these tests are all about; without the spouse or other family, the patient may then be ushered in to a very brief meeting with the professor, who gives the bad news rather bluntly, announces that there is nothing further to be done, and often advises the patient to simply go home and take to bed, "to conserve the remaining strength." There may also be advice to visit the family attorney on the way home in order to settle affairs. No return appointment is made, so the patient (not to mention the family) leaves uninformed and with the feeling that a "don't call me, I'll call you" attitude prevails. We have encountered patients of a few neurologists who were actually told that they should *not* come back again because there was nothing to be done (which completely ignores all the available symptomatic treatments discussed later in this chapter). We have encountered many cases in which not only the bad news about the diagnosis of ALS is given at this time, but also a prognosis that the patient would be dead within a year, for which there is absolutely no scientific basis anywhere in the literature. Many ALS patients are psychologically devastated by this approach.

Admittedly, some extremely difficult problems for the physician occur as a result of ALS. Some doctors are so appalled that they do not think "it is right to embark on measures likely to prolong distress . . . (such as) gastrostomy or tracheostomy . . ." (1). This attitude can be accepted when death is imminent, but some ALS patients live longer than forecast, even for decades (2). Withholding supportive and symptomatic treatments adds significantly to the suffering. We advocate a broad range of symptomatic treatments to increase the victim's quality of life, whether the remaining time be six months, six years, or sixteen years.

ALS is usually a fatal illness and, like any of the other major fatal disorders, the patient merits the attention of a senior specialist in the area in addition to very careful attention to the diagnostic workup in hope of finding some other condition that can be treated successfully, or at least one that gives a better prognosis. During this early stage of investigation, the patient and the family can get to know this neurologist, just as the physician can acquire more understanding of them as individuals and of their likely reactions and capacities for managing the diagnosis of ALS when it is finally given. Many clinics in the United States today operate on a rather tight schedule of about twenty minutes per patient, which is simply inadequate for the type of acquaintanceship necessary in a disease such as ALS. A physician in such a practice or clinic should make arrangements for the patient to be seen at the nearest specialty clinic or ALS center where the necessary time, attention, and expertise are available.

For example, at the San Francisco ALS Research Center, most of the patients are referred after investigation by one or two other neurologists, but it is very common in our experience for such patients to have had no spinal fluid examination. We strongly urge that the spinal fluid be evaluated in every case because of the "long shot" possibility of multiple sclerosis or some other process. The magnetic resonance (MR) brain scan is of great value in making the diagnosis of multiple sclerosis, but it is not always positive and is usually not done in ALS unless there are bulbar symptoms. It is also true that in MS there may be completely normal spinal fluid, including absence of oligoclonal bands. Nevertheless, the effort should be made to detect an atypical case of MS mimicking ALS. The spinal fluid should also be examined with regard to the possibility of some other dysimmune process, syphilis, or Lyme disease.

Another problem arises from the physician's well-intentioned use of related diagnoses, such as progressive muscular atrophy (PMA) in a case where the typical upper motor signs of ALS are not evident. PMA certainly shares many of the signs and symptoms of ALS and offers a much better prognosis (2,3), but in the great majority of those cases there is fairly rapid progression to the full-blown picture of ALS, from which the patient dies after a few more years of progressing paralysis. Unless the possibility of an error in diagnosis has been very carefully explained to the patient, it does no good to come to a more benign diagnosis and to close off other avenues of investigation when the patient will soon be suffering from much more extensive and serious problems. Another example is progressive bulbar palsy (PBP), a common early manifestation of ALS that is very rare as a "pure" disorder (2). Confused patients may become frightened and lose confidence in the physician when such other diagnoses prove wrong. Also, there is less information available about those disorders should the patient wish to investigate on his own. We have always found that the fully informed, intelligent patient is the best one to deal with and have made every effort to keep our patients as informed as possible.

Chapters 1 and 2 outline a practical differential diagnosis for ALS, "practical" in that some extremely rare, dubious, or uncertain conditions have not been listed. Table 3-1 lists the tests that we carry out routinely in every new patient unless they have already been obtained earlier in the workup. Notice that not all the tests are applicable or necessary in every case. For example, hexosaminidase need not be evaluated if there is a large family that is clearly negative for any other cases of motor neuron disease. On the other hand, if the family is small, or if even in a large family there are some possible but vague motor neuron problems, then the hexosaminidase should be measured. Excluding a heavy metal intoxication does not involve a single simple lab test but a more complex series

Table 3-1. Routine Diagnostic Tests in ALS

General physical by general practitioner
Neurologist's examination
Electromyogram (EMG), plus motor and sensory nerve conduction measurements, plus test of neuromuscular transmission
MR scans: head and neck (cervical spine)
Blood tests for cell counts, standard chemistry panel, creative kinase (CK), sedimentation rate, anti-nuclear antibodies, ganglioside antibodies, IgA, IgG and IgM levels, hexosaminidase, fluorescent treponemal antibody absorption (FTAabs, also detcts Lyme disease antibodies), Lyme titer (if FTAabs not available), parathormone level, thyroid panel
Cerebrospinal fluid (CSF) tests for cell counts, total protein level, oligoclonal bands or an "MS panel," VDRL
Urine tests for cells, bacteria, protein, and glucose excretions
(Plus any further tests suggested by abnormalities in the above)

of tests and procedures, including a bone biopsy, which have been described elsewhere (4).

Even after an exhaustive, apparently negative workup, the attending physician should maintain the possibility, however slight, of some other diagnosis, such as multifocal motor neuropathy when there is mainly lower motor neuron involvement. We have one patient who was atypical in that his progression ceased for several years, and then some improvement began. In earlier workups, ganglioside antibodies had been within the normal ranges on two occasions. In light of his improvement, a third ganglioside antibody titer was obtained, and markedly increased levels indicated a diagnosis other than early ALS or PMA, which had been the main possibilities considered up to that time. This is a very rare occurrence and might be written off as insignificant by those dealing with a large number of patients, yet it completely reversed the outlook for the patient in whom this abnormality was detected.

This is the first stage in the care of an ALS patient: making the diagnosis with great care and coming to the definite conclusion only after the physician has demonstrated to the patient his interest in the case by means of a careful workup, and both patient and physician (and preferably the family as well) have become more acquainted from multiple visits for these tests than is possible in the ordinary clinic setting. The unfortunate aspect of this approach is that no managed health care system provides the necessary time, and at least in the United States private insurance schemes do not reimburse. An inadequate solution, which is resorted to by many large clinics particularly at universities, is that the patient is seen by a multitude of junior or less experienced workers, e.g., interns, social workers, physical therapists, and so on, none of whom bring to bear the necessary experience with motor neuron problems.

Family Involvement

It should be emphasized at this point that we make every effort to include the family in all evaluations, including the physical examinations. This increases their understanding of the magnitude of the problem and demonstrates to them our desire to have them participate actively, which will eventually become essential if the diagnosis turns out to be the malignant motor neuron disease, ALS.

Symptomatic Treatment Cramps, Spasms, Secretions

During this time or shortly afterward, it is desirable to start the patient on any indicated symptomatic medication or treatment to relieve as best we can some of the more troublesome symptoms caused by the disease (5), such as painful

Table 3-2. Medications Useful in Relieving Spastic Symptoms

Medication	Dosage, Schedule*
Diphenhydramine	50–100 mg q4H or 50–200 mg HS
Quinine sulfate	200–600 mg q4H
Quinidine	200–400 mg q4H
Procainamide	250–500 mg q6H
Baclofen#	5–50 mg q4H**
Diazepam	2–20 mg q4H
Phenytoin	200–800 mg qd***

    * Usual adult dosages, all to be used PRN ("as needed") except phenytoin.
    ** Some ALS patients have had no benefit from the usually recommended dosages (up to 80 mg per day) but have obtained significant relief from higher doses.
    *** Phenytoin for this purpose seems to be potentiated by the addition of calcium gluconate 0.5 to 1.0 gm q4 to 6H. Phenytoin action is dependent on a stable blood level and so it should be taken regularly, not PRN.
    # Drug of choice.

muscle cramps. Table 3-2 provides a list of the medications useful in the treatment of cramps and disabling muscle spasms, such as clonus at knee and ankle tending to precipitate the patient forward when going down stairs.

    Table 3-3 lists the medications useful in the management of excessive salivation and drooling. Some ALS patients accumulate oropharyngeal secretions that periodically spill over into the airway and produce laryngospasm and/or episodes

Table 3-3. Medications Useful in Control of Secretions and Drooling

Medication	Dosage, Schedule*
Methantheline	50–100 mg q4H
Propantheline	15–30 mg q4H
Glycopyrrolate	1–2 mg q4H
Amitriptyline	10–50 mg q4H
Imipramine	50–200 mg HS
Methyl phenidate	10–20 mg q6H
Trihexyphenidyl	2–10 mg q4H
Scopalamine	transdermal "patch" applications

    * Usual adult dosages, all to be used PRN ("as needed") except the scopalamine patch.

of severe coughing. Baclofen (Table 3-2) and one or more of the anticholinergics (Table 3-3) often give substantial benefit for this problem. The use of a cough suppressant is usually *not* advisable because the coughing is a normal reaction to avoid the dangers of aspiration.

The scopalamine patch (Table 3-3) is listed last, because ALS affects an older age group, some of whom develop paranoid ideation or other mental abnormalities from chronic daily use of atropine derivatives. Constipation is a frequent problem in any paralyzing illness, and any such medication will surely increase that problem.

Reflex hyperactivity of cranial nerve-supplied muscles as well as excess secretions are frequent causes of dysarthria in ALS patients. Speech may be impaired by spontaneous jaw clonus that develops with attempted speech, and the involuntary gargling from excessive pooled secretions can also interfere with speech, in addition to causing the episodes of laryngospasm and coughing mentioned previously. Such symptoms often fluctuate significantly from day to day or week to week. We advise the patient to try a given medication on a regular basis for two or three weeks, both to assess its tolerance and to find the necessary dosage, and then reduce the frequency to use as needed, such as taking baclofen only at bedtime if painful cramps or other spasms are mainly a nocturnal problem, or not using an anticholinergic at all on days when secretions are not greatly increased.

Continence

It is commonly stated that bowel and bladder sphincters are not affected in ALS, so that incontinence does not occur, but in fact a sizable minority of patients do develop such difficulty, which in the early to intermediate stages is always almost an "urgency incontinence" of urine. Of course, men and women should have a yearly prostate or pelvic examination, and if that has been done in recent months we do not pursue further investigation. Rather, we try oxybutynin 5 mg from once in the morning to three or four times during the day, or at bedtime if the urgency problem is confined to the hours of sleep. Oxybutynin has been very successful in controlling this troublesome symptom in the majority of our patients who have such a problem. Earlier in our experience, thorough urological investigations were carried out in such patients, and no primary disorder of the urinary tract was ever discovered.

Pseudoincontinence of feces is common in advanced ALS due to partial impaction from severe chronic constipation. Careful attention to hydration, diet, and laxatives is the solution to this problem, which arises from inadequate hydration due to dysphagia and from the requirement for daily physical activity to promote normal bowel contractility. In advanced paralysis (from any cause), this normal bowel stimulus is reduced or absent. As bulbar involvement increases, many patients reduce their fluid intake in order to reduce aspiration. Autonomic dysfunction may be a contributing factor.

Several patients became truly incontinent of both bowel and bladder but only after developing far advanced generalized paralysis. Perhaps in such tragic circumstances some patients become so depressed, even psychotic, that incontinence develops through inattention or regression to infantilism, although I have seen three patulous anal sphincters, indicating organic neuromuscular involvement, among several thousand cases of ALS. Fortunately, the average patient and family can be reassured that this is a very rare complication of ALS.

Dysautonomia

Cold, swollen, cyanotic feet and toes, made worse by dependency, are quite common in ALS and primary lateral sclerosis (PLS). Elevation of the legs may not reverse these symptoms completely, and another indication of dysautonomia is the occasional development of similar alterations in the hands and fingers. One patient had it first in one forearm and later in the other, resembling the old comic book character Popeye. This dysfunction may also contribute to the bladder and bowel continence symptoms just described, as well as to the initial bulbar symptom. In rare cases there is reduction of tears and oropharyngeal secretions, and then, of course, the workup for autoimmune disorders should be repeated. The sensitivity to cold reported by many ALS patients may also indicate autonomic involvement in ALS, to which the studies reported by Daube et al. (6) lend support.

Fatigue: Myasthenic State

Fatigue is a very common (and usually very early) symptom in ALS. In early stages, it responds to brief rest periods, as in myasthenia gravis. As the disease progresses, the fatigue usually becomes more severe, even to the point where an overnight rest fails to restore the previous level of strength, and sometimes every exertion seems to cause more weakness. Several studies have shown that this is indeed a "myasthenic state" (7,8), but with significant differences from myasthenia gravis. As would be predicted, the response is not as gratifying as it usually is in myasthenia gravis, but at least some ALS patients obtain transient benefit from anticholinesterase medication to varying degree and for varying times. Such benefit often fades after several months, although one patient obtained maximum benefit every day for eighteen months, even though the disease continued to progress otherwise.

Of the available anticholinesterases, we have used pyridostigmine most frequently. The major problems encountered have been lack of any benefit, or some benefit but at the cost of major gastrointestinal disturbances leading to cessation of such a treatment effort. We usually start with 30 mg once a day and advance over several weeks to 120 mg with each meal. If pyridostigmine is ineffective or poorly tolerated, neostigmine can be tried.

In patients with the greatest involvement in the muscles of respiration, aminophylline can be tried instead, as it has been shown to have a direct effect on strengthening diaphragm contractility (9). Sometimes this also seems to benefit arm and leg muscle strength and fatigability.

At the present time, many ALS patients have been practicing the evil habit of cigarette smoking for many years and have the pulmonary changes of emphysema, so when there is significant weakness of the respiratory muscles, there may be additional reason to use aminophylline or a derivative. At this stage of the illness, quantitative spirometry (10) should be carried out frequently in order to closely observe for impending critical loss of respiratory function. Spirometry also serves as an objective measurement of the value of any medication. In our experience, the forced vital capacity (FVC) and the maximum voluntary ventilation (MVV) have been the most useful parameters (10), although recently others have shown that the FEV_1 also provides a good index of the pulmonary neuromuscular function (11).

Physical Therapy

The use of physical therapy is very important in the care of the ALS patient (12), particularly as the paralysis progresses and the patient becomes unable to move the major joints, which then become painful when moved by those in attendance. Passive "range of motion" (ROM) treatment should be administered at regular intervals several times each day. Early in the illness, particularly with evolving finger flexion contractures, the intelligent patient can usually perform his own stretching exercises to keep these small joints mobile and reduce the risk of permanent contractures, but as the disease progresses there is usually need for assistance from those in attendance. Fortunately, these are simple treatments that can be learned quickly and administered satisfactorily by family and friends.

A major cause of pain in ALS is sublaxation of the shoulder joint with development of periarthritis. On this account it is particularly important that the range of motion maneuvers include the shoulder joint. If sublaxation has already developed to a severe degree, it may be necessary for an orthopedist to inject the joint with a steroid combined with local anesthetic and for the patient to have professional physical therapy attention for several weeks in order to restore a relatively normal range of motion without pain. In a case of far advanced paralysis, particularly when death seems near, pain control alone (a major narcotic is usually needed) is probably better than efforts to restore motion.

Assist Devices

Assist devices (splints, corrective braces, grab bars, elevated toilet seats, reach devices, and so on) are also essential for this treatment (12). Insurance carriers in the United States frequently contest prescriptions for this equipment on the ground that ALS is progressive and such devices do not prevent death. This attitude, of course, further reduces any hope the sufferer may have summoned and accelerates the original self-defeating prophecy. Refusal of assist devices seems unjustified, and indeed may actually cause psychological deterioration in a patient. Even simple devices such as a foot lift can make a great difference for some patients. At the minimum, a lift can prevent a disastrous fall. A neck brace can help maintain a stance permitting ambulation, conversation, and so on.

Communication aids must be included among the devices that have made an important difference for patients with ALS. For those who lose speech but maintain use of the hands, writing or typing are rapid and effective means of making needs known. More severely handicapped persons can employ simple devices such as the Etran Communication Board or microcomputer-based instruments. Software is available to allow patients to operate a computer. Rapid developments in computers for the handicapped will permit ALS patients to become even more independent. Current technology makes it possible to control appliances such as a light switch, telephone, and word processor.

Sleep Disorders

Sleep disorders are very common in ALS patients, because paralysis reduces or prevents the customary daily physical activities and interferes with nighttime postural adjustments. Complicating psychological problems such as depression may interfere with sleep. A contributing factor in our society may be the myth inculcated since childhood that fixed hours of sleep each night are essential to preserve health. Worry about sleeplessness last night may reduce sleep tonight. We open this aspect of treatment by searching for such other problems, amelioration of which can improve sleep. Another example is the painful cramps many ALS patients suffer; suppression of nocturnal cramps improves sleep substantially. Patients with a sleep disorder resulting from inability to move may obtain relief from use of an electrically powered bed, in which pushing a button to elevate the knees or lower the upper body may substitute for the natural body movements.

ALS patients tend to be older and if a sleep medication is actually required, care must be taken that it be well tolerated. Another concern in ALS is that sedative medication not depress respiration. Potentially all of the benzodiazepine medications may depress respiration, particularly diazepam. Flurazepam, however, has been relatively safe as a sleeping medication for many patients. A particularly useful medication is diphenhydramine, which suppresses cramps and also safely promotes sleep in older people.

Dysphagia

Dysphagia and aspiration usually occur hand in hand in ALS. The latter may be manifest only as a dry cough increased at meal times. At least early in bulbar involvement, judicious use of blenderized food and drink is by far the best way to approach this problem. The physician can prescribe medications in liquid form or advise pulverization of medications. Many different food-drink combinations can be mixed in the blender to achieve both palatability and less dysphagia.

When there is severe dysphagia and secondary malnutrition requiring bypass of the oropharyngeal mechanism, a nasogastric feeding tube is the simplest approach. If that is refused or poorly tolerated, we recommend percutaneous gastrostomy or cervical esophagostomy. Esophagostomy, once the preferred method of feeding dysphagic patients, has the disadvantage of requiring general anesthesia and much longer hospitalization. Recent application of percutaneous catheter gastrostomy (13) has been a simple, safe, effective procedure for malnourished, dysphagic patients, especially when severe pulmonary muscle weakness greatly increases the risk of anesthesia. Even when all seems lost and death appears imminent, we recommend at least intravenous fluids. Although many doctors discourage such treatment (1), is the amelioration of constant gagging and choking not a reasonable therapeutic outcome? Is adequate hydration likely to prolong life more than a few days or weeks? Is it preferable to die of starvation and thirst, as well as ALS, because the doctors do not think it is ''right'' to prolong suffering?

Emotional Lability

Loss of emotional control is one of the most demoralizing problems from upper motor bulbar involvement, affecting patient, family, friends, and medical attendants. Everyone is demoralized by sustained weeping or laughter, or laughter making a transition to frustrated weeping. In a small series, we have observed significant amelioration from administration of lithium carbonate 300 mg given once to three times a day. Sporadic serum lithium levels were always less than 0.6 mEq/L, so this effect is not likely to involve the neural pathways affected by lithium in manic-depressive psychosis. Levodopa has also been reported to help (14).

Other Treatments

Most patients want to take vitamins, which objectively give no benefit, and many seek unorthodox therapy. It is probably wise to acquiesce, at least when the proposed therapy is not obviously risky or inordinately expensive. An important factor in every illness, particularly in progressive paralytic diseases like ALS, is patient morale. In the era of heart transplantation, it is probably asking too much for ALS patients to rely completely on their physicians, who do not even know the cause of the disease! Acupuncture has had an appeal in the past decade. Hundreds of our patients have tried it without noticeable benefit, although four became jaundiced afterwards, presumably from contaminated needles.

Terminal Care

The terminal state is heralded by increasing somnolence from hypercarbia due to increasing respiratory paralysis. There may also be frontal headache and a slow strong pulse. The hypercarbia is probably increased by secondary atelectasis at the bases from hypoventilation. There are usually also increasing episodes of aspiration, and in about half our patients an actual aspiration pneumonitis precipitates the terminal state. Hypoxemia is actually infrequent in such patients until the very end, but the hypercarbia may develop weeks or even months before and slowly increase as the respiratory muscles undergo further paralysis.

In exceptional cases, we have advised tracheostomy and artificial ventilation at this time, particularly if the patient has a fair amount of strength in most other muscle groups and if the aspiration seems to be an unusual event and not a daily occurrence. For most ALS patients, however, at this stage the quality of life is so low, if not actually negative, that we advise the administration of a major narcotic (15, 16) such as meperidine or morphine, administered either orally or subcutaneously. The latter is preferable because the dysphagia usually increases in parallel with the pulmonary weakness. The subcutaneous injection is very easy for the family and other attendants to learn quickly and administer at home. It is essentially painless, as in the case of the daily insulin dose for diabetics. When hospitalized, the terminal patient will probably have an intravenous line, and the narcotic can then be given intermittently by that route. Addiction has not occurred in any of our patients and in any event should not be a concern at this time, as patient comfort is paramount (15,16).

Some patients will have heard about artificial respiration and may want to try that approach to prolong life as long as possible. We do recommend that for patients when other muscle functions have been significantly less affected, particularly if the patient has been able to ambulate up to the time of the aspiration or other respiratory catastrophe. In those cases, the first intubation is usually by nasotracheal or orotracheal tube, converted after several days to a tracheostomy. In combination with one or more of the strongest modern antibiotics (depending on the cultures), frequent deep tracheobronchial suctioning, chest massage, and so on, we find that about half of these patients can be retrieved, and perhaps half of those may regain enough strength to become only partially dependent on the ventilator in subsequent weeks or months, using it at night and only intermittently during the day for fatigue. The management of these problems has been discussed elsewhere (11) and is also the subject of Chapters 10–12 in this volume.

Morale: "Burn Out"

It is important that the patient know early in the illness that there is still room for hope, even if the evolving disorder proves to be ALS. In a minority of cases, perhaps 10–15 percent, the disease seems to cease progressing (2). Investigation of many cases over the years has not turned up any clue as to what happens when the "burn out" occurs. The progression usually begins to slow very subtly, and it is only after another year or two that the patient and the physicians in attendance realize that a significant slowing is underway. For patients in whom the paralysis stabilizes with considerable function preserved for more than a year or two, there is a distinct tendency for this to evolve into a permanent state of arrested disease, which we term "benign ALS" (2,3). In patients with more severe involvement when such stabilization occurs, as in the case of Professor Stephen Hawking, there is nothing benign about the residual disability, but the same stabilizing mechanism has probably also occurred, although unfortunately with much more severe paralysis.

In our ignorance of the exact cause and a specific treatment of the primary pathophysiologic process in ALS, perhaps the best we can hope for at this time is amelioration of major troublesome symptoms and the preservation of patient and family morale. The saddest cases we have attended are those who were wrongly counseled that death would occur early and there was nothing at all to be done, whereupon they became despondent, took to bed, and avoided all use of their muscles; disuse atrophy and depression then compounded all the essential problems of ALS. On the other hand, the cases with the best outcomes have been characterized by an optimistic mental attitude throughout the illness and frequent use of the muscles as much as possible, together with a good general state of health. The patients are asked to come for evaluations at least every three months, whether there is any real need or not, simply because this concretely demonstrates the physician's interest in the case and thus serves to encourage the patient and the family to come in or call more frequently if new or troublesome problems develop.

The generous application of treatments to relieve symptoms, particularly those that cause pain, is a further concrete demonstration of the dedication of the physicians and also promotes patient morale. Most of these patients will then consent to enter double-blind scientific trials of experimental medication, which may one day prove of actual value to them or to others. Such trials also demonstrate that the physician is in touch with the worldwide network of physician-scientists who are actively studying and attempting experimental treatments of the disease—a further boost to morale.

Home Care

"Be it ever so humble, there's no place like home" (17). We actively encourage home care throughout the illness, even in the terminal stage (18,19), rather than hospitalization or even hospice care, as good as the latter is in some health systems (16).

There are many difficult problems in nursing, such as the patient with second and third degree burns over 90 percent of the body, but surely one of the most difficult problems is in preterminal or terminal ALS, when mentation and the special and somatic senses are usually intact but the cognizant, intelligent patient is imprisoned in his own body from supraquadriplegia, fully perceptive and aware, but only able to communicate by eye movements or blinks, otherwise unable to notify others of the filling bladder, the itching nostril, the need for quiet, the pain of aspiration, or the pain of being paralyzed and no longer able to contribute to the family, indeed the pain of depleting the family's resources, both material and spiritual. Moreover, the nursing problem usually lasts not for a few days or weeks, while the sufferer hovers between life and death as in a severe burn, but for months or years unless untreatable pneumonia or another complication intervenes. Our experience in many such cases is that it is not only the patient who becomes demoralized, but also all the medical attendants, especially the nurses.

In these rather desperate circumstances, we have received encouragement from many ALS patients and their families and friends who elected to fight ALS and its complications and disabilities at home. Some failed dismally, others struggled to hold their ground, but a minority not only managed to maintain themselves but also occasionally regained some ground. From the latter cases, assuming that we are seeing the same disease, we all gain hope and the necessary encouragement to attempt to treat new cases (18,19).

In most cases, rather than in rare atypical cases, a useful life of good quality is possible on a ventilator at home; continued hospitalization is not essential and may even be detrimental. Family and concerned friends may rapidly learn the essential nursing care. Case illustrations have been published elsewhere (11,18, 19). The results generally have been good and particularly appreciated by the patients. Home restores the patient's control: meals come on request, not at predetermined institutional times; friends and family visit at will, not at institutional visiting hours; familiar sights and sounds are restored; and the germ environment of the hospital is replaced. Finally, morale is greatly improved at home.

Acknowledgments

Many collaborators over many years contributed to this work, particularly neurological colleagues Drs. R.A. Smith, E.H. Denys, and P.R. Calanchini, and nurses D. Holden and L. Elias. Much more has been learned from patients, particularly T. Anderson, K. Billa-Shannon, P. Harrington, P. Seidelhuber, and M. Wiliams, than we ever learned formally or read in standard texts.

References

1. Newrick PG, Langton-Hewer R. Motor neurone disease: can we do better? *Brit Med J* 1984, 289:539–542.

2. Norris FH, Shepherd RM, Denys EH, et al. Onset, natural history and outcome in subtypes of idiopathic adult motor neuron disease. *Neurology* 1992 (in press).
3. Norris FH. Amyotrophic lateral sclerosis: the clinical disorder. In: Smith RA, ed. *Handbook of Amyotrophic Lateral Sclerosis*. New York: Dekker, 1992.
4. Conradi S, Ronnevi L-O, Norris FH. Motor neuron disease and toxic metals. In: Rowland LP, ed. *Human Motor Neuron Diseases*. New York: Raven Press, 1982.
5. Norris FH, Smith RA, Denys EH. Motor neurone disease: towards better care. *Brit Med J* 1985, 291:259–262.
6. Daube JR, Litchy WJ, Low PA, Windebank AJ. Classification of ALS by autonomic abnormalities. In: Tsubaki T, Yase Y, eds. *Amyotrophic Lateral Sclerosis: Recent Advances in Research and Treatment*. Amsterdam, Excerpta Medica, ICS 769, 1988: 189–191.
7. Mulder DW, Lambert EH, Eaton LM. Myasthenic syndrome in patients with amyotrophic lateral sclerosis. *Neurology* 1959, 9:627–631.
8. Denys EH, Norris FH. Amyotrophic lateral sclerosis: impairment of neuromuscular transmission. *Arch Neurol* 1979, 36:74–80.
9. Aubier A, De Troyer M, Sampson P, Macklem T, Roussos C. Aminophylline improves diaphragmatic contractility. *New Engl J Med* 1981, 305: 249–252.
10. Fallat RJ, Jewitt B, Bass M, et al. Spirometry in amyotrophic lateral sclerosis. *Arch Neurol* 1979, 36:74–80.
11. Norris FH, Fallat RJ. Respiratory function in motor neurone disease. In: Williams A, ed. *Motor Neurone Disease*. London: Chapman & Hall (in press).
12. Janiszewski DW, Caroscio JT, Wisham LH. Amyotrophic lateral sclerosis: a comprehensive rehabilitation approach. *Arch Phys Med Rehab* 1983, 64:304–307.
13. Russell TR, Brotman M, Norris FH. Percutaneous gastrostomy: a new simplified and cost-effective technique. *Am J Surg* 1984, 148:132–137.
14. Udaka F, Yamao S, Magata H, Nakamura S, Kameyama M. Pathologic laughing and crying treated with levodopa. *Arch Neurol* 1984, 41:1095–1096.
15. Norris FH. Motor neurone disease: treating the untreated. *Brit Med J* 1992, 304: 458–459.
16. O'Brien T, Kelly M, Sanders C. Motor neurone disease: a hospice perspective. *Brit Med J* 1992, 304:471–473.
17. Payne JH. Home sweet home. In: *Clari: The Maid of Milan*, 1823.
18. Norris FH, Holden D, Kandal L, Stanley E. Home nursing care by families for severely paralyzed ALS patients. *Adv Exp Med Biol* 1987, 209:231–238.
19. Norris FH, Smith RA, Denys EH, et al. Home care of the paralyzed respirator patient with amyotrophic lateral sclerosis. In: Charash L, Lovelace R, Wolf S, Kutscher A, Roye D, Leach C, eds. *Realities in Coping with Progressive Neuromuscular Diseases*. Philadelphia: Charles Press, 1987.

4

Therapeutic Trials in Amyotrophic Lateral Sclerosis

Sany T. Khabbaz, M.D., and Raymond P. Roos, M.D.

Amyotrophic lateral sclerosis (ALS) is a progressive degenerative neurologic disease. There is no known cure and no treatment regimen that slows the progression. In this chapter, we present several proposed etiologies for ALS and a number of therapeutic trials that have been planned or conducted based on these hypotheses. Although none have yielded definitive beneficial effects, some trials have had provocative results suggesting the need for more extensive studies.

Several important principles should be kept in mind with respect to the design of treatment trials in ALS. One must be careful to plan the trial to ensure sufficient numbers of patients in order to reliably evaluate the efficacy of the drug. The inclusion of an adequately sized control group is of value since the natural history of ALS is still not well defined. In order to evaluate the efficacy of treatment, the availability of good, consistent quantitative muscle testing is essential since an effective drug may not cure ALS, but only slow the progression of disease. Unfortunately, reliable quantitative testing may be more available for testing some muscle groups, but not others, such as those involving brainstem function.

Therapeutic trials have been targeted in several directions.

Immunological Factors and ALS

Several studies have suggested that immunologic factors play an important role in the pathogenesis of ALS. For example, there are a number of old as well as newer observations that suggest the serum of ALS patients contains antibodies

43

to motorneurons (MNs). Wolfgram et al. (1) and Roisen et al. (2) reported that sera from ALS patients cause damage to cultured MNs. Oldstone et al. (3) found that the renal glomeruli of ALS patients have evidence of immune complexes. Kletti (4) reported that ALS sera contain antibodies directed against MN antigens. More recently, Gurney et al. (5) claimed that ALS patients have antibodies against a MN growth factor called "neuroleukin." Unfortunately, these reports have generally not been reproduced and are no longer pursued.

The relationship between the immune system and the pathogenesis of ALS was put on a firmer foundation with the description of a treatable multifocal motor neuropathy syndrome associated with anti-GM_1 ganglioside antibody (6). This syndrome, probably first described by Freddo et al. (6), was given greatest attention after the report of Pestronk et al. (7) describing effective treatment with cyclophosphamide. Although the syndrome is primarily a lower motor neuron one, some patients do have brisk reflexes, raising the possibility that ALS may also be an immune-mediated process. These ideas prompted Drachman and Kuncl (8) to propose that ALS was caused by an unconventional T cell-independent immune response that is difficult to treat with conventional immunosuppressive therapy.

A variety of immunosuppressive treatments have been tested in ALS. Plasmapheresis alone or in combination with azathioprine failed to produce any improvement (9). A combination of azathioprine and prednisolone did not produce a beneficial effect in a study of twenty-one patients (10). Appel et al. (11) found that cyclosporin A appeared to be of some benefit for men who entered the study within eighteen months of the onset of symptoms, although the overall rate of progression in the thirty-eight patients included in the study was not altered.

There are a number of ongoing trials with immunosuppressive treatments. In a trial at Johns Hopkins Hospital (R. Kuncl, personal communication), patients received total lymphoid irradiation (TLI) with a maximum of 3,000 rads given five days a week for eight weeks, while a control group received sham TLI. A third arm of the study will involve patients who receive intravenous followed by oral cyclophosphamide according to the protocol used by Pestronk et al. (7).

Neurotoxins and ALS

Neuroexcitotoxic amino acids, such as glutamate and aspartate, have been hypothesized to play a role in the pathogenesis of ALS or in the final common pathway of MN damage. One of the glutamate receptors, the N-methyl-D-aspartate (NMDA) receptor, has been proposed to play a central role in glutamate neurotoxicity (12). NMDA receptors are decreased in amount in affected brain tissue from patients with Alzheimer's disease (13) and Huntington's disease (14), suggesting that neurons with this receptor may be preferentially damaged, perhaps through the action of an excitotoxic amino acid. Additionally, the overall metabolism of glutamate has been reported to be altered in patients with ALS (15). There are claims of a reduction in glutamate dehydrogenase (GDH) activity in patients with motor neuron degeneration (16), with increased plasma (17) and spinal fluid (18) and decreased central nervous system (especially spinal cord) levels of glutamate (19,20). Other related compounds such as aspartate, N-acetylaspartate, and N-acetylaspartylglutamate have also been noted to be reduced in ALS spinal cord (21). Serum aspartate has been reported to correlate inversely with the severity of ALS (22).

Normally, glutamate that is released from nerve terminals into the synaptic cleft is eliminated by an uptake system that is mainly present in the surrounding glial cells. The glutamate is either metabolized to glutamine or α-ketoglutarate, which could serve as a precursor of glutamate in the nerve terminal (23,24). Any abnormality that disrupts this process may increase the extracellular glutamate in the synaptic cleft, which in turn could overexcite the NMDA receptor and cause cell death. This could occur by a decreased uptake secondary to a defective energy transporter, a defective metabolism of glutamate within the glial cells, or leakage of glutamate from nerve endings through a defective membrane. Additionally, there is evidence to suggest that the presence of glycine in the spinal cord and brainstem renders them increasingly susceptible to the potential neurotoxicity of glutamate. Glycine has been shown to potentiate the NMDA response in cultured mouse brain neurons by acting in a strychnine-insensitive allosteric site (25); this seems to be important with repeated activation of the receptor. Thus, the presence of glycine in increased amounts coupled to the increased synaptic glutamate levels could play a role in the neuronal degeneration.

Further support for a relationship between excitatory neurotoxic amino acids and ALS comes from investigations of lathyrism. This disease is a spastic paraparesis from upper motor neuron involvement thought to be a result of toxicity from the seed of *lathyrus sativus*, the chickling pea. Spencer et al. (26) have postulated that beta-N-oxyalylamino-L-alanine, a potent neuroexcitatory aminoacid in the chickling pea, induces the disease.

In 1988, Plaitakis performed a pilot study using branched chain amino acids (BCAA) in ALS (27). The BCAA are believed to stimulate GDH (activating GDH in brain) and lead to increased oxidation of synaptic glutamate (which is found by some to be increased). BCAA were found to produce a significant benefit in ALS patients with respect to maintenance of muscle strength and a continued ability to walk. A more recent study, however, failed to demonstrate any benefit (28). Additional studies of BCAA are ongoing.

The data suggesting that glutamate may play a role in ALS has led to a number of clinical therapeutic trials involving NMDA receptor antagonists. Appelbaum et al. (29) used low dose dextromethorphan, an NMDA antagonist, in eighteen patients with ALS; fifteen patients reached the six-month crossover point with no side effects. There was no statistically significant improvement in the drug-treated patients (perhaps due to the small number of patients); further studies using high dose dextromethorphan are presently in progress. Future studies may benefit from the co-administration of quinidine with dextromethorphan. Cyto-chrome P4502D6 enzyme in humans is responsible for the o-demethylation of dextromethorphan, a major route for its elimination. Zhang and his colleagues (30) have shown that the administration of quinidine, a cytochrome P4502D6 inhibitor (31,32), with dextromethorphan in ALS patients resulted in higher dex-tromethorphan plasma concentrations compared to levels obtained with adminis-tration of dextromethorphan alone, even when higher dosages of dextromethor-phan were used. A phase III double-blinded placebo control clinical trial of riluzole, which is believed to inhibit glutamate release and antagonize the gluta-mate receptor, is presently underway.

Lastly, studies aimed at modulating glycine have also been carried out. These studies have involved treatment with L-threonine, a glycine precursor. Blin and coworkers (33) reported that this treatment caused short-term, but not long-term, benefit in ALS patients.

It may be relevant to discussions of neurotoxins to also discuss trials of selegi-line (deprenyl) in ALS. There are at least two rationales for this treatment. First, the observation that Guamanians have an increased incidence of ALS and Parkin-son's dementia syndrome and of both of these syndromes has suggested a relation-ship between ALS and Parkinson's disease. Since selegiline is a selective, non-competitive inhibitor of the monoamine oxidase type B enzyme, an enzyme primarily responsible for the degradation of dopamine in the striatum, this drug was predicted to be effective in treating the symptoms of Parkinson's disease and "related diseases." The second rationale involves the concept that excessive formation of toxic free radicals from oxidative reactions leads to neurodegenera-tion. Selegiline has been claimed by some to protect against neurodegeneration by reducing the formation of free radicals and oxidative stress. One clinical dou-ble-blind crossover trial involving a treatment trial of twenty-five ALS patients with deprenyl found some possible benefit of the drug, suggesting the desirability of further study (34).

Growth Factors and Hormones

Ciliary Neurotrophic Factor (CNTF)

A recently described growth factor that has generated a great deal of interest is CNTF, first identified as a factor that sustained the survival of chick embryo ciliary nerve ganglia. It has also been found to support the survival of chick embryo spinal cord motor neurons in culture (35); prevent degeneration of facial nucleus motor neurons *in vivo* (36); and prevent about 50 percent of denervation-induced atrophy of the soleus muscle after adult rat sciatic nerve section (37). Its richest source is intraocular tissue, but it is found in other tissues, including sciatic nerve. CNTF was purified, and the rabbit, rat, and human genes were cloned and sequenced (38,39). The successful cloning led the way for expression in bacteria and the production of large amounts for therapeutic testing. Treatment efficacy was first tested on mouse genetic mutant models: the wobbler mouse, motor neuron degeneration (mnd) mouse, and the pmn/pmn mouse (40–42). These studies demonstrated statistically significant benefits following the treatment (40–42), suggesting that CNTF may have a potentially beneficial effect on ALS; a multicenter phase III clinical trial is underway.

Thyrotropin Releasing Hormone (TRH)

TRH is released by the hypothalamus, which then stimulates the release of thyrotropin stimulating hormone (TSH) from the pituitary. TRH has a direct effect on the nervous system and may play a role as a neurotransmitter. TRH receptors are distributed throughout the central nervous system, especially in the dorsal and ventral horns of the spinal cord. Schmidt-Achert et al. (43) and Banda et al. (44) demonstrated that TRH has a trophic effect on lower motor neurons; TRH increases the area of neurite growth in cultured fetal rat ventral spinal cord tissue, resulting in an increased number of axosomatic synapses (45). Additionally, TRH causes an increase in contraction frequency of cultured motor neuron-innervated human muscle (46). Based on these data, high doses of TRH have been administered to patients with ALS in therapeutic trials. Despite the fact that initial uncontrolled trials showed a beneficial effect, controlled studies have generally failed to support these findings (47–50); one saline-controlled treatment trial, however, did claim improvement (51). There is at least one center still involved in a trial using TRH and analogues in ALS.

Growth Hormone and Insulin-Like Growth Factor

Insulin-like growth factor 1 (IGF-1), which mediates growth hormone effects, has been shown to be present in satellite cells of regenerating muscle (52). Despite the latter observation, serum IGF-1 levels in ALS patients are not significantly different from levels in controls (53); this finding suggests that IGF-1 may play a role locally as a trophic or growth factor for regenerating muscle fibers and the nerves innervating them. IGF-1 has also been shown to play a role in the growth and differentiation of muscle cells (54) and in the development of oligodendrocytes (55). These reports led to a therapeutic trial using human growth hormone in ALS (56). This study failed to find clinical improvement in the patients following treatment.

Brain-Derived Neurotrophic Factor (BDNF)

Recent evidence suggests that BDNF, a member of the neurotrophin family, is normally transported from skeletal muscles to alpha motor neurons and is upregulated with respect to its expression in muscle following denervation (57). BDNF prevents naturally occurring motor neuron cell death in chicken embryos (58) and also prevents death of motor neurons in neonatal rats following axotomy of the sciatic (59) and facial nerves (57,60). Clinical trials of BDNF in ALS are planned in the future.

Treatment of Familial Amyotrophic Lateral Sclerosis (FALS)

The therapy of autosomal dominantly inherited familial ALS (FALS) received new direction recently with a report that mutations in the gene for superoxide dismutase type 1 (SOD1) are found in patients with this disease (61). SOD1 is a homodimeric enzyme that "breaks down" superoxide, a toxic free radical. The mutated SOD subunit may cause disturbed function of the normal subunit of the enzyme dimer (a dominant "negative" effect) and thereby lead to free radical accumulation; the reason for the motor neuron selectivity of the disease remains unclear. Since SOD1 is cloned and is even available through genetic engineering, FALS patients are candidates for treatment with the enzyme; unfortunately, there may be difficulties in delivering SOD1 to motor neurons. Additionally, gene therapy of FALS will undoubtedly become an option in the future. Investigators presently wonder whether sporadic ALS may also result from free radical damage. For this reason, a number of trials are anticipated in the near future involving treatment of both familial and sporadic ALS patients with varied free radical scavengers.

Conclusion

The last decade has seen an increase in the number of therapeutic trials in ALS and an improvement in our ability to assess patients by means of quantitative muscle testing. We look forward to the identification of treatment modalities that will positively influence the clinical course. These modalities may have to await a better understanding of the pathogenesis of the disease.

An up-to-date list of ongoing therapeutic trials can be obtained from the ALS Association, 21021 Ventura Boulevard, Suite 321, Woodland Hills, CA 91364 (818–340–7500).

Acknowledgment

We thank Lee Baksas for her help in preparing this chapter. Supported in part by NIH Grant #1PO1NS21442-08.

References

1. Wolfgram F. Blind studies on the effect of amyotrophic lateral sclerosis sera on motor neurons in vitro. In: Andrews JM, Johnson TR, Brazier MAB, eds. *Amyotrophic Lateral Sclerosis: Recent Research Trends*. New York: Academic Press, 1987: 145–451.
2. Roisen FJ, Bartfeld H, Donnenfeld H, Baxter J. Neuron specific in vitro cytotoxicity of sera from patients with amyotrophic lateral sclerosis. *Muscle Nerve* 1982, 5:48–53.

 3. Oldstone MBA, Perrin LH, Wilson CB, Norris FH. Evidence for immune-complex formation in patients with amyotrophic lateral sclerosis. *Lancet* 1976, 2:269–272.
 4. Kletti NB, Marton LS, Antel JP, Stefansson K. Antibodies against neural antigens in sera of patients with amyotrophic lateral sclerosis. *Neurology* 1984, 34 (Suppl. 1): 238.
 5. Gurney ME, Belton AC, Cashman N, Antel JP. Inhibition of terminal axonal sprouting by serum from patients with amyotrophic lateral sclerosis. *N Engl J Med* 1984, 311: 933–939.
 6. Freddo L, Yu RK, Latov N, et al. Gangliosides GM_1 and GD_{1b} are antigens for IgM M-protein in a patient with motor neuron disease. *Neurology* 1986, 36:454–458.
 7. Pestronk A, Cornblath DR, Ilyas AA, et al. A treatable multifocal motor neuropathy with antibodies to GM_1 ganglioside. *Ann Neurol* 1988, 24:73–78.
 8. Drachman DB, Kuncl RW. Amyotrophic lateral sclerosis: an unconventional autoimmune disease? *Ann Neurol* 1989, 26:269–274.
 9. Kelemen J, Hedlund W, Orlin JB, et al. Plasmapheresis with immunosuppression in amyotrophic lateral sclerosis. *Arch Neurol* 1988, 40:752–753.
10. Werdelin L, Boysen G, Jensen JS, Mogensen P. Immunosuppressive treatment of patients with amyotrophic lateral sclerosis. *Acta Neurol Scand* 1990, 82:132–134.
11. Appel SH, Stewart SS, Appel V, et al. A double-blind study of the effectiveness of cyclosporine in amyotrophic lateral sclerosis. *Arch Neurol* 1988, 45:381–386.
12. Choi DW. Glutamate neurotoxicity and diseases of the nervous system. *Neuron* 1988, 1:623–634.
13. Young AB, Greenamyre JT, Hollingsworth Z, et al. N-MDA receptor losses in putamen from patients with Huntington's disease. *Science* 1988, 241:981–983.
14. Maragos WF, Greenamyre T, Penney JB, Young AB. Glutamate dysfunction in Alzheimer's disease: an hypothesis. *Trends Neurosci* 1987, 10:65–68.
15. Plaitakis A, Caroscio JT. Abnormal glutamate metabolism in amyotrophic lateral sclerosis. *Ann Neurol* 1987, 22:575–579.
16. Plaitakis A, Berl S, Yahr MD. Neurological disorders associated with deficiency of glutamate dehydrogenase. *Ann Neurol* 1984, 15:144–153.
17. Perry TL, Kriegger C, Hansen S, Eisen A. Amyotrophic lateral sclerosis: amino acid levels in plasma and cerebrospinal fluid. *Ann Neurol* 1990, 28:12–17.
18. Rothstein JD, Tsai G, Kuncl RW, et al. Abnormal excitatory amino acid metabolism in amyotrophic lateral sclerosis. *Ann Neurol* 1990, 28:18–25.
19. Perry TL, Hansen S, Jones K. Brain glutamate deficiency in amyotrophic lateral sclerosis. *Neurology* 1987, 37:1845–1848.
20. Plaitakis A, Constantakakis E, Smith J. The neuroexcitotoxic amino acids glutamate and aspartate are altered in the spinal cord and brain in amyotrophic lateral sclerosis. *Ann Neurol* 1988, 24:446–449.
21. Constantakakis E, Plaitakis A. N-acetylaspartate and acetylaspartyl glutamate are altered in the spinal cord in amyotrophic lateral sclerosis. *Ann Neurol* 1988, 24:478.
22. Patten BM, Harati Y, Acosta L, Jung SS, Felmus MT. Free amino acid levels in amyotrophic lateral sclerosis. *Ann Neurol* 1978, 3:305–309.
23. Fonnum F. Transmitter glutamate in mammalian hippocampus and striatum. In: Kvamme E, ed. *Glutamine and Glutamate in Mammals*, vol 2. Boca Raton, FL: CRC Press, 1988.
24. Shank RP, Aprison MH. Glutamate as neurotransmitter. In: Kvamme E, ed. *Glutamine and Glutamate in Mammals*, vol 2. Boca Raton, FL: CRC Press, 1988.

25. Johnson JW, Ascher P. Glycine potentiates the N-MDA response in cultured mouse brain neurons. *Nature* 1987, 325:529–531.
26. Spencer PS, Roy DN, Ludolph AC, Hugon J, Dwivedi MP, Schaumburg HH. Lathyrism: evidence of the role of neuroexcitatory amino acid BOAA. *Lancet* 1986, 2: 1066–1067.
27. Plaitakis A, Smith J, Mandeli J, Yahr MD. Pilot trial of branched-chain amino acids in amyotrophic lateral sclerosis. *Lancet* 1988, 1:1015–1018.
28. Testa D, Caraceni T, Fetoni V. Branched-chain amino acids in the treatment of amyotrophic lateral sclerosis. *J Neurol* 1989, 236:445–447.
29. Appelbaum JS, Salazar-Grueso EF, Richman JG, Shanahan M, Roos RP. Dextromethorphan in the treatment of ALS: a pilot study. *Neurology* 1991, 41 (Suppl. 1):393.
30. Zhang Y, Britto MR, Valderhaug KL, Wedlund PJ, Smith RA. Dextromethorphan: Enhancing its systemic availability by way of low-dose quinidine-mediated inhibition of cytochrome P4502D6. *Clin Pharmacol Ther* 1992, 51:647–655.
31. Brosen K, Gram LF, Haghfelt T, Bertilsson L. Extensive metabolizers of debrisoquine become poor metabolizers during quinidine treatment. *Pharmacol Toxicol* 1987, 60: 312–314.
32. Brinn R, Brosen K, Gram LF, Haghfelt T, Otton SV. Sparteine oxidation is practically abolished in quinidine-treated patients. *Br J Clin Pharmacol* 1986, 22:194–197.
33. Blin O, Pouget J, Aubrespy G, Guelton C, Crevat A, Serratrice G. A double-blind placebo-controlled trial of L-threonine in amyotrophic lateral sclerosis. *J Neurol* 1992, 239:79–81.
34. Norris FH, Tan Y, Fallat RJ, Elias L. Trial of deprenyl in amyotrophic lateral sclerosis. Submitted.
35. Wong V, Arraiga R, Panayotatos N, Lindsay RM. Ciliary neurotrophic factor (CNTF) supports survival of motor neurons in culture. *Neurology* 1991, 41(Suppl. 1):312.
36. Sendtner M, Kreutzberg GW, Thoenen H. Ciliary neurotrophic factor prevents the degeneration of motor neurons after axotomy. *Nature* 1990, 345:440–441.
37. DiStefano PS, Yancopoulos GD, Squinto SP. Ciliary neurotrophic factor (CNTF) prevents degeneration-induced atrophy of rat skeletal muscle. *Neurology* 1992, 42(Suppl.3):336.
38. Stöckli KA, Lottspeich F, Sendtner M, et al. Molecular cloning, expression and regional distribution of rat ciliary neurotrophic factor. *Nature* 1989, 342 (6252): 920–923.
39. Masiakowski P, Liu H, Radziejewski, et al. Recombinant human and rat ciliary neurotrophic factors. *J Neurochem* 1991, 57:1003–1012.
40. Holmlund T, Mitsumoto H, Greene T, Wong V, Cedarbaum JM, Lindsay RM. The effect of ciliary neurotrophic factor (CNTF) on spontaneously degenerating motor neurons in Wobbler mice. *Neurology* 1992, 42(Suppl. 3):369.
41. Helgren ME, Wong V, Kennedy M, et al. Ciliary neurotrophic factor (CNTF) slows the progression of motor dysfunction in the Mnd mouse. *Works in Progress. American Academy of Neurology*, 1992.
42. Sendtner M, Schmalbruch H, Stöckli KA, Carroll P, Kreutzberg GW, Thoenen H. Ciliary neurotrophic factor prevents degeneration of motor neurons in mouse mutant progressive motor neuropathy. *Nature* 1992, 358:502–502.
43. Schmidt-Achert KM, Askanas V, Engel WK. Thyrotropin-releasing hormone enhances choline acetyltransferase and creatine kinase in cultured spinal ventral horn neurons. *J Neurochem* 1984, 43:586–589.

44. Banda R, Means ED, Samaha FJ. Trophic effect of thyrotropin-releasing hormone on murine ventral horn neurons in culture. *Neurology* 1985, 35 (Suppl 1):93.
45. Askanas V, Engel WK, Egleson K, Micaglio G. Influence of TRH and TRH analogs RGH-2202 and DN-1417 in cultured ventral spinal cord neurons. In: Metcalf G, Jackson I, eds. *Recent Advances in the Biomedical Significance of Thyrotropin-releasing Hormone (TRH)*, vol. 553. NY: Acad Sci, 1989.
46. Askanas V, Engel WK, Kobayashi T. Thyrotropin-releasing hormone enhances motor neuron-evoked contractions of cultured human muscle. *Ann Neurol* 1985, 18:716–719.
47. Imoto K, Saida K, Iwanmura K, Saida T, Nishitani H. Amyotrophic lateral sclerosis: a double-blind crossover trial of thyrotropin-releasing hormone. *J Neurol Neurosurg Psychiat* 1985, 47:1332–1334.
48. Caroscio JT, Cohen JA, Zawodniak, et al. A double-blind placebo-controlled trial of TRH in amyotrophic lateral sclerosis. *Neurology* 1986, 36:141–145.
49. Brooke MH, Florence JM, Heller SL, et al. Controlled trial of thyrotropin-releasing hormone in amyotrophic lateral sclerosis. *Neurology* 1986, 36:146–151.
50. Mitsumoto H, Salgado ED, Negroski D, et al. Amyotrophic lateral sclerosis: effects of acute intravenous and chronic subcutaneous administration of thyrotropin-releasing hormone in controlled trials. *Neurology* 1986, 36:152–159.
51. Brooks BR, Sufit RL, Montgomery GK, Beaulieu DA, Erickson LM. Intravenous thyrotropin-releasing hormone in patients with amyotrophic lateral sclerosis. Dose-response and randomized concurrent placebo-controlled pilot studies. *Neurol Clin* 1987, 5:143–157.
52. Jennische E, Skottner A, Hansson, HA. Satellite cells express the trophic factor IGF-1 in regenerating skeletal muscle. *Acta Physiol Scand* 1987, 129:9–15.
53. Braunstein GD, Reviczky AL. Serum insulin-like growth factor-1 levels in ALS. *J Neurol Neurosurg Psych* 1987, 50:792–794.
54. Florini JR. Hormonal control of muscle growth. *Muscle Nerve* 1987, 10:577–598.
55. McMorris FA, Smith TM, DeSalvo S, Furlanetto RW. Insulin-like growth factor-1/Somatomedin C: a potent inducer of oligodendrocyte development. *Proc Natl Acad Sci USA* 1986, 83:822–826.
56. Festoff BW, Melmed S, Smith R. Therapeutic trial of recombinant human growth hormone in amyotrophic lateral sclerosis. *Myelopathles, Neuropathles, Myopathies—Acquisitions Recentes: Advances in Neuromuscular Disease*. Paris: Expansion Scientifique Francaise, 1988:117–126.
57. Koliatsos VE, Clatterbuck RE, Winslow JW, Cayouctte MH, Price DL. Evidence that brain-derived neurotrophic factor is a trophic factor for motor neurons in vivo. *Neuron* 1993, 10:359–367.
58. Oppenheim RW, Qin-Wei Y, Prevette D, Yan Q. Brain-derived neurotrophic factor rescues developing avian motoneurons from cell death. *Nature* 1992, 360:755–757.
59. Yan Q, Elliott J, Snider WD. Brain-derived neurotrophic factor rescues spinal motor neurons from axotomy-induced cell death. *Nature* 1992, 360:753–755.
60. Sendtner M, Holtmann B, Kolbeck R, Thoenen H, Barde Y-A. Brain-derived neurotrophic factor prevents the death of motoneurons in newborn rats after nerve section. *Nature* 1992, 360:757–759.
61. Rosen DR, Siddique T, Patterson D, et al. Mutations in Cu/Zn superoxide dismutase gene are associated with familial amyotrophic lateral sclerosis. *Nature* 1993, 362:59–62.

5

Amyotrophic Lateral Sclerosis: Unorthodox Treatments

Mark R. Glasberg, M.D.

Patients should be strongly encouraged to participate in valid clinical research. Although many may not choose to do so, ample time should be spent with each patient, discussing experimental therapeutic options available within one's own institution as well as elsewhere. Patients may choose not to participate in clinical drug trials for many reasons. In placebo-controlled studies, patients do not want to take a 50 percent chance of receiving placebo rather than the active pharmaceutical agent. Even for open-ended trials, without placebo, there are many reasons patients choose not to participate. These include psychological aspects, such as denial and hopelessness, that may make it difficult to recruit ALS patients into clinical trials. Therefore, it is often helpful to have a clinical psychologist work within the protocol trial to help forestall compliance problems. Additionally, a patient's degree of physical impairment may make frequent visits to the clinic difficult. If the financial resources of the family are limited, travel expenses and time off from work, for either the patient or the caregiver, may be a big concern. Also, lack of understanding of the importance of clinical trials on the part of the patients and families is a frequent reason that patients choose not to participate. Investigators must thoroughly explain the purpose of the trial and the procedures to ALS patients and their families.

Patients often tend to choose unorthodox treatments. One reason is the lack of the constraints found in a scientifically approved study. It will continue to be hard to discourage our patients from obtaining alternative treatments when we do not have any treatment available to either cure or significantly alter the course of the disease. Unorthodox treatments change with time and consist of such items as megadose vitamin treatment, pancreatic enzymes, wheat germ, snake venom, or bee pollen. Although one perhaps feels that these treatments can do no harm, they may be very expensive, and their eventual failure may lead patients to either withdraw from health care professionals completely or seek one unorthodox treatment after another.

Besides advocating participation in valid research, physicians taking care of ALS patients need to counsel their patients regarding unorthodox treatment that could be considered as quackery. One clue is a treatment promoted for a number of unrelated diseases, such as cancer, heart disease, and multiple sclerosis, as well as ALS. Also beware of treatments for which no formal protocol is available for either patients or referring physicians and for which controls are lacking. Rather than a formal protocol, the supporting literature often relies on patient testimonials. This nonsponsored research has not undergone any form of peer review, and there are high costs that are all borne by the patients, who often have to pay thousands of dollars before even starting the treatment protocol (1). However, as long as a devastating disease like ALS remains without any treatment that either cures or significantly improves the disease, it will be difficult to dissuade patients from undergoing unorthodox treatments.

Snake Venom

In the 1970s, there was particular interest, accompanied by a great deal of public controversy, in the purported effectiveness of modified snake venom mixture (2, 3). Based on observations that certain snake venoms block the action of polio virus on the anterior horn cells, patients were treated with an inactivated venom from the cobra (*Naja siamensis*) and krait (*Bungarus multicinctus*), and significant benefit was purported to be observed. After an average treatment of fourteen months, 52 out of 113 ALS patients were reported as stabilized and 13 as improved.

During the later 1970s, many ALS patients went to Florida for treatment with snake venom. To evaluate the benefit of this unconventional therapeutic agent more carefully, Tyler completed a carefully controlled, double-blind study (4). No therapeutic benefit occurred with snake venom. Of considerable interest was the observation that over one-third of the patients had temporary improvement whether they were on placebo or the ineffective experimental drug.

Snake venom is an example of how an unorthodox treatment may have some rationale, i.e., blocking the action of polio virus on anterior horn cells, plus a major placebo effect that produces what seems like a significant clinical response. This was an unorthodox treatment that bordered on medical respectability, and subsequently led to an NIH-funded clinical trial.

In reviewing many of the treatments for ALS in the past, there have been a number of agents that one might consider to have even less rationale, and perhaps be even more unorthodox than snake venom. Nonetheless, looking back over fifteen years, snake venom still stands out as the prototype of an unorthodox treatment that not only received much publicity, but for which ALS patients spent a good deal of valuable time and money.

Calcium-EAP

An example of an unorthodox treatment that ALS patients are currently taking is Calcium-EAP. This is one of the key staples in Hans Nieper's arsenal for fighting many diverse diseases, including cancer, cardiovascular disease, and neurological diseases, especially multiple sclerosis. He is a German physician who practices "eumetabolics." Calcium-EAP is the key repair substance for the myelin sheath around nerve pathways, according to Dr. Nieper. It is the modern alternative to ineffective drugs with many side effects, Nieper stresses, and its mechanism is to protect "the myelin sheath along the nerve paths, the cells of the so-called oligodendroglia and the so-called blood brain barrier" by using substances that seal off the sheath surface and guard against "immune aggression." While several compounds are said to achieve this, the most important is Calcium-EAP. Although originally used in neurological disease therapy for multiple sclerosis, the same rationale, that of myelin protection, is advocated for the use of Calcium-EAP in ALS. The first ALS patients were started on this treatment in about 1975.

Calcium-EAP may be taken either orally or by injection. The range of healthful activity attributed to Calcium-EAP is impressive. According to the Hans Nieper Foundation newsletter, "it is helpful in capillary flow, cerebellar activation, against chronic gastric disturbances, against inflammation and allergic reactions initiating disturbances on the skin. It is soothing to high fever, combats bacterial infection of mucous membrane, helps stop water retention (edema) and helps stop osteoporosis as well as bleeding gums. In other words, it helps a person's continuous battle against calcium metabolism deficiency."

Dr. Nieper claims to be world-renowned for his work in cancer, multiple sclerosis, mineral and electrolyte metabolism, aging, and the prevention of cardiac infarction. He is also said to be well known for his research in gravity, physics, and energy fields, "a beloved avocation which serves to complement his biochemistry and physiology studies." Dr. Nieper's newsletter claims that his influence in the United States has reached all the way to the White House, and that he has established firm friendships with many top American scientists. Thanks to Dr. Nieper's influence, there is claimed the introduction of selenium therapy for heart protection, introduction of deshielding or deblocking therapy of cancer with pineapple enzymes (bromelaine) and beta-carotene and "desodification" (expulsion of sodium) of cancerous tumors, not to mention the enzyme-based cleaning of coronary and leg arteries using serrapeptase, an enzyme produced by bacterium found in silkworms. In the 1970s, Dr. Nieper dared to champion the controversial substance, laetrile. He discovered a compound found in laetrile that acts as a "gene repair substance." Today, Dr. Nieper is said to be the "world leader in therapies involving gene repair" substances such as squalene, derived from shark livers, and carnivora derived from the Venus's-flytrap, a carnivorous plant.

Needless to say, Dr. Nieper's therapies have been very controversial. A copy of a letter sent to an ALS patient for prospective treatment showed the cost of the initial three days of treatment as an outpatient would be from $1,000 to $1,500, plus travel expenses to and from Germany, and hotel and food. Additionally, a three-month supply of medication, which the patient would take home, would cost from $1,000 to $2,000.

In l986 the U.S. Food and Drug Administration halted the import of drugs from Hans Nieper, including Calcium-EAP for multiple sclerosis and ALS, Laetrile (Amygdalin), Iscador, "fresh cell therapy," and "Wobe-Mugos enzymes," offered for treatment of cancer, as well as bromelin, carnitine, selenium, magnesium orotate, and potassium orotate for heart disease. The U.S. Customs Service has detained some one hundred fifty shipments of these drugs, while many other shipments have been entering the country illegally. The FDA is concerned not only that these unproven remedies may be unsafe, but also that they will deter patients from undergoing potentially beneficial and accepted lifesaving treatments.

Live Cell Therapy

Live cell therapy consists of injections of animal fetal cells (5). The rationale is to confer innumocompetence on lymphoid cells, endocrinological stabilization, and treat protein dysmetabolism and degenerative processes, by using the corresponding organospecific RNA. Regeneresen, especially, promoted the latter. It is composed of organospecific ribonucleic acids (RNA) from organs and tissues of young cattle or fetuses and from yeast. A specific treatment given to an ALS patient in 1987 used the following formula:

> 5 amp. RN
> 3 amp. Großhirnhemisphare (cerebral hemisphere)
> 4 amp. Stammganglien (brain stem)
> 4 amp. Medulla oblongata
> 6 amp. Ruckenmark (spinal cord)

Aztec Institute in the Philippines also offers live cell treatment, derived from embryos of animals, usually a lamb; thus, they termed this treatment "lamb cell therapy" (LCT). They claim that this is a "wonder drug" and that the efficacy of utilizing lamb cells for paralysis and other related genetic disorders has been proven beyond doubt. Basic fees for on-site treatment in the Philippines are the following:

1. 3 weeks outpatient treatment (cancer) $5,300.00
2. 10-day treatment (in- or outpatient) for live-centered therapies $4,000.00
3. 5-day treatment for rejuvenation, regeneration $2,700.00
4. Diagnostic workup alone $ 500.00

However, specific diagnostic testing such as CAT scan, ultrasound, accelerated charge neutralization, metabolic food testing, herbal tumor removal, ozone, and live cells (when not part of a live cell program) are not included in this fee. Also, the cost of take-home medications is not included, because "it may vary greatly from case to case." Payment is due one week in advance by any secured form of payment, but not by personal check. The ten-day treatment is applicable to all forms of cardiac and circulatory disorders, all forms of arthritis, autoimmune diseases, neurological disease including Parkinson's, primary lateral sclerosis and ALS, genetic defects including Down's syndrome, inborn errors of metabolism, sexual disorders, chronic kidney and lung diseases, and multiple allergies.

Interferon and Sandostatin

Dr. Rajko Medenica is a controversial physician (oncologist, hematologist, and immunologist), who is currently treating patients with ALS, along with a number of other disorders, with interferon (an antiviral agent) and sandostatin (a growth hormone). One of his famous patients is Mohammad Ali, whom he is treating for posttraumatic Parkinsonism syndrome. He was highlighted on the television program "Inside Edition" in 1989, and since then there have been many inquiries from patients about his treatment. Dr. Medenica's work was started in Switzerland, and he has been in the United States since 1984. His work is unpublished

His program consists of treatment with escalating doses of interferon by intramuscular injection for three days. He begins with three million units of interferon and may increase the dose to six million units. Prior to giving interferon, he does blood work to test patients for the interferon inhibitor factor, and if this factor is present, he gives higher doses. Along with interferon, he gives sandostatin, a growth hormone that is supposed to increase the metabolism of nerve fibers and help decrease atrophy. This is given by subcutaneous injection three times a day for four days. The cost of this regimen is $2,000.

Dr. Medenica claims that this treatment appears to slow the progression of the disease, with the responses being varied in each patient. Some of the responses include improved speech and swallowing, decreased fasciculations, ability to walk again, and increased energy. The most remarkable changes were observed in a man who was bedridden and ventilator-dependent. After three to four months of treatment, he was able to walk with assistance and to be off the ventilator for short periods of time. Dr. Medenica did not confirm the diagnosis of ALS with any additional studies, and no double-blind studies were planned.

Ayurvedic Medicine

Treatment programs have been proposed for a variety of neurological disorders, including ALS, by the American Association of Ayurvedic Medicine. By 1991, they had seen in their clinic a total of seven patients with a definite diagnosis of ALS. A standard ALS severity scale was administered to all patients, and improvement in all patients was noted.

The treatment program consists of neuromuscular and neurorespiratory integration programs, an internal purification program, and three to four treatments of total body immersion in sesame oil during a period of massage. The oil temperature is increased slightly during the course of the treatment, as the oil is constantly being recirculated with pumps and massage by trained technicians. Additionally, and possibly more importantly, all patients have complemented this program with the practice of transcendental meditation (TM). Patients are then also given a number of different kinds of Ayurvedic herbal preparations based on specific imbalances. Overall results are said to have been quite successful (6).

The patients with ALS vary in severity from minimally to extremely debilitated and wheelchair-bound. Seventeen patients with MS have also been treated, with significant improvement. Patients with multiple sclerosis received a slightly different program because of the often negative effect of heat treatments on that disorder.

Edgar Cayce Foundation

Foundations such as the Edgar Cayce Foundation in Virginia advocate an approach to healing of the whole person—body, mind, and soul. They provide both patients and physicians with explanations of different diseases, such as a commentary on amyotrophic lateral sclerosis written in 1968 by Dr. William McGarey. The commentary provides an explanation of Edgar Cayce's rationale of treatment, which involves both divine influences, karmic aspects, the necessity of mental activity bringing about a change before physical application of therapy is begun, and deficiency of a specific mineral, i.e., gold. A suggested therapeutic regimen is divided into five parts: 1) Change in mental attitudes, which includes specific verses of scripture that are to be read; 2) Use of wet cell therapy, which is a battery solution consisting of distilled water, copper sulfate, sulfuric acid-CP, zinc, and willow charcoal. The plates of the battery are then attached to the individual's body; 3) After the wet cell treatment, massage for a period of thirty to forty-five minutes is done using a mixture of olive oil, peanut oil and lanolin; 4) Every third day, one of the following solutions should be added to half a glass of water and taken immediately: gold chloride solution, 1 grain per ounce of distilled water; and bromide of soda solution, 2 grains per ounce of distilled water; 5) Finally, there should be an alkaline-forming diet, low in carbohydrates, without alcohol.

Dietary Treatment

Dietary treatments have been advocated for ALS for a number of years. Dietary treatments often start with a reasonable rationale, such as avoidance of excessive amounts of aluminum, which are noted in the neurofibrillary tangle in Alzheimer's disease and in Guamanian ALS. Sources of aluminum in the diet consist of the following (per Pfeiffer):

1. Aluminum in baking powders.
2. Aluminum sulfate used to purify drinking water.
3. Naturally occurring aluminum in water supplies; varies by location.
4. Aluminum from cooking utensils.
5. Some free-flowing salt contains aluminum.
6. Most antacids and buffered aspirin contain aluminum compounds.
7. Some toothpastes and dental amalgams utilize aluminum.
8. Some cigarette filters.
9. Food additives and food wrappers.
10. Cosmetics and deodorants.
11. Amphogel and Gelusil.
12. Some cheeses emulsified with aluminum compounds.
13. Some white flour bleached with potassium alum.

Therefore, according to the *Clinical Nutritionist* newsletter, a nutritional support schedule as an adjunct to primary medical care should be directed not only to supplying nutrients known to biochemically support nerve repair, but also to stopping all ingestion, physical and respiratory exposure to all aluminum compounds possible. At the same time, specific nutrients that assist the body in excreting aluminum residuals should be given. However, since aluminum is so ubiquitous, this diet is almost impossible to adhere to. Many other dietary approaches to ALS treatment have been employed, including megadoses of multivitamins, vitamin E, pancreatic extract, and amino acids.

Allergy Injections

Various health care professionals and others send letters to the ALS Association (ALSA) promoting their own individual treatments. A Las Vegas physician claimed in a 1991 letter that he has put ALS into remission with his own specific combinations of allergy injections. The letter is as follows:

"I am sure that I can put multiple sclerosis into remission. I have done it several times before, along with amyotrophic lateral sclerosis and many other immune abnormality diseases. Please don't throw this letter down in complete disbelief. Please read it. I have been working in this field about twenty-five years. I use no cortisone or any harmful habit-forming drugs. Those who are on these drugs are carefully weaned off. I use FDA approved antigen (allergy shots). These same antigens are used everyday by doctors all over the world, but the specific combination of these antigens is mine. It is this specific combination that makes the difference, just like a specific combination of notes makes a particular song. The shots do not hurt and they are not harmful. A great problem has been, people shut me off in complete disbelief without even talking to the patients or examining the facts. Also, there has been nothing written in the medical literature on these discoveries. For this reason doctors have made authoritative negative comments without knowing anything of the immunology involved or do they have the slightest idea of what I am doing. To make authoritative derogatory remarks about something that is critical to millions of lives without having knowledge of the facts is cruel. If what I say is too good to be true please talk to my patients. There are many who will talk to you or your representative. There is no risk or harmful side effects, only improvement."

Multiple Unorthodox Treatments

Next I will detail the history of a patient I have seen, who has taken, almost continuously, one unorthodox treatment after another. He is a man in his early fifties who first developed leg weakness in 1982. He is currently wheelchair-bound, although he still has moderately good strength in the upper extremities. Bulbar and respiratory impairment is minimal. His clinical diagnosis is that of the lower motor neuron form of ALS, progressive muscular atrophy.

He began acupuncture treatments in 1984 and went to Boston for "deep" acupuncture. In 1985 he went to Mexico for the Gershon treatment, which consisted of a vegetarian diet with high doses of vitamins and liver juice, raw calves' liver, and five coffee enemas daily. After a few months of that treatment, he was started on the macrobiotic diet in Philadelphia for one year. This consisted primarily of vegetables, sea weed, whole grain brown rice, and soup. During that time, he lost forty lbs. He also saw a physician in Philadelphia for a homeopathic treatment plan that included application of oils both in baths and with towels. Furthermore, he went to New England for an intensive bee venom regimen, which included applications of thirty to fifty bees daily for six to seven months. During the last five to six years, he has been receiving TRH, first by injection and now one drop daily sublingually. He also took L-threonine for six months and is considering going for malaria therapy in Panama (a regimen devised as "fever" therapy for Lyme disease).

Conclusion

Throughout the years, unorthodox treatments for ALS have had a markedly negative effect on patients and families, who can deplete not only their financial resources but also their valuable time in undergoing these treatments. Even worse, a feeling of hopelessness may set in to make patients avoid treatment at multidisciplinary ALS clinics. These clinics not only improve an ALS patient's quality of life with symptomatic treatment and psychosocial support, but also provide information about legitimate treatment trials.

Acknowledgment

I am indebted to Lynn Klein, Vice President for Patient Services of the ALS Association, and the Association for making available to me both correspondence and materials sent to them regarding unorthodox treatments. This information provides the basis for a substantial portion of this chapter.

I also wish to thank Joyce Brown for technical preparation of the manuscript.

References

1. Kunel RW, Clauson LL. Amyotrophic Lateral Sclerosis. In: Johnson RT, ed. *Current Therapy in Neurologic Disease*, 3rd ed. Philadelphia: B.C. Decker, 1990, pp. 291–300.
2. Sanders M, Fellowes ON. A therapeutic approach to neuromuscular disease. *Proc 3rd Internat Cong Neuromuscular Dis*. Newcastle-Upon-Tyne: 1974.
3. Sanders M, Fellowes ON. Use of detoxified snake neurotoxin as a partial treatment for amyotrophic lateral sclerosis. *Cancer Cytol* 1975, 15:26–30.
4. Tyler HR. Modified snake venom therapy in motor neuron disease: a double-blind study. *Neurology* 1979, 29:77–81.
5. Kuhnau Wolfram W, Aites G. *Live Cell Therapy: My Life with a Medical Breakthrough*. Tijuana, Mexico: 1983.
6. Chopra D. *Perfect Health: Complete Medical Body Guide*. New York: Harmony Books, 1991.

6

Dysphagia and Dysarthria: The Role of the Speech-Language Pathologist

James M. Mancinelli, M.S., CCC-SLP/L

Introduction

A defining characteristic of ALS is its variable clinical presentation within a general framework of more or less continuous neuromuscular debilitation. Specific to the concerns of the speech-language pathologist (SLP) are the effects of the disease on the patient's oral mechanism, communicative abilities, and deglutition. Furthermore, the SLP quickly discovers the powerful influence on the family dynamic engendered by these effects and is obligated to address the familial and psychosocial issues surrounding speech and swallowing compromise. All of these particular manifestations—oral mechanism compromise, communicative disorder, dysphagia, and family issues—are more dramatic in clinical presentation and become more crucial when confronted with a patient presenting with bulbar symptomatology either initially or progressively. Paradoxically, it is the progressively bulbar nature of ALS that has fostered innovative and adaptive diagnostic and therapeutic methods, resulting in improved quality of life throughout the remaining life span.

As vigorous research continues to look for the cause(s) of ALS and to find a cure, managing the symptoms of the disease remains the only option for clinicians at this time. For ancillary health care professionals, this is both challenging and highly rewarding.

The purpose of this chapter is to present a model for the diagnosis and treatment of the ALS patient dealing with the issues within the scope of practice of the

SLP, based on the author's weekly clinical experience at the Hahnemann University Hospital ALS Clinic in Philadelphia, Pennsylvania. It is hoped that the reader will find the information presented here realistic, practical, and clinically sound.

Diagnostic Evaluation

The Oral Mechanism

The oral peripheral speech mechanism is the best place to start. The goal of this assessment is to determine functional competency for speech, deglutition, and secretion management. Any traditional method(s) for assessing the strength, force, tone, and range of motion of the labial, velar, and lingual structures can be used. With the ALS patient, one must be sure to examine for the presence of fasciculations, as well as signs of lingual atrophy. Typically, fasciculations are observed in the tongue—throughout the lingual body or in isolated locations (apex and lateral edges are common sites). Of course, they are not limited to the tongue and may be appreciated in the face. The exact relationship between fasciculations of the oral and peripheral speech musculature and speech production needs to be addressed experimentally.

Lingual atrophy is characterized by an irregular topography, with a "hill and valley" appearance of the tongue. In my experience, patients presenting with significant lingual fasciculations without atrophy do not necessarily present with concomitant speech disorders or oral stage dysphagia, although the variability of ALS may offer surprises. On the other hand, severe lingual atrophy is usually associated with both speech disorder and an oral stage dysphagia.

The extent and symmetry of velar excursion elicited by having the patient phonate "ah" should be noted. One could also stimulate the gag reflex (which may not be present in some patients) to assess these features. Adequate velopharyngeal competency is necessary during deglutition to prevent nasopharyngeal reflux and during speech production to eliminate hypernasality and nasal air emission. The examiner may find a variety of velar anomalies, depending on the stage of the disease process, using either one of these assessment techniques.

Of crucial importance over the course of the disease process is a continuous evaluation of the muscles of mastication. Masticatory inefficiency and fatigue are common in the bulbar ALS patient. Monitoring the progression and rate of deterioration assists in planning for future nutritional and swallowing needs. The simplest and quickest test of the muscles of mastication is to have the patient bite down on the back teeth while the examiner feels for the bulging of the masseter muscles in the area of the temporal-mandibular joint (TMJ) bilaterally.

Secretions and the patient's ability to manage them pose a persistent problem in this population, and the oral examination should address this issue.

Normal salivary secretion is 1000–1500cc per day, with 70 percent of the normal flow supplied by the submandibular and sublingual glands (1). In the

ALS population, the problem is thought to be not increased salivary flow, but an inefficient or absent transport mechanism, i.e., incoordinated buccal, lingual, and palatal muscles (1). Furthermore, the patient's saliva may thicken due to a chronic open-mouth posture causing evaporation. This results from the weakening of the muscles maintaining jaw closure.

An examination of the oral cavity in patients with sialorrhea, excessive secretions, reveals pooled saliva in the buccal cavities or in the anterior sulcus, but only if the secretions are still thin. In the more compromised bulbar patient, thick stringy secretions bridging the tongue and palate as well as the entrance to the oropharynx are commonly seen. Patients often report secretions so thick that they can be scooped out of the pharynx with their fingers. It is obvious that the patient presenting with a secretion management problem most likely has a dysphagia. An excellent source of information on this issue is the family/primary caregiver(s). Since they are typically with the patient throughout the day, they can comment on the thickness of the secretions, at which times of the day they are more or less problematic, and how this problem is handled in the home environment.

The ALS patient may also present with xerostomia, or dry mouth. Many patients complain of nocturnal xerostomia, which may indicate that they are mouth breathing, commonly reported by family members. As mentioned previously, this is due to compromise of the mandibular elevators. Other patients experience xerostomia as a pharmacologic side effect. The immediate concern of the SLP is the effect on verbal communication and deglutition. Some ways to help the patient deal with xerostomia are discussed in the treatment section.

Finally, the oral mechanism examination must include an evaluation of volitional and reflexive coughs. Asking the patient to cough volitionally produces variable results within this group, from the nonexistent to the robust. Also, a weak volitional cough does not preclude the presence of a more effective reflexive cough, which is the patient's protective mechanism against airway penetration. Again, family members are a good source of information.

The oral mechanism examination is a very significant component in the clinical evaluation of the ALS patient. It provides information about the functional competency of these structures, as well as a baseline with which one can compare changes in these structures as the disease progresses. The status of the oral mechanism also provides a preliminary impression of the patient's capacity for verbal communication, to which we now turn our attention.

Communication Assessment

ALS patients present with spastic, flaccid, or a mixed spastic-flaccid dysarthria. On the initial visit, the patient may present with any one of the above or no dysarthria at all. The variability of the disease process becomes evident with each new patient. However, in a study of speech disorder in motor neuron disease, Carrow et al. (2) found that 83.33 percent of patients with moderate to severe loss of intelligibility demonstrated dysphagia and signs of lingual atrophy. She also reported that pulmonary function and difficulty breathing played a negligible role in loss of intelligibility. This is the type of broad generalizability one finds with ALS. The role of the SLP is to:

(1) Determine if a dysarthria or some other communication disorder exists.
(2) Determine the type and level of severity if a dysarthria is identified.
(3) Administer appropriate diagnostic testing if another type of communication disorder exists concomitant with the dysarthria, and make referrals as indicated.
(4) Provide communication counseling to the patient and family members about the evaluation and your recommendations.

It is very possible, although rare in my experience, to meet a patient with a coexisting dementia, aphasia, fluency or voice disorder, especially if one considers that ALS predominantly manifests in the sixth decade of life. At the Hahnemann University Hospital ALS Clinic, I have encountered two cases of dysfluency post-onset of the disease in patients with no history of stuttering. The precise etiology remains mysterious, but one is tempted to attribute it to a dyscoordination between the respiratory, laryngeal, and articulatory valves. Whether it remains a peripheral dysarthric event or a more central one is a fascinating subject for future research.

In the ALS population, any evaluation of communication skills does not stop with the verbal modality, but it most naturally begins there. The factors affecting speech intelligibility are rate of speech, prosody, articulatory accuracy, and phrase groupings, and each of these is evaluated according to the Valving Model (3). The vocal parameters assessed are pitch (habitual and range), intensity, quality, resonance, and respiration. The methods of evaluation are dependent on type(s) of communication disorder(s), time available within the clinician's schedule, patient cooperation and tolerance of testing, and patient/family goals. For instance, if one is in a clinic setting, the traditional methods of formal speech/voice testing are not time-efficient, and necessity has become the mother of invention. On the other hand, if one does not have time constraints and formal testing can provide valuable information, one should proceed with that approach. I do not advocate abandoning the traditional evaluation for more informal ones, especially in these times of more stringent accountability guidelines; I do support informal methods of assessment in clinic settings, where time constraints are a reality.

My approach to assessment begins with greeting the patient and family. She is asked to state her name and address and is then asked if the speech that she is presenting is her best, worst, or typical. It is very important to remember that the variability of ALS is not only intersubject but also intrasubject. Because this is a progressively deteriorating neuromuscular process, what you are seeing may be very different from what you will see in one hour, one day, or one week, especially in the more advanced bulbar patients. Muscles fatigue with use, and the speech musculature is no exception, accounting for patient and family reports that intelligibility varies throughout the day, usually worse by day's end. The next level of assessment is to have the patient read one of the traditional diagnostic reading passages familiar to most SLPs, e.g., the "Rainbow Passage" or the "Grandfather Passage." Based on these findings, as well as on family report, a diagnosis of the type of dysarthria and its severity is made. If anarthric, the status of natural alternative communication modalities is then assessed.

Not everyone wants to be or is a candidate for the most advanced, computerized augmentative system. Most ALS patients are in their fifth, sixth, or seventh decade and feel uncomfortable with such devices. When confronted with the anarthric patient, I first observe how she communicates with her family. The effectiveness of that method is noted and recommendations are made accordingly. The nonverbal modalities we see most often include facial expression, gesture (when the upper extremities are functional), body language, and writing. Even the most severely dysarthric and some anarthric patients usually pair a nonverbal modality with the remnants of verbal language. If communication is still not effective and the impact of the patient's nonverbal status on the family is significant, then candidacy for an augmentative device is addressed.

In order to successfully and effectively use the computerized augmentative systems, the patient must demonstrate supportive motor abilities and motivation and must have a supportive family network. Careful discussion and evaluation with the occupational and physical therapists must take place before any recommendations can be made. Once that patient is evaluated and deemed a suitable candidate for a device, system selection is initiated. The following are criteria for selecting the most appropriate system to accommodate the patient's skills (not in order of importance):

1. Level of complexity matched to level of need.
2. Regressive capability.
3. Transportability.
4. User friendly.
5. Iconic vs. alphabetic?
6. Cost.
7. Training time needed for patient/family.
8. Amount of follow-up needed.
9. Compatibility with environmental systems and/or PC.
10. The significance of text-to-speech capability and sex-appropriate synthesized voice.

The SLP is then responsible for locating the device that meets the criteria for the patient, and a training program is implemented.

The oral peripheral/speech mechanism examination and the communication assessment have been presented.

Swallowing Assessment

The typical Stage I (oral stage) swallowing dysfunctions seen in the ALS population include incohesive bolus formation, prolonged oral transit time, posterior lingual leakage to the valleculae and pyriform sinuses prior to swallow initiation, oral residual after the swallow, and nasopharyngeal reflux. These Stage I anomalies are manifestations of oral mechanism compromise. Pharyngeal symptomatology includes a delayed swallow initiation, reduced pharyngeal contraction, glottal incompetency, inability to coordinate respiration and swallowing, and cricopharyngeal dysfunction. The results of the oral mechanism examination can provide information regarding the competency of Stage I deglutition. However, pharyngeal dysfunction can only be grossly addressed with videofluoroscopic assessment.

In a clinic setting, where time with each patient is limited, the interviews, patient report, and liquid swallow screening form a first-line dysphagia evaluation. It is not meant to substitute for a clinical dysphagia evaluation and/or videofluoroscopic assessment. This information does, however, provide the clinician with preliminary findings on which to base a request for further assessment. Furthermore, one can provide interim textural, positioning, and quantity guidelines for the patient/family until more refined tests can be conducted.

The liquid swallow screening gives fundamental information for Stage I and Stage II deglutition, but cannot address any covert pharyngeal symptomatology. I use water to challenge the patient's lingual function, since controlling such a neutral, rapidly moving substance requires optimal lingual function and efficient transfer-swallow coordination. This screening provides information regarding lingual and labial function as well as pharyngeal strength (repetitive swallows?) without the support of radiographic assessment. The liquid swallow screening affords the clinician the opportunity to observe the patient's typical approach to liquid ingestion, i.e., positioning, rate of ingestion, and quantity control. Furthermore, one can also observe whether the patient has begun to independently implement any compensatory techniques to facilitate the liquid swallow. Based on these findings, recommendations are made to the physician regarding further diagnostic needs or, in some cases, for alternative nutritional support. Although I rarely recommend an alternative nutritional device without a videofluoroscopic assessment, it is occasionally necessary due to the clinical presentation of some patients upon initial contact.

The videofluoroscopic swallowing study can be used as part of the workup for patient's presenting with bulbar symptomatology or just beginning to do so. This would provide a baseline for future comparison and is a very useful addition to the physician's data base. Although there are other forms of assessment in use, e.g., ultrasound, manometry, and manofluorography, videofluoroscopy is usually the method most accessible to the majority of SLPs. For a more detailed review of procedures for assessment, see Sonies (4).

The purpose of the videofluoroscopic evaluation in the dysphagic ALS patient is:

1. To assess the status of the deglutition process.
2. To document aspiration.
3. To assess the effectiveness of any compensatory strategies.
4. To determine the appropriate diet level for the patient's level of functioning.
5. To document the patient's skill as the diet level changes.

The results should be reviewed with the patient and family members. In a clinic setting, results should be reviewed with all team members, since swallowing is a quality of life issue and may require further support/input from other personnel. The patient and caretakers are then provided with guidelines and trained in their implementation. In the event that an NPO recommendation is made and the patient is reluctant to accede to an alternative nutritional device, the role of the SLP is to insure that the patient and family are aware of the ramifications of continued oral feeding. Chronic aspiration with possible pulmonary compromise, nutritional depletion, dehydration, and possible asphyxiation by choking must be explained and discussed in a sensitive but realistic manner. On the other hand, if the patient requires and agrees to an alternative nutritional device, the role of the SLP is to inform the physician and nursing staff; to determine if oral feeding for supplementary or pleasure purposes is possible; to direct the patient to the clinical nutritionist for clarification of the surgical procedure and the mechanics of tube feeding.

The assessment of the oral peripheral/speech mechanism, communication status, and deglutition of the ALS patient have been described. It must be stressed that these diagnostic methods may not be generalizable to all clinical settings. It is true that certain assessment paradigms are universal; however, the clinic setting in which the described approach evolved demanded that more traditional forms occasionally be suspended. This was primarily a result of time constraints and patient availability. I encourage other clinicians to find other creative and effective ways to assess this patient population, improving on this model to better serve those entrusted to our care.

Family Issues

A licensed psychologist, psychiatrist, and/or psychiatric nurse are the professionals to diagnose any dysfunction. However, the SLP cannot leave untouched the serious disruptions to family life caused by communication and swallowing disorders. Any counseling that is offered by the SLP should address only those two issues.

The typical problems include denial of deficits, anger, anxiety (especially about oral feeding), frustration, hostility directed toward caregivers, depression, and self-imposed isolation. A wealth of information can be obtained through observation of the patient and family during the initial interview. Being direct with my questions has been a fruitful approach. For example, "Mr. Smith, have you noticed that people are pretending to understand you when you know that they don't?" often stimulates vigorous verbal and nonverbal responses from everyone present. The SLP can then use those as a springboard for a comment such as, "I see that provoked a difference of opinion among you. Why doesn't someone tell me about that." The diagnostic goals for family issues would be:

1. To uncover any disruptions in the family dynamic caused by the communication and swallowing disorders.
2. To determine family receptivity to possible intervention to resolve these issues.
3. To suggest the appropriate referrals to mental health professionals, as indicated.

Interventional approaches are discussed in the next section.

Treatment Strategies

Due to the progressive nature of ALS, *remediation* of speech, swallowing, and oral muscular deficits is not possible. *Compensation* is the best we can do at the moment. Despite this bleak prognosis, I offer our patients this advice: one lives with ALS by flowing with ALS. If a patient makes the necessary adaptations throughout the course of the disease, he can have quality of life. It is when the patient and/or caretaker resist the progressive nature of the disease that frustration, anxiety, and anger can supplant the possibilities for a more pleasurable existence. Furthermore, one must always stress to the patient that daily goals must be compatible with the level of functioning. For example, to successfully call the dog in the backyard from a distance with compromised respiratory support for speech is unrealistic. The role of the SLP in this case is to help the patient adjust to this component of his dysarthria and then provide a compensatory strategy to accomplish his goal. It is always a question of equilibrium: balancing ability with the intended goal. This is the basic principle for optimal therapeutic intervention for the ALS patient in all areas within the SLP's scope of practice.

The Oral Mechanism

The effectiveness of exercises to increase or stabilize the range of motion and/or strength of the lingual, labial, and velar structures has no support in the clinical literature (5). Unfortunately, the clinical research in this area, like most areas of rehabilitative ALS management, is sparse to nonexistent. Prescribing oro-motor exercises in the case of weakness or debilitation due to inactivity may be indicated.

However, in ALS where the transmission of neural information to muscle is failing or absent, I believe that no amount of exercise can facilitate improvement.

Communication Therapy

Communication therapy for the still verbal ALS patient entails optimizing any residual physiologic functions related to the speech production process. The goal is to enhance intelligibility and thus increase effectiveness of communication, while decreasing frustration, isolation, anger, and anxiety. Human beings are driven to communicate, so that even the most severely dysarthric patients and even some anarthric patients will have already discovered the most effective means to do so. If they have not independently devised their own strategies, your communication evaluation will have provided information needed to intervene. As mentioned previously, we believe that if a patient has a natural modality for communication, it is the role of the SLP to refine and optimize its use. In my experience, it is rare to find a patient who is unable to communicate a message in a manner of his own design. Problems arise when the speaker-listener dyad does not support the chosen method. For example, one ALS patient has a deaf spouse. She refused to accommodate to her reduced intelligibility. Although her husband is deaf, she continued to call him from another room, did not wait for eye contact to initiate conversation, and blamed him for being insensitive. In this case, communication therapy consisted of:

1. Demonstrating the importance of eye contact.
2. Counseling the patient on the combined effects of her dysarthria and his hearing loss on his ability to perceive the message.
3. Demonstrating the use of overarticulation to optimize visual cues for the listener.
4. Having them commit to trying the "new" way of communicating.

After all the tears were over, an agreement was reached to make a new start. This scenario may appear maudlin, but ALS can be so devastating to the family dynamic that such situations are more typical than atypical.

There are some instances in which short-term outpatient speech therapy is indicated, especially for mildly dysarthric professionals still in the work force. The basic therapeutic goals for this type of patient are:

1. To instruct the patient in the use of overarticulation.
2. To instruct the patient in the use of appropriate breath support for speech purposes.
3. To provide training in optimal phrase groupings to enhance communication.

Since ALS patients are typically cognitively intact and are usually very motivated to improve their speech, goal achievement can be quick.

For the anarthric patient without an alternatively efficient, natural modality of communication, the therapeutic goals are:

1. Appropriate selection of the device based on the criteria of the evaluation.
2. Ongoing family/caregiver training throughout the course of the disease.
3. Training the patient in switch use when applicable.
4. Training the patient in scanning, since this can be difficult for the ALS patient with limited cervical range of motion.
5. Continual consultation with the PT/OT services regarding changes in the patient's motor skills.
6. Monitor the patient's use of the device with phone calls, treatment sessions, and/or home visits.

In clinic settings where patients are seen at predetermined intervals, e.g., every three months, the role of the SLP who staffs that clinic may be primarily diagnostic and consultative to the managing SLP. Regardless of clinical settings, treatment schedules must remain sensitive to the patient's mobility, tolerance, and need, as well as fiscally responsible.

Swallowing Therapy

Swallowing therapy, like communication therapy for the verbal ALS patient, is based on compensation. The fundamental principle is:

> If one controls the texture, quantity, and the body position, feeding by mouth is still possible, as long as other medical factors do not contraindicate it.

Unfortunately, this was not always the approach to management of dysphagia in ALS. Cricopharyngeal myotomy was tried for dysphagia in ALS (6,7,8). The risks of respiratory problems and general anesthesia in the ALS population are higher, and the results reported in the literature do not support surgery as the optimal solution. Gagic (6) reported that patients with neuromuscular processes had "poorer results" after cricopharyngeal myotomy compared with patients with vagal injuries and stroke. However in this study only one ALS patient was included. Lebo et al. (7) found that 64 percent of ALS patients who underwent cricopharyngeal myotomy improved short-term, while 36 percent showed no significant change. Although these figures seemed encouraging, long-term experience was not (8), and cricopharyngeal myotomy is not recommended by my team.

After the results of the diagnostic evaluation are reviewed by the neurologist, the SLP, and the clinical nutritionist, the goals for swallowing rehabilitation are established. In the case of the ALS patient, they are:

1. To optimize hydration.
2. To facilitate nutritional maintenance via oral feeding, according to the fundamental principle.
3. To monitor changes in the oral stage of swallowing and propose textural adaptations as indicated to accommodate those changes.
4. To reevaluate videofluoroscopically if pharyngeal stage changes are overt or suspected based on report or clinical observations.
5. To provide supportive counseling/education to patient/family throughout the course of treatment.

Any of the therapeutic techniques specific to Stage I and Stage II anomalies may be implemented, but as the patient develops increasing bulbar problems, even compensatory techniques lose their effectiveness. Generally, any patient with a ten pound weight loss between visits is considered for an alternative nutritional device, once it is established that the loss is secondary to dysphagia and not self-feeding issues.

The most treacherous body positions for the dysphagic ALS patient include supine and hyperextension. These reduce bolus control even more, increasing the probability of severe complications during oral feeding. If a patient is unable to sit during meals, we recommend the side-lying position. Prolonged sitting is typically problematic for ALS patients because they are often unable to shift their weight without assistance. Subsequently, meals should be arranged for the times when the patient is sitting most comfortably, since this will prevent somatic distractions and increase oral intake.

It is common to encounter an ALS patient whose Stage II function is supportive for oral feeding, but whose Stage I function is so impaired that feeding by mouth is precluded. If a patient is known to be headed in this direction, it is recommended that they keep a "Can/Can't" list. The patient can fold or divide a sheet of paper in half and for one week list every item that poses no problem in Stage I or Stage II on one side and on the other side every item that presents even the most negligible difficulty. At the end of the week, the patient and caregiver review the list and determine if a trend is present. Are all the items on the "Can't" side sticky, stringy, crumbly, liquid, and so on? If such a trend is identified, they should contact the clinical nutritionist who helps them to adjust their diet level or instructs them in ways to alter the substance instead of eliminating it completely. This is a crucial interventional component since ALS patients with compromised deglutition begin to eliminate items that pose problems, leading to nutritional depletion and/or dehydration. Furthermore, by having the patient confront dysphagia in this way, little room is left for denial of deficits, opening the door to effective management.

Finally, the problems of sialorrhea, excessive secretions, and xerostomia (dry mouth) must be addressed. As with early approaches to dysphagia management, surgical solutions to secretion management, such as transtympanic neurectomy, were proposed (9). Unfortunately, nerve regeneration occurs rapidly so this procedure must be repeated.

Secretion management is the most tenacious symptom of ALS. The most typical complaint is that secretions feel "stuck" in the distal pharynx, causing a persistent annoying sensation. These secretions can become thicker and dried out due to mouth breathing. The neurologist may prescribe a tricyclic antidepressant, e.g., amitriptyline, to dry up the secretions since that is a known side effect of this family of cholinergic drugs. However an effective nonpharmacologic treatment can be a lemon and water solution. The ratio is one tablespoon of lemon juice to two ounces of warm water; the patient drinks the solution until he feels relief, *if and only if* the pharyngeal swallow is supportive. It works amazingly well in some patients and not at all in others, consistent with the intersubject variability common in ALS. An alternative is to substitute Italian lemon ice, again more facilitative for some patients than others. Sialorrhea can be extremely severe in ALS and can actually lead to social isolation. Xerostomia is secondary to mouth breathing during sleep, chronic open-mouth posture due to muscle weakness, or side effects from drugs. Patients seem to tolerate xerostomia much better than sialorrhea. Of course, if it is relentless, it can affect the oral stage of deglutition and a recommendation for more moist foods is in order. For xerostomic episodes during waking hours, one could try spraying the oral cavity with ice cold water and have the patient "swish," then expectorate. Of course, this is only advisable if the oral mechanism is supportive of such an approach. Lemon-glycerine swabs may help.

Family Counseling

Once the effects of the communication and/or swallowing disorders have manifested themselves in the family dynamic, it is the role of the SLP to help the family identify the issues and begin discussion around willingness to improve the existing situation. For example, it is crucial to be sensitive but direct when addressing denial of deficits and the patient's feelings of hostility toward family members because they cannot understand her speech or want to feed her. These are very common scenarios within the ALS population, and the SLP must consider everyone's position in any discussion. Since communication is a "fifty-fifty" event, i.e., equal responsibility on the part of the listener and the speaker, all parties have legitimate grievances. It is very helpful to explain the communication dyad in this way since it promotes equal justice. Whenever the family dynamic appears especially complex, a psychiatric and/or psychological consultation is the most rational and beneficent intervention.

The role of the SLP in the diagnosis and treatment of the ALS patient is a very challenging one in that he is confronted with a progressively deteriorating clinical picture. Above all, the SLP must always keep in mind that the management of the ALS patient is symptomatic in nature. Adjusting diagnostic and therapeutic methods to the ever-changing needs of the patient helps provide the quality of life that they so justly deserve.

References

1. Hillel AD, Miller RM. Management of bulbar symptoms in amyotrophic lateral sclerosis. *Adv Exp Med-Biol* 1987, 209:201–221.
2. Carrow E, Rivera V, Maudlin M, Shamblin L. Deviant speech characteristics in motor neuron disease. *Arch Otolaryngol* 1974, 100:212–218.
3. Darley FL, Aronson AE, Brown JR. *Motor Speech Disorders*. Philadelphia: Saunders, 1975.
4. Sonies BC. Instrumental procedures for dysphagia diagnosis. *Sem Speech Lang* 1991, 12:185–198.
5. Dworkin JP, Hartman DE. Progressive speech deterioration and dysphagia in amyotrophic lateral sclerosis: case report. *Arch Phys Med Rehab* 1979, 60:423–425.
6. Gagic NM. Cricopharyngeal myotomy. *Can J Surg* 1983, 26:47–49.
7. Lebo CP, Ü KS, Norris FH. Cricopharyngeal myotomy in amyotrophic lateral sclerosis. *Laryngoscope* 1976, 86:862–868.
8. Ü KS, Norris FH, Denys EH. *Surgery for ALS Patients*. Amsterdam: World Congr Neurol, 1977.
9. Smith RA, Goode RL. Sialorrhea. *N Eng J Med* 1970, 283:917–918.

7

Nutritional Maintenance in Amyotrophic Lateral Sclerosis

Eileen M. Carr-Davis, R.D., L.D.

Introduction

Amyotrophic lateral sclerosis can be nutritionally devastating to patients. Weight loss can occur as muscles atrophy and dietary intake decreases as a result of weakness in the arms and hands, difficulty in swallowing, fear of choking, embarrassment over drooling, or depression. The nutritional deficiencies incurred by poor intake can result in impairment of functioning and reduced self-esteem.

Patients can be best helped if nutritional issues are recognized in the early stages of the disease and are handled with a practical and positive approach. Patients may be able to maintain oral intake longer if they are counselled as difficulties arise rather than after they have become severely depleted. They may also be more receptive to suggestions if they are given enough time to consider their options.

This chapter describes the effects of ALS on nutrient intake and nutritional status, nutritional assessment, strategies for maintaining adequate nutrient intake, supplementation with specific nutrients, tube feeding, and options for feeding.

Effects of ALS on Nutrient Intake and Nutritional Status

Dysphagia

Dysphagia, or difficulty swallowing, is probably the most commonly recognized symptom affecting dietary intake in ALS patients. Patients with early ALS may have dysphagia and dysarthria, but eventually all patients show swallowing dysfunction (1).

By definition, dysphagia results from impaired function of the jaw, lips, tongue, velum, larynx, pharynx, upper esophageal sphincter, or esophagus (2). These structures are innervated by the lower motor neurons of cranial nerves VII, IX, X, XI, and XII, which are often affected by neurological disorders such as ALS (3). Nine to thirty percent of patients with ALS initially present with difficulty swallowing or speech production. In nearly 100 percent, the mouth, the pharynx, or both are eventually involved (4).

Swallowing occurs in four phases: 1) the preparatory phase, during which food is manipulated in the mouth, chewed, and, if necessary, pulled together into a cohesive bolus; 2) the oral phase, during which the tongue propels the bolus posteriorly to the anterior faucial arches; 3) the pharyngeal phase, during which the bolus is propelled through the pharynx; and 4) the esophageal phase, when esophageal peristalsis moves the bolus to the stomach (4).

Any impairment of the tongue muscles or dysfunction of its innervator (cranial nerve XII) compromises the oral phase. A patient whose tongue is atrophied, partly paralyzed, or otherwise difficult to control has trouble forming and containing a bolus and often coughs or chokes before swallowing. Food can fall over the base of the tongue and into the open airway. Some patients compensate for the lack of control by tilting the head backward, thus relying on gravity to move the bolus, or by pushing the bolus to the back of the throat manually (3).

The success of the oral preparatory phase of the swallow depends on proper functioning of cranial nerves V, VII, and XII, and the facial, oral, and tongue muscles they innervate. Patients who cannot negotiate this phase avoid solid foods and complain that they cannot control or move food in their mouth (3).

The pharyngeal phase involves the pharyngeal constrictors, the soft palate, and the group of laryngeal structures that protect the lower airway, which are innervated by cranial nerves IX, X, and XI. Patients who have trouble with this phase complain of food catching in the throat, nasal regurgitation, coughing or choking during or after swallowing, and hoarseness after swallowing (3).

Typical manifestations of oropharyngeal dysphagia include inefficient oral control and mastication of liquid and food boluses; delayed initiation of the swallowing reflex; residue in the pharynx after swallowing; and aspiration into the trachea before, during, or after swallowing (2).

In a study comparing lip, jaw, and tongue muscle involvement, DePaul et al. (5) reported that ALS affects the hypoglossal motor neuron cells earlier and to a greater extent than it affects facial or trigeminal motor neuron cells. This pattern was observed in the bulbar ALS group and also in patients with symptoms confined to the limbs.

Research has examined the sequence with which individual muscles are affected in ALS. A review of initial complaints by patients seen at the University of Wisconsin Neurodysphagia Clinic and an early report in the literature reveal that early difficulty with swallowing affects solids at least as often as liquids, with liquids becoming more difficult later. Robbins (4) notes the frequent initial complaint of "solids sticking in my throat." Difficulty chewing, liquids leaking from the lips, eating more slowly, increased saliva production, thick saliva, or postnasal congestion are also common complaints.

Bulbar palsy is secondary to involvement of the cranial nerve musculature. Classically, bulbar palsy is a later event, but it may be an initial complaint in up to one-fourth of patients. Carpenter et al. (6) found dysphagia to be among the first symptoms in 13 percent of 123 patients diagnosed between 1970 and 1972. Of secondary symptoms, which were noticed one month to five years after onset of initial symptoms, dysphagia was the second symptom in 48 percent of the patients (6).

Because dysphagia varies with the severity of the disease, management must be individualized. In all patients, the main causes for concern about swallowing are malnutrition and aspiration (3). Aspiration may not be identified at a bedside evaluation nearly 40 percent of the time, even by experienced clinicians (7).

Defining the severity of dysphagia helps both in tailoring dietary recommendations and in the timing of further intervention. Speech pathologists evaluate swallowing ability by visual inspection and radiologic studies or by modified barium swallow. These studies help to assess the location and severity of swallowing dysfunction using various bolus consistencies (1). This approach can help identify those patients who aspirate small amounts of food that are not easily detected on visual inspection. Nutrition therapy for ALS patients should not only meet the energy, fluid, vitamin, and mineral needs of the patients, but should also be aimed at preventing aspiration. Speech pathologists and dietitians work closely with patients to determine which types of foods and beverages can be safely consumed and to recommend proper positioning for eating and drinking.

Decreased Dietary Intake

Some patients report not having eating or swallowing difficulties when questioned, but still appear to lose weight and are unable to maintain a constant nutritional status. The poor prognosis of ALS may cause many emotional changes that must also be considered carefully. Patients may become depressed and hopeless, which may lead to lack of interest in eating and resistance to the suggestions to eat. Patients may become embarrassed about their disability if weakness causes drooling or choking at mealtimes. Many times they prefer to eat alone to avoid social eating occasions. Some even stay at home for meals rather than eat with relatives. Loss of upper extremity strength can also be frustrating as patients cannot feed themselves and become more dependent on caregivers. As eating becomes more of a struggle, the time taken to eat meals becomes longer and overall intake drops.

Nutritional Assessment

Assessing the nutritional status of the ALS patient can be difficult because of the muscle wasting that characterizes the disease. Weight loss from the disease is difficult to distinguish from weight loss as a result of poor intake. Therefore, prevention of weight loss is not always possible. However, it may be minimized with dietary counseling. In general, weight loss of greater than 20 percent is usually considered severe. Because of the progressive nature of ALS, however, any uncontrolled weight loss warrants attention, especially if seen in conjunction with signs of dysphagia.

In general nutritional assessment, body weight, nitrogen balance measurements, skinfold fat measurements, and mid-arm muscle circumference are the most commonly measured anthropometric variables (8). All of these measurements have limitations, however.

Weight

Weight is probably the most common measure of nutritional assessment. A more useful standard than the "ideal body weights," specified by sources such as the Metropolitan Life Insurance Company, is the percentage of usual, healthy body weight (9). The percentage of healthy weight helps to determine changes in nutritional status and how well a patient is able to maintain usual body weight. Patients often have never weighed the amount recommended by the life insurance charts or the ideal weight-for-height calculated by common formulas. Therefore, comparing a person to a standard that is not individualized does not help to assess changes during the disease.

Nitrogen Balance

Nitrogen balance measurements are often obtained to document the effects of nutritional support, but such measurements are difficult to perform and are associated with a large measurement error. Additionally, nitrogen balance is a measure of the effect of nutritional support and is not a measure of a patient's nutritional state (10).

Skinfold Fat Thickness

Skinfold fat thickness is another measure that must be considered with caution. It is unknown whether internal and subcutaneous fat masses change proportionally with more acute changes in nutritional status from illness or stress or whether changes in total body water, particularly in subcutaneous tissues, introduce serious errors in the measurement of skinfold thickness (9). The accuracy of skinfold measurements depends on the skill of the person taking the measurement and varies from person to person. Separating skinfolds from severely atrophied muscle can be difficult, as can interpreting the results of the test.

Mid-Arm Muscle Circumference

Mid-arm muscle circumference is a measurement of the muscle component of the fat-free body mass. Arm circumference is converted to arm muscle circumference with a formula that corrects for skinfold thickness (arm muscle circumference = arm circumference − 0.314 triceps skinfold) (9). However, the conversion introduces a systematic measurement error, and arm circumference varies with activity level as well as with nutritional status.

Biochemical Measures

Several biochemical variables can also be measured. Although no single variable has proven to be completely reliable, serum albumin concentration is the most commonly used. The synthesis of albumin is depressed during malnutrition. Semistarvation causes albumin to move from the extravascular to the intravascular space, artificially elevating serum albumin concentration. This movement contrasts with the decrease in albumin that is usually seen in stress when albumin shifts from the intravascular to the extravascular space (9).

Finally, over- or underhydration can alter serum albumin concentration by changing blood volume without changing total body albumin. Thus, overhydration decreases serum albumin concentration (10). These factors make albumin, or any other biochemical variables that may fluctuate with hydration, difficult to interpret.

Continual monitoring of weight along with subjective information from the patient and family and input from other services, such as speech pathology, are often the most practical method of assessing the adequacy of nutritional intake.

Strategies for Maintaining Nutritional Intake

Food

Nutrition care plans should be based on the patient's symptoms. Patients who are losing weight need suggestions for maximizing intake through high-calorie and high-protein supplements. Nutrition counseling can help the patient identify household food items that are nutrient-dense (see Table 7-1). Patients may be filling up on "empty calories" or even on low-calorie beverages, such as coffee, tea, or diet soda. Commercial products are available if patients are unable or unlikely to make homemade supplements. They are convenient to use and are fortified with vitamins and minerals. A balance of regular foods and supplements can be suggested by a dietitian.

The patient with dysphagia is likely to have lost weight. Therefore, supplemen-

Table 7-1. Increasing Calories of Common Foods

Regular Food Item	Calories	Supplemented Food Items	Calories
Hot cereal (plain)	100	Hot cereal with butter or margarine, cream and honey or sugar	300
Boiled potato (plain)	115	Potatoes mashed with cream plus butter and sour cream and dry milk powder	250
Fresh apple	80	A peeled, cored apple baked with brown sugar and butter, topped with cream	250
Milk, 8 oz., whole	150	Add one cup dry milk powder to one quart milk, or make thick milkshakes with ice cream, syrup, and instant breakfast mix	225 or 500–700

tation needs to provide maximum calories and protein while minimizing aspiration.

Textures must be soft and usually smooth (see Table 7-2). Patients need to be advised to avoid dry, crumbly foods and tough meats. These textures may make food difficult to manipulate into a smooth bolus for swallowing, and a weakened tongue complicates moving foods in the mouth. Once mixed with saliva, breads may be too gummy to be transferred to the back of the mouth. Unmoistened or unchewed small particles can then be aspirated on swallowing. Meats and other foods may need to be pureed to an appropriate texture (11). Bread can be made easier to eat by toasting it and then dunking it in a beverage. Soft canned fruits, especially applesauce, work well. Fruits and vegetables can be pureed. Gravies and butter or margarine provide extra moisture to help puree foods and provide extra calories as well.

Liquids

Thin liquids can be transferred through the mouth faster than the patient is able to control them. Liquids can also enter the airway, causing coughing or choking, and they can be aspirated. Liquids may be difficult if lip weakness is present, because drooling often occurs; the lips may not be able to seal around a cup or straw.

Foods of multiple consistencies, such as cold cereal with milk or broth-based chunky soups, can be difficult to eat because of the control needed to keep the liquid portion from being aspirated while the solid portion is chewed. Patients find that soft, moist, smooth solids and thickened liquids are best tolerated. Examples of this are hot breakfast cereals, like farina, and cream soups.

Table 7-2. Guidelines for Choosing Appropriate Textures

	Use	Avoid
Fluids	Nectars, sherbets, ice cream, milkshakes, pudding, yogurt, pureed fruit	Water, coffee, tea, soft drinks, thin juices, hot chocolate, thin soup, chunky soup, broth
Meats	Moist, ground, or pureed meat and poultry, tender fish without bones, eggs	Tough dry meats, dry poultry or dry fish, peanut butter
Starches	Toast, cold cereal well-soaked in milk or cream, cooked cereal, pancakes, pasta, casseroles, rice with gravy/sauce, moist cookies, baked, mash, or boiled potato with gravy, cream, or margarine	Crumbly bread, hard rolls, bread with nuts, seeds, coconut, or fruit, bread with cracked wheat particles, dry cereal flakes, dry toast, crackers, melba toast, dry rice, dry cookies
Vegetables	Soft canned vegetables or well-cooked fresh or frozen vegetables, scalloped tomatoes	Raw vegetables, firm-cooked vegetables, stringy vegetables such as corn, spinach, or firm peas

Patients need specific instructions on how to meet their fluid needs safely. Fluid needs are usually two to three liters per day (12). Suggestions for thickening liquids with regular household items and commercial thickeners are helpful. Liquids may need to be taken in very small sips or from a spoon, with the chin tipped forward during the swallow. Fluids lost from drooling need to be replaced. Pudding, applesauce, and mashed potato-type consistencies may be the most easily manipulated and swallowed. Foods need to be well moistened. These foods, as well as thick milkshakes, yogurt, and ice cream, provide the much needed fluid, calories, and protein.

Patients who complain of excessive phlegm may notice that milk products aggravate this problem. Suggestions for non-milk containing supplements, such as thickened frozen ices and modular carbohydrate, fat, and protein products, need to be provided.

Encouraging Adequate Intake

Some patients are more willing to adjust their diets than others. If meals take progressively longer to complete, smaller, more frequent, nutrient-dense meals should be served. Family members should be encouraged to stay at the table longer to help encourage the patient to eat (11). Although patients should not be forced to eat, a variety of foods should always be available, recipes provided by the dietitian should be tried, and a pleasant, positive atmosphere should be maintained.

If dietary intake has been compromised, multivitamin and mineral supplementation may be necessary. Many patients can take chewable supplements. Liquid vitamin and mineral supplements may be too thin to be swallowed safely. However, if added to a small amount of thicker liquids, they may still be tolerated better than tablets (12).

Constipation

Patients may become constipated when they decrease physical activity, when the voluntary muscles involved in defecation weaken, when fluid intake diminishes, or when fiber intake is decreased as foods with certain textures are dropped from the diet (12). Activity is encouraged to keep bowels moving. Fluid intake needs to be maintained; soft, fiber-containing foods need to be recommended; and bulking agents may need to be tried.

Supplementation with Specific Nutrients

Nutrients do more than meet basic nutritional requirements. Due to their role as metabolic pathway regulators, the potential therapeutic effects of several nutrients in the treatment of ALS have been investigated. Norris and Denys (13) reviewed the literature pertaining to high doses of multiple vitamins, organ extracts, and other nutrients, specifically vitamin E, and found no benefit in the use of any of these products. Abnormal calcium metabolism has been suspected as playing a role in ALS, but detailed metabolic studies of calcium and vitamin D metabolism show no significant abnormalities (14).

Octacosanol

Norris et al. studied the effects of octacosanol in ALS patients for three months. Octacosanol refers to the long-chain alcohols C-28 through 36, isolated from wheat germ oil, that are present in the central nervous system, but absent in the usual diet (13). The mean results of breathing tests and a weighted 100-point "ALS Score" showed no difference between octacosanol and placebo (15).

Branched Chain Amino Acids

Investigators have suggested that a systemic defect in the metabolism of glutamate, possibly involving both the neurotransmitter and the metabolic glutamate pools in the central nervous system, may underlie ALS (16). Glutamate, the primary excitatory neurotransmitter in the brain, can exert specific neurotoxic effects and can induce neuronal degeneration in vivo and in vitro, so excitatory neurotoxins may be responsible for motor neuron degeneration. Therefore, Rothstein et al. (17) hypothesized that metabolism of excitatory amino acids might be altered in patients with ALS. They examined the concentrations of glutamate, aspartate, and the excitatory neuropeptide N-aspartyl glutamate (NAAG) in the cerebrospinal fluid (CSF) and spinal cords of patients with ALS and found significant increases in the concentrations of these excitatory compounds (17).

Measurements of the cerebrospinal fluid (CSF) of ALS patients have shown conflicting results, including increased concentrations of lysine and leucine; no significant alterations in any amino acid levels; and elevated concentrations of glutamate, glycine, alanine, threonine, isoleucine, and phenylalanine (16).

Because elevated levels of glutamic acid in CSF might reflect increased synaptic concentrations of this excitatory neurotransmitter in ALS patients, and because glycine potentiates the N-methyl-2-aspartate (NMDA) excitatory amino acid receptor on neurons, Perry measured these and other amino acids in the CSF and fasting plasma of patients with ALS. Glutamate or glycine concentrations were not elevated in the CSF of patients with ALS, nor was glutamate concentration frequently elevated in their fasting plasma (16).

Plaitakis et al. (18) did find glutamate levels significantly decreased in the frontal and cerebellar cortex and in the cervical and lumbar cord of ALS patients on autopsy. Because tissue glutamate levels represent primarily the intracellular component and plasma levels may reflect the extracellular fluids, these data suggest the possibility of an altered distribution of glutamate in the central nervous system (CNS) of ALS patients (18).

Additionally, data from studies by Plaitakis et al. (18) showed that human brain glutamate dehydrogenase (GDH) can be activated by physiological concentrations of L-leucine, suggesting that dietary supplementation with branched chain amino acids (BCAA) may provide a new therapeutic approach to human neurodegenerative disorders in which modification of glutamate metabolism might prove beneficial (19). The rationale for this therapeutic approach is based on the ability of BCAA to activate GDH and thus to modify glutamate metabolism, which is altered in ALS (19). Research continues as to the effectiveness of this therapy.

Tube Feeding

In spite of all efforts, patients may lose the ability to eat as a result of the increased time required to eat or from more frequent episodes of coughing or choking.

A study by Slowie et al. (20) showed caloric intake below recommended dietary allowances in 70 percent of ALS patients. Patients reporting the lowest caloric intakes experienced the greatest weight loss. As intake by mouth becomes difficult and often insufficient, alternative methods of feeding should be considered. When the patient with bulbar palsy is losing weight and can no longer eat without the risk of aspiration, the decision of whether to begin tube feeding must be made (21).

Tube Feeding Versus TPN

Total parenteral nutrition is not indicated for patients with ALS, because beyond the swallowing mechanism, the gastrointestinal (GI) tract is functional. Norris and Denys (13) found no abnormalities in nutrient absorption through the GI tract of six patients with ALS. In most patients, the gastrointestinal tract is at least partially functional, and enteral feeding, therefore, should be prefered to intravenous feeding. Enteral nutrition is physiologically more natural and has beneficial effects on intestinal structure and function (22). Additionally, it is safer and less costly. In patients with severe dysphagia, enteral nutrition should be part of routine care (22).

Various forms of tube feeding are available, including nasogastric or nasointestinal tubes, gastrostomy tubes placed surgically or endoscopically, and jejunostomy tubes.

Nasogastric and Nasoduodenal Tubes

Nasogastric tubes have been used by physicians since at least 1790. Unfortunately, the nasogastric tube is satisfactory only when the duration of feeding is relatively short. Long-term use is complicated by septal and esophageal erosion, gastroesophageal reflux with peptic stricture formation, and aspiration pneumonia (23). Nasogastric and nasoduodenal feeding tubes can be used in cooperative and alert patients, preferably for the short term, when anorexia, severe odynophagia, and temporary dysphagia are present (22).

Nasogastric tube feedings and gastrostomy both involve the risk of gastroesophageal reflux and aspiration. Nasoenteric tubes are capable of transversing the pylorus and thereby avoid the problems associated with larger nasogastric tubes (24).

Although the soft silastic nasogastric and nasojejunal tubes are more comfortable than the stiffer polyvinyl nasogastric tubes, they have the disadvantages of increased clogging and the inability to check gastric residual volumes as a result of a smaller internal diameter (25).

Some patients find the nasogastric tube intolerable but may accept a feeding gastrostomy to maintain nutrition and to avoid aspiration (21).

Percutaneous Endoscopic Gastrostomy

In 1979 Ponsky et al. developed a technique for creating a feeding gastrostomy through a percutaneous puncture of the stomach under endoscopic guidance (26):

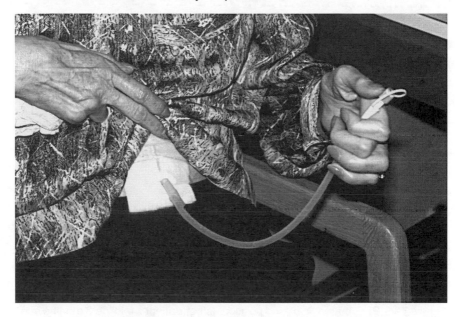

Figure 7-1. Patient showing regular PEG tube. Entrance to the stomach is covered by gauze dressing.

percutaneous endoscopic gastrostomy (PEG). PEG tubes are available in tube and button form (Figures 7-1, 7-2, and 7-3). There are several techniques for PEG placement, as described by Cogen and Weinryb (23) and Russell et al. (27). The PEG tube should be placed by an experienced gastroenterologist or surgeon in cooperation with the dietitian and nurse, who then arrange for patient instruction and supplies.

Larson et al. (28) report that PEG is safe and has a low mortality, even in patients who are medically debilitated secondary to the underlying disease. In 314 patients, 75 percent of whom had neurological disorders, PEG tube placement was successful in 95 percent.

Steffes et al. (29) reviewed their 32-month experience of 115 PEG placements in 112 adult patients with a mean follow-up of 59.4 days. Placement was unsuccessful in 12 patients and difficult in another 6. Minor postoperative complications not requiring intervention occurred in 11 patients and major complications in 24. Infection was the most common postoperative problem. Although 30-day mortality was 24 percent, no patient died as a direct result of the procedure. Five of the 12 unsuccessful and 3 of the 6 difficult placements involved partially or nearly completely obstructing pharyngeal tumors. Other placement difficulties were caused by thickened gastric and abdominal walls, adhesions, or ascites (29).

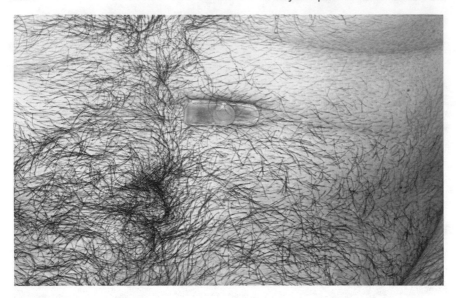

Figure 7-2. PEG button, in closed position, left of patient's midline 3 months after placement. Tube is used by inserting a feeding adapter, into which liquids are poured via syringe or bag.

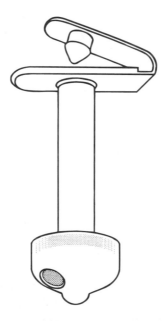

Figure 7-3. Button tube seen in its entirety.

Surgical Gastrostomy and Jejunostomy

Surgical gastrostomies are reserved for complicated cases today because it is generally unnecessary to subject patients to the risk of general anesthesia. Percutaneous gastrostomy placement under local anesthesia is preferred (22). Physical tolerance of the gastrostomy procedure depends on an adequate vital capacity, usually more than 50 percent of the predicted value with no upper airway obstruction (21). Gastrostomy in ALS patients carries the immediate (but not protracted) risk of enhancing pulmonary failure in patients with weak respiratory muscles (21). Ideally, the operation should be performed as early in the course of the disease as possible, when vital capacity is almost normal, but the need is seldom realized until the patient has serious difficulty with swallowing (21). Unfortunately, some patients will not accept the assistance of a feeding tube until their nutritional status has deteriorated severely. It may be wise to offer tubes requiring invasive procedures for placement only up to a certain point in the disease. After that point, nasogastric feeding tubes would be the only option.

When considering tube feeding, it is important to remember that the desire to eat may still be present. For some patients, psychological well-being can be improved by small amounts of oral feedings of an appropriate consistency, even though tube feeding must be continued to provide adequate hydration, nutrient intake, or both (30).

Patients who elect tube feeding need assistance with formula selection, volume, and scheduling. Tubes terminating in the stomach usually allow bolus feedings, whereas those entering the small intestine require a slower continuous infusion. Dietitians calculate calorie, protein, vitamin, mineral, and fluid needs and help train patients in feeding procedure and tube care. Arrangements for follow-up should be made so that the feeding schedule can be adjusted as needed and to provide the patient assistance with any problems that develop.

Considering Patient Options/Choices in Feedings

Patients accept recommended dietary changes with varying degrees of enthusiasm. Dietary intervention should begin at diagnosis so that nutritional inadequacies can be detected and addressed early. Because of the progressive nature of the disease, it is reasonable to assume that difficulties with eating will worsen with time and that nutritional status will almost certainly deteriorate if adjustments are not made. Many patients find it difficult to accept the need to change lifelong eating habits.

The frustration of losing the ability to perform such activities of daily living as eating, chewing, and swallowing can lead to a feeling of hopelessness. Patients need to be encouraged to allow family members to help them, to try adaptive feeding devices and modifications in diet, and to realize when they are unable to meet their needs by oral diet alone. The positive aspects of tube feeding should be emphasized; it reduces the risk of aspiration, eliminates the dangers of malnu-trition and dehydration, and avoids the frustration of trying unsuccessfully to consume sufficient amounts of food and fluids.

A discussion of tube feeding options should include a description of the place-ment of the tube, training procedures, and feeding schedules. The final decision should rest with the patient and family. If the patient decides against tube feeding, that decision should be respected by those involved in his or her care. The goal of nutritional therapy, whether by oral diet alone or in combination with tube feeding, is to help patients maintain the best comfort, pleasure, and overall quality of life that they are able to attain.

Conclusion

Nutritional assessment, intensive counseling, diet supplementation, and tube feeding are important and useful weapons for fighting the nutritional devastation ALS patients often experience. Dysphagia, weakness, weight loss, and depression are common problems for ALS patients. Nutrition needs to be fully addressed in properly caring for these patients. Early intervention is required to help patients adjust their life-styles to make eating a satisfying, pleasurable, and fulfilling activity, as well as providing for nutritional needs.

References

1. Chen MYM, Peele VN, Donati D, Ott DJ, Donofrio PD and Gelfand DW. Clinical and videofluoroscopic evaluation of swallowing in 41 patients with neurologic disease. *Gastrointest Radiol* 1992, 17:95–98.
2. Horner J and Massey EW. Managing dysphagia. *Postgrad Med* 1991, 89:203–213.
3. Price ME and DiIorio C. Swallowing: A practice guide. *Amer J Nurs* 1990, July: 42–46.
4. Robbins J. Swallowing in ALS and motor neuron disorders. *Neurol Clin* 1987, 5: 213–229.
5. DePaul R, Abbs JH, Caligiuri M, Gracco VL and Brooks BR. Hypoglossal, trigeminal, and facial motoneuron involvement in amyotrophic lateral sclerosis. *Neurology* 1988, 38:281–283.
6. Carpenter FJ, McDonald RJ and Howard FM. The otolaryngologic presentation of amyotrophic lateral sclerosis. *Otolaryngology* 1978, 86:479–484.
7. Logemann J. *Evaluation and Treatment of Swallowing Disorders.* San Diego: College-Hill Press, 1983.
8. Dionigi R, Dominioni L, Jemos V, Cremaschi R and Monico R. Diagnosing malnutri-tion. *Gut* 1986, 27:5–8.
9. Grant JP. Nutritional assessment in clinical practice. *J Parent Ent Nutr* 1986, 86: 3–11.
10. Forse RA and Shizgal HM. Serum albumin and nutritional status. *J Parent Ent Nutr* 1980, 4:450–454.

11. Welnetz K. Maintaining adequate nutrition and hydration in the dysphagic ALS patient. *Canad Nurse* 1983, 79:30–34.
12. Asbeck C and Burns BL. Nutritional management of amyotrophic lateral sclerosis. *Dietitians in Nutrition Support* 1988, 10:9–10.
13. Norris FH and Denys EH. Nutritional supplements in amyotrophic lateral sclerosis. *Adv Exp Med Biol* 1987, 209:183–189.
14. Mitsumoto H, Hanson MR and Chad DA. Amyotrophic lateral sclerosis: Recent advances in pathogenesis and therapeutic trials. *Arch Neurol* 1988, 45:189–202.
15. Norris FH, Denys EH and Fallat RJ. Trial of octacosanol in amyotrophic lateral sclerosis. *Neurology* 1986, 36:1263–1264.
16. Perry RL, Krieger C, Hansen S and Eisen A. Amyotrophic lateral sclerosis: Amino acid levels in plasma and cerebrospinal fluid. *Ann Neurol* 1990, 28:12–17.
17. Rothstein JD, Tsai G, Kuncl RW, et al. Abnormal excitatory amino acid metabolism in amyotrophic lateral sclerosis. *Ann Neurol* 1990, 28:18–25.
18. Plaitakis A, Constantakakis E and Smith J. The neuroexcitotoxic amino acids glutamate and aspartate are altered in the spinal cord and brain in amyotrophic lateral sclerosis. *Ann Neurol* 1988, 24:446–449.
19. Plaitakis A and Shashidharan P. Branched-chain amino acids in amyotrophic lateral sclerosis. *Lancet* 1988, September:680–681.
20. Slowie LA, Paige MS and Antel JP. Nutritional considerations in the management of patients with amyotrophic lateral sclerosis. *J Amer Diet Assn* 1983, 83:44–47.
21. Hudson AJ. Outpatient management of amyotrophic lateral sclerosis. *Semin Neurol* 1987, 7:344–351.
22. Ganger D and Craig RM. Swallowing disorders and nutritional support. *Dysphagia* 1990, 4:213–219.
23. Cogen R and Weinryb J. Tube feeding: Providing the most nutrition with the least discomfort. *Postgrad Med* 1989, 85:355–359.
24. McWey RD, Curry NS, Schabel SI, and Reines HD. Complications of nasoenteric feeding tubes. *Amer J Surg* 1988, 155:253–257.
25. Clarkston WK, Smith OJ and Walden JM. Percutaneous endoscopic gastrostomy and early mortality. *Southern Med J* 1990, 83:1433–1436.
26. Gauderer MWL, Ponsky JL, and Izant RJ. Gastrostomy without laparotomy: A percutaneous endoscopic technique. *J Pediat Surg* 1980, 15:872–875.
27. Russell TR, Brotman M and Norris F. Percutaneous gastrostomy: A new simplified and cost-effective technique. *Amer J Surg* 1984, 148:132–137.
28. Larson DE, Burton DD, Schroeder KW and DiMagno EP. Percutaneous endoscopic gastrostomy: Indications, success, complications, and mortality in 314 consecutive patients. *Gastroenterology* 1987, 93:48–52.
29. Steffes C, Weaver DW and Bouwman DL. Percutaneous endoscopic gastrostomy: New technique—old complications. *Amer Surg* 1989, 55:273–277.
30. Henderson C. Safe and effective tube feeding of bedridden elderly. *Geriatrics* 1991, 46:56–66.

8

Physical Therapy Interventions in the Management of Amyotrophic Lateral Sclerosis

Catherine M. Howell, M.S., P.T.

Physical therapy (PT) management of the patient with amyotrophic lateral sclerosis presents the challenge of dealing with progressive functional losses over a relatively short course of life expectancy. The inexorable pace of deterioration dictates that the physical therapist be mindful of future loss as well as the current functional status of the patient when designing the treatment plan.

Due to the deteriorating course of this illness, the ALS patient presents with accelerated needs for ongoing assessment and frequent reassessment of functional status. The initial PT evaluation is no different from that for other patient populations, but management of this patient group requires a knowledge of predicted loss of function in order to intelligently prescribe orthoses and durable medical equipment.

The skills of the physical therapist often required for the treatment of the ALS patient involve methods of pain control, treatment or prevention of contractures, gait analysis, orthotic recommendations, provision of durable medical equipment (DME), home assessment, and family or attendant teaching. Of special benefit to the patient is the therapist's knowledge of financial resources and insurance coverage for durable medical equipment and orthoses. Experience with drafting letters of medical necessity also assists in justifying the acquisition of medically necessary equipment to the insurance claims reviewer.

Evaluation

Evaluation should include all usual parameters of objective measurement, such as manual muscle testing, range of motion (ROM), pain diagrams, sensation, skin integrity, edema, balance, tone, coordination, transfers, bed mobility, gait analysis, and home assessment. Expected dysfunction may be found in the categories of ROM, strength, tone, transfers, bed mobility, and gait. ROM may be limited in patients with interfering spasticity or in those with capsular tightness secondary to loss of functional use of the involved limb. Pain may be present in patients with secondary orthopedic problems. Dependent edema is a common problem in the less active limbs. Coordination and balance may be affected by spasticity. Disturbances of sensation and cerebellar dysfunction are not found in cases of ALS. If present, they indicate the existence of a concomitant condition.

The unique presentation of symptoms in each patient and the seemingly random pattern of progression makes prediction of future losses very difficult. Varieties of the disease have been recognized, such as bulbar onset, respiratory onset, progressive muscular atrophy (lower motor neuron involvement), spinal ALS (mixed upper and lower motor neuron involvement), and spastic (upper motor neuron involvement). Each form tends to have specific pathological involvement and therefore differing clinical features. (1) The referring physician may not specify the exact form of ALS with which the patient presents, but the form may be useful for the physical therapist to note because it may enhance the therapist's ability to predict speed of progression of the disease, patterns of weakness, development of interfering spasticity, likelihood of respiratory involvement, and likelihood of bulbar involvement.

Interventions for Pain

Pain problems require immediate, aggressive intervention. The most frequent site of pain is the shoulder. Common problems encountered are adhesive capsulitis, bursitis, and tendinitis. These problems occur when weakness or spasticity prevent full use of the shoulder, and joint limitation and pain ensue.

The author has treated one ALS patient with severe shoulder-hand syndrome. This patient had a predominance of upper motor neuron involvement, which may have precipitated development of this syndrome as can other central nervous system disturbances such as strokes and tumors (2). Shoulder-hand syndrome involves capsular restriction in the shoulder, edema and contracture in the wrist and metacarpophalangeal joints, and variable involvement of the sympathetic nervous system, which may include pain and swelling of the hand, trophic skin changes, vasomotor instability, pain, and limited ROM in the shoulder (2).

Treatment of these problems in the ALS patient is the same as for any other orthopedic patient. Treatment considerations revolve around the stage, i.e., acute, subacute, chronic, or chronic-recurring. These stages refer to the state of the tissues in the injured areas (2).

Following any insult to the tissues, there are changes that occur in a characteristic pattern of healing. The acute stage involves inflammation, with a predominance of vascular changes (2). Clinical signs include redness, edema, heat, and pain with loss of function. Treatment of the acute stage of injury should involve the use of ice, elevation, and rest to control edema. Compression garments may be helpful in reducing limb edema. Passive range of motion exercises help prevent loss of motion without increasing inflammation. Gentle massage and intermittent isometric exercises help to increase blood flow and decrease muscle spasms. The patient with inadequate motor power to perform isometric exercises may use negative polarity electrical stimulation to augment or substitute for isometric efforts.

The subacute stage begins as pain and inflammation subside. The tissues in this stage are still delicate and prone to formation of adhesions. Exercises may progress to active range of motion. The therapist may use mobilization techniques as dictated by patient response and joint end-feel. Ice may be used following exercise sessions to prevent recurrence of edema.

The chronic and chronic-recurring stages of pain involve scar formation and scar remodeling whose fiber direction and pliability are directly related to the stresses applied to them during this phase of healing. When loss of ROM is still present, joint mobilization may be preceded by use of heat and ultrasound. Exercises should be used to gain and maintain ROM, regain loss of strength caused by the acute pain problem, and teach mechanically efficient methods of substituting for weakened muscles in order to avoid injuring adjacent joints.

A valuable adjunct in the treatment of painful conditions is the use of transcutaneous electrical nerve stimulation (TENS). These units can be used with effectiveness during all stages of healing, although the recommended settings may differ depending on the actual syndrome present (tendinitis, reflex sympathetic dystrophy, adhesive capsulitis), and the stage of healing (acute, subacute, chronic, or chronic-recurring).

TENS units differ in complexity and availability of current modes between manufacturers. The best advice for the use of a particular model can come from the manufacturer. The articles provided by Empi Corporation* listed the keys to successful use of TENS as being early intervention; optimal electrode placement; parameter adjustment of the modality to identify the most effective mode of TENS; use in combination with physical therapy modalities and exercises; and appropriate use of anti-inflammatory and antidepressant medications as advised by the patient's physician.

The author found good long-term control of pain by TENS in an ALS patient with severe shoulder-hand syndrome. The use of brief-intense settings (high frequency, wide pulse width, high intensity) to control acute pain episodes, in combination with a bimodal setting for long-term use, was helpful in this case. The bimodal setting allows one channel of the TENS to supply 100 Hz current for quick onset anesthetic effect while the second channel supplies 4 Hz current for long duration (acupuncture-like) pain control. The brief-intense setting should be

---

* 1275 Grey Fox Road, St. Paul, Minnesota 55112, (612) 636-6600.

used for less than fifteen minutes per treatment session to avoid skin irritation and muscle fatigue. The bimodal setting can be used for longer periods with comfortable intensity settings.

Basic Principles for Exercise Programs

Recommended exercise intensity and duration should always be related to the patient's endurance level. The oft repeated tenet of exercise prescription for the neuromuscular patient is to "avoid overfatigue." Patient compliance with this advice is a particular problem in the earlier stages of motor involvement.

Energy Conservation As Applied to Exercise

The patient's emotional reaction to the disease and the impact of that reaction on compliance with exercise programs can range from apathetic avoidance of activity due to feelings of hopelessness and depression to near maniacal absorption in rigorous exercises as a means of atoning for prior neglect (imagined or real) of their health. The latter group is often following a program outlined in a book or magazine article aimed at physical conditioning for healthy adults. The therapist is left with the challenge of convincing these two groups that moderate expenditures of energy and specific stretching and strengthening routines are healthier for them than either inactivity or vigorous, fatiguing exercise.

Education regarding disuse atrophy, formation of contractures, and the positive effects of frequent changes in body position on pulmonary hygiene may help motivate the inactive patient. Educating the overzealous patient about differences in response to exercise between healthy and diseased nerves and muscles may help to create a rationale for the observance of energy conservation instructions. Education builds patient confidence in the therapist's advice and encourages continued participation in the prescribed exercise program. It also gives the patient a foundation from which to critically evaluate and discard unsound advice from future readings and lectures.

In the early stages of involvement, most activities, such as walking, swimming, cycling, and aerobics, can be continued if the patients monitor and adjust to their fatigue level. If weakness or spasticity during weight-bearing activities makes balance precarious, then aerobics or cycling a road bike may be dangerous. Walking on an uneven surface may require the use of an assistive device such as a cane or a walking stick.

Range of Motion and Strengthening Exercises

A common question posed to the physical therapist is whether strengthening exercises will help the patient regain the use of weakened, atrophied muscles. The answer requires some delicacy in presentation to avoid creating a feeling of hopelessness with an unqualified negative response or creating a set of unrealistic expectations with an unqualified positive response. The response of "yes and no," while probably truthful and accurate, requires some explanation for the patient to grasp.

Clinical observation leads one to notice that severely involved muscle groups do not respond well to strengthening regimens. Loss of strength in overfatigued groups can be rapid and often irreversible. Relatively uninvolved muscle groups may show a training effect and a subsequent gain in strength with a specific strengthening program. Bohannon (3) reported a patient who improved his static strength in fourteen muscle groups but lost strength in four muscle groups after seventy-five days of upper extremity resistance exercise. While the actual cause for the differing response to training is not proven, a hypothesis for future study would be that responses differ depending on the degree of motor neuron involvement in the respective muscle groups.

Even in the early stages of ALS, range of motion exercises for the shoulders should be routinely performed in order to avoid the insidious onset of adhesive capsulitis. Patients with lower tolerance for aerobic activities should be encouraged to independently perform active exercises to maintain their ROM and prevent disuse atrophy.

Patients with less than fair (3/5) muscle strength grades need to have a passively assisted exercise program designed for them, and family members or attendants should be instructed in its proper execution. Two instructional sessions should be adequate to teach and then check on retention and proper performance of the skills.

Illustrated handouts are essential for correct follow-through at home. A well-illustrated guide entitled *Managing Amyotrophic Lateral Sclerosis, MALS Manual II, Managing Muscular Weakness* is available through the Amyotrophic Lateral Sclerosis Association (ALSA)(4). The Muscular Dystrophy Association also has published an excellent illustrated book, *ALS: Maintaining Mobility* (5).

Gait Disturbances

The most frequent referrals to physical therapy are for correction of gait deviations. The most commonly encountered deviations include inadequate dorsiflexion in swing phases (foot-drop); ankle instability with possible varus during initial contact and midstance; foot slap and inadequate knee flexion at loading response; knee extension thrust at loading response; knee wobble, contralateral drop of the pelvis (noncompensated Trendelenburg limp), compensated Trendelenburg limp with trunk lean, and trunk collapse into flexion at midstance; inability to advance body weight onto the forefoot and lack of heel rise at terminal stance; inadequate knee flexion in preswing; toe drag and inadequate hip and knee flexion at initial swing; circumduction, vaulting on stance limb, or trunk lean during initial swing to advance the limb.

The major causes of gait deviation in the ALS patient are weakness, spasticity, or both. Occasionally there is a soft tissue contracture at the ankle or toes. Central balance deficits (cerebellar dysfunction, impaired upright motor control, lack of proprioception) do not usually play a role in gait disturbances of the ALS patient.

Assistive Devices

The choice of assistive devices is influenced by the level of hip and trunk instability and functional ability in the arms. Mild balance deficits due to weak hip abductors or interfering spasticity can be corrected with a single point cane.

A quad cane is an advantage for a patient who uses the cane for sporadic assistance during activities of daily living such as cooking. The cane's wide base allows it to remain standing on the floor within easy reach while the patient engages in two-handed activities. For routine use, however, the quad cane is seldom a prudent choice for the ALS patient.

Hand and wrist weakness is a common presenting sign of ALS, and control of the eccentrically weighted base of the quad cane is awkward and leads to early hand and wrist fatigue. The other drawback of the quad cane is its paradoxical instability during gait. All four tips can be in contact with the ground only when the shaft of the cane is perfectly perpendicular to the ground. During initial contact, the cane strikes the ground at an acute angle directly related to the step length, and thus the degree of hip flexion and pelvic rotation in the contralateral leg. When the cane strikes the ground at an angle, the best contact it can achieve is with only two of its four tips. As the patient moves toward midstance, the cane rocks toward a vertical position and the remaining tips contact the ground only if the ground is perfectly level. On uneven surfaces, the cane may wobble and never achieve a position of balance and stability. To compensate for the instability of the quad cane, patients tend to shorten their stride length to minimize the shaft-ground angle and prolong their midstance phase in order to maximize the feeling of stability.

A unique piece of equipment that may substitute for the quad cane in patients with good arm strength and a fair grip is the flexible-base quad cane with a Lofstrand crutch attachment (Gatorade) (Figs. 8-1–8-3). The flexible attachment between the base of the cane and the shaft allows all four tips to come in contact with the ground even when the shaft of the cane is angled away from a perpendicular position. The Lofstrand top helps to reduce hand fatigue and allows the patient to substitute for a weakened wrist by shifting control of the cane's base to the elbow and shoulder.

Bilateral hip weakness or moderate trunk weakness combined with mild hand or wrist weakness is usually best aided by a front-wheeled walker (Figure 8-4). A large variety of attachments are available at additional cost to best suit the patient's walking environment.

Routine use on sidewalks is best tolerated with the use of rubberized front

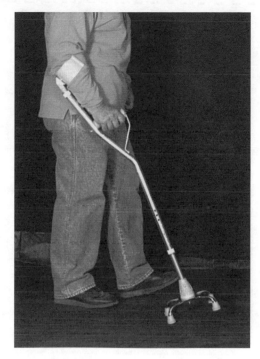

Figure 8-1. The Galorade is a flexible-base quad cane with a Lofstrand top.

casters to absorb the vibrations (Figure 8-5). Mobile patients with good side-to-side stability often prefer swivel front casters. These casters make changing direction less laborious. Patients with spastic gait patterns do not tolerate well the swivel casters due to frequent loss of balance to the side.

Drag of the rear walker legs on carpeting can be minimized by the use of spring-loaded retractable rear glides or retractable wheels. These devices glide or roll along the floor unless the patient loads his/her body weight on the walker and drops the rear walker legs to the ground, thus providing a braking action (Figs. 8-6, 8-7).

Modification of the walker may be necessary if upper extremity weakness is present. Forearm troughs are a useful addition to the walker to allow control of the walker via the shoulders, with the weakened forearms supported in the troughs (Figure 8-8).

Patients with very good arm strength and moderate bilateral hip weakness or spasticity may prefer the use of bilateral crutches (either axillary or Canadian style) to allow for easier stair management.

A very simple piece of equipment that should be recommended to the family is a safety belt for use during assisted gait, stair management, or transfers. Instruction and practice sessions should be offered to train all responsible parties.

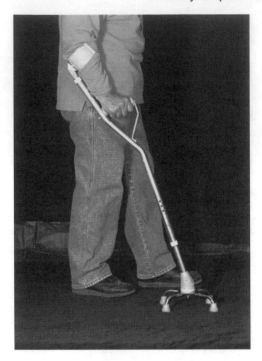

Figure 8-2. The base of the Gatorade can move independently from the cane shaft, thus allowing all four cane tips to be in contact with the ground even when the cane shaft is angled away from a vertical position.

Orthotic Recommendations

Ankle Foot Orthoses

Orthotic control of ankle and knee instability should reflect combined input from the physical therapist and the orthotist. The goal of all bracing should be to allow the greatest amount of normal movement while preventing unwanted deviations. A general rule of thumb is to allow the deviations seen in stance to determine the type of brace recommended. One must remember that for the ALS population continued loss of strength is expected at the ankle and invariably at the knee. The prescribed brace should be adequate to control the deviations seen during the initial gait analysis and should be capable of later modifications.

An early sign of lower extremity involvement is distal loss of strength. The most common presenting deviations are inadequate dorsiflexion at initial contact and ankle varus. Specific muscle testing of inversion, eversion, dorsiflexion, plantar flexion, and knee extension should give the most valuable data for deciding the type of brace to be fabricated.

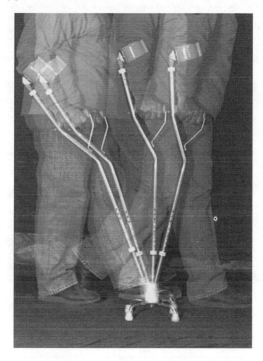

Figure 8-3. This time-lapsed photograph of the Gatorade shows the flexible positioning of the shaft and the base throughout the gait cycle.

The posterior leaf spring AFO, which only provides dorsi-assist in swing, is seldom a suitable brace for the ALS patient due to the usual progression of the disease. This brace is not designed to provide medial-lateral support to the ankle or knee control.

Medial and lateral instability of the ankle must be stabilized by either a solid ankle AFO that is rigid at all phases of gait or an AFO with a hinged joint to allow varying degrees of plantar flexion and dorsiflexion but prevent all inversion and eversion. Several joints are available for use with subtle differences in fit and function (Figure 8-9).

Solid ankle AFOs are a good choice for patients who present with ankle instability and knee extensor weakness. The solid ankle AFO is rigid at all times and can thus stabilize the knee in stance by preventing forward collapse of the tibia. The disadvantage of this AFO is that the passive ankle dorsiflexion used when rising from sitting, ascending stairs, and ascending inclines is prevented, and use of this orthosis makes these activities more difficult to perform.

If the patient with medial-lateral ankle weakness is fortunate enough to have adequate knee extensor strength to prevent knee wobble or collapse during gait,

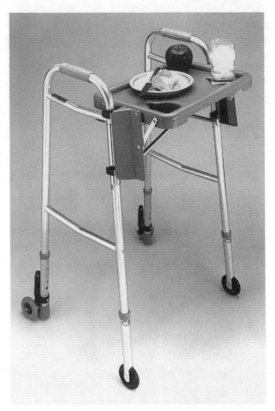

Figure 8-4. Folding walkers are available with a variety of attachments. This walker is equipped with standard front casters, rear wheel brakes, and a food tray.

a hinged AFO can be provided to allow free dorsiflexion, and a plantar-stop may be added, if needed, to control foot drop. Examples of ankle joints currently available are the Gillette joint, the Oklahoma joint, and the Gaffney joint.

The Gillette joint is made of flexible rubber vacuformed into a polypropylene AFO (Figure 8-10). The flexibility of the hinge material allows minute amounts of motion at end-range plantar flexion and when large amounts of rotational torque are applied to the ankle. This feature adds a more flexible feel to the function of the joint and seems to allow a more fluid gait pattern. Heavier patients or patients with clonus are not well suited to this joint because of the possibility of structural failure for the heavy patient and of elastic feedback into ankle clonus (Figure 8-9).`

The thinner Oklahoma joint is made of polypropylene vacuformed into a poly-propylene AFO. Its size varies to accommodate pediatric and adult patients and it provides firm control of inversion-eversion (Figure 8-11).

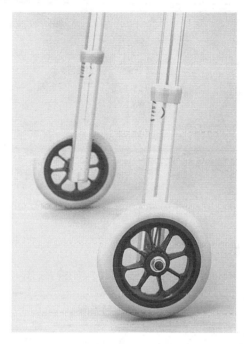

Figure 8-5. Rubberized front casters allow for smoother propulsion on concrete sidewalks.

The Gaffney joint is made of stainless steel vacuformed into the polypropylene AFO (Figure 8-12). It comes in different sizes to accommodate heavy and light duty use and for differing body weights. This joint tends to last longer than the rubber or plastic joints and provides firm control of inversion-eversion.

All the hinged AFOs can be modified to provide both a plantar-stop and a dorsi-stop. A plantar-stop is formed by molding the rear of the articulating surfaces of the shaft and foot portions of the AFO to approximate at a desired angle—usually neutral in the ALS patient. It can be stopped in a small amount of dorsiflexion to prevent knee hyperextension. An adjustable posterior strap can be attached to span the rear articulation and thus be used to provide a dorsi-stop if knee collapse becomes a problem. Small rubberized cords can be riveted by studs anterior to the joint line to provide dorsi-assist if desired (Figure 8-9).

The hinged AFOs are more readily accepted by the patient with early loss of ankle strength because desired ankle motions can still be permitted. The possibility of making future brace modifications to provide control of dorsiflexion, plantar flexion, and knee collapse allows these braces to remain functional throughout the ambulatory phase of this disease.

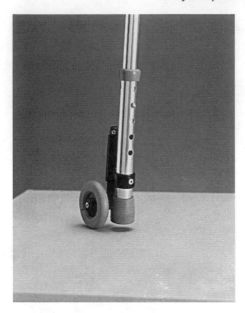

Figure 8-6. The rear wheel brake suspends the rear walker strut off the ground via a spring-loaded chamber. It is designed to be used with front wheels to allow near normal walking speeds on a variety of surfaces. If the patient begins to lose balance and presses down on the walker for support, the struts lower to the floor to brake forward motion.

Cervical Orthoses

Neck weakness in the ALS patient frequently occurs rather early in the disease process. The earliest signs of cervical weakness occur while the patient is still ambulatory. Patients may initially complain of neck stiffness or of feeling "heavy-headed" after reading or writing. Early neck weakness may also cause a feeling of general fatigue and poor tolerance for walking. Other early symptoms of neck instability are usually noticed by the patient while a passenger in a car. Unanticipated movements of the car tend to accelerate the head and quickly overwhelm the ability of the weakened cervical muscles to stabilize the head.

Comfortable orthotic control of cervical weakness is difficult to obtain in the ambulatory patient. The variety of body positions that the active patient assumes in a day usually requires that the orthosis provide multiple points of control for anterior, posterior, and lateral movements. An orthosis that is adequate to control these motions frequently produces a multitude of complaints from the patient about discomfort from pressure on areas of bony contact or hindrance of desired motions. Looking downward to read is difficult in a more rigid collar. Patients can use a raised slanted surface for reading to compensate for the restricted

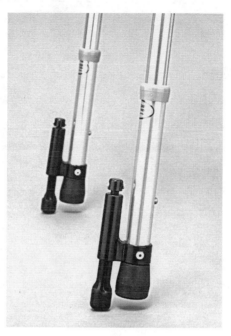

Figure 8-7. The rear glide brake Is a slick plastic glide that suspends the rear walker strut off the ground to allow for easier propulsion of a front-wheeled walker on carpet. Pressure on the walker will lower the rear struts to the ground to provide braking action.

cervical flexion. A more difficult problem to solve involves the dysphagic patient who must use cervical and capital flexion while swallowing to aid in preventing aspiration. It is usually easier to remove the collar while eating to facilitate correct body posture for swallowing and to eliminate interference of the collar with opening the mouth. When neck fatigue is the main patient complaint, a soft cervical collar provides a mild assist for the weakened muscles and is very well tolerated due to its relative comfort (Figure 8-13). Due to its compressibility, its useful time span is limited to the earliest periods of cervical weakness, prior to the onset of less than fair (3/5) muscle strength.

Rigid collars provide very firm control of the head and are useful for patients with severe neck weakness (Figure 8-13). These collars are usually made of padded rigid plastic or leather. They are somewhat heavy and tend to be quite warm due to the large amount of surface area they enclose. When patients use the collars to support the entire weight of their head, they often experience discomfort at the points of bony contact along the inferior surface of the mandible and over the clavicles. These collars also restrict access to the front of the throat and cannot be used by the patient with a tracheostomy tube.

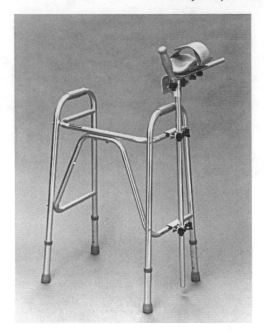

Figure 8-8. The walker in the above photograph is equipped with a forearm trough platform to support a weakened arm.

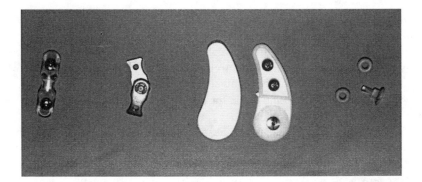

Figure 8-9. A variety of ankle joints can be attached to an ankle-foot orthosis to allow dorsiflexion and/or plantar flexion. Illustrated above are the Gillette joint, the Gaffney joint, inside and outside views of the Oklahoma joint, and rubber rings and rivets that can be used to provide dorsiflexion assistance.

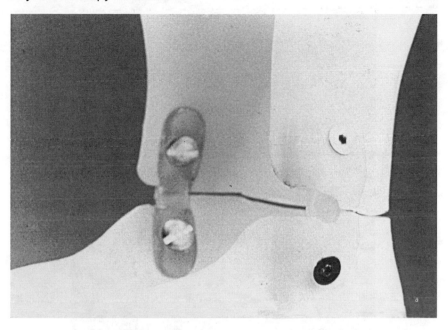

Figure 8-10. The Gillette ankle joint is made of a relatively flexible rubber vacu-formed into the AFO. It allows minute amounts of motion at end-range plantar flexion or when rotational torque is applied to the brace. This flexibility allows a more natural feel to the patient and can allow a smoother gait pattern.

Wire frame collars and their molded plastic cousins, such as the Executive collar, are much lighter and cooler than the rigid collars and provide quite firm control of head motion (Figure 8-14). Their open design allows them to be used by the patient on a ventilator. These collars have the same problems with bony contact discomfort. Posterior pillars of varying height are available to provide varying degrees of extension control.

A compromise in comfort and control between the soft collars and rigid or wire frame collars are the semirigid thermoplastic foam collars such as the Philadelphia collar (Figure 8-13). The soft foam causes fewer bony contact problems due to its slight compressibility. The Philadelphia collar encompasses the neck in the same manner as the rigid collar and thus provides multiple points of control to stabilize the head in all directions. The only complaint about this collar is that it tends to be quite warm.

A cooler alternative to the Philadelphia collar is provided by the Malibu neck brace (Figure 8-15). The contact areas are made of resilient foam. An open plastic frame provides anterior and posterior support. Height adjustments can be made for both the occipital and chin supports. The foam chin cup can be trimmed to allow more chin movement and less restriction of cervical rotation. Although the

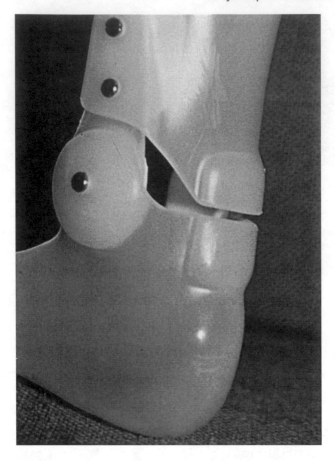

Figure 8-11. The Oklahoma ankle joint is made of polypropylene vacuformed into the AFO. The relatively thin components give the finished AFO a slimmer mediolateral profile.

open frame allows access to a tracheostomy site, the brace does not allow room for placement of ventilator tubing.

Patient Lifts

Patient lifts such as the well-known ''Hoyer'' lift are commonly seen in hospitals or long-term care facilities that have a high population of physically dependent patients. A patient lift is often recommended for home use for the nonambulatory ALS patient when he or she becomes too difficult to transfer by other means.

A patient lift that can reach to the ground, such as the ''Transaid'' lift, can be

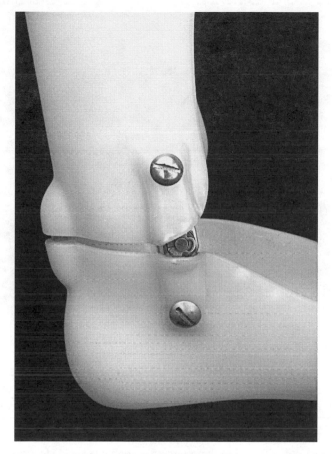

Figure 8-12. The Gaffney ankle joint is made of stainless steel vacuformed into the AFO. It provides firm control of the subtalar joint. This joint is very durable and can be used for heavier patients. It is also valuable for patients with plantar flexion spasticity and/or clonus because of its strength and because the joints do not give elastic feedback.

a valuable tool for those patients who are still ambulatory on a limited basis. Patients who walk in the home with assistive devices and/or orthoses have a history of occasional falls in the house. Those with significant proximal weakness require maximal assistance to rise from the floor. The spouse or caregiver often is not strong enough to move them without the assistance of another person. The availability of a device that can lift the patient from the floor can provide unmeasured peace of mind to the family and can allow the patient who is a marginally safe ambulator to continue walking in the home. It can also be used by patients

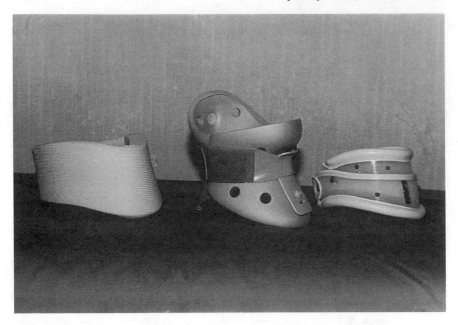

Figure 8-13. A soft cervical collar, the Philadelphia collar, and a rigid, adjustable height cervical collar.

who insist on performing exercises on the firm surface of the floor, but are too weak to rise independently.

The lifts are usually available with a variety of stationary bases for specialized uses, such as bathtub or pool transfers, or with a mobile base. A single mast and boom can be used with any of these interchangeable bases. One word of caution should be given to families for safe use of a patient lift with a mobile base. Although laws mandate that they be sold with wheel brakes, it is safer to always leave the brakes unlocked during use. If the patient moves in the sling and places their center of gravity outside the lift's base of support, the lift is designed to roll under the patient to restore balance. If the wheels are locked, this safety mechanism cannot work and the lift may tip over.

The patient lift that has been most beneficial for home use is the "Transaid" lift (Figure 8-16). Several design features, such as its aforementioned ability to lift from the floor, make it preferable over the institutional standard, the "Hoyer" lift.

The "Transaid" lift has a C-shaped base that is more maneuverable than the spreadable U base of the "Hoyer" lift. The base can be ordered with a low clearance height to allow passage under standard bed frames. The sling is attached to the boom via four separate chains or webs, thus allowing the patient to be placed in relatively upright or reclined positions depending on need.

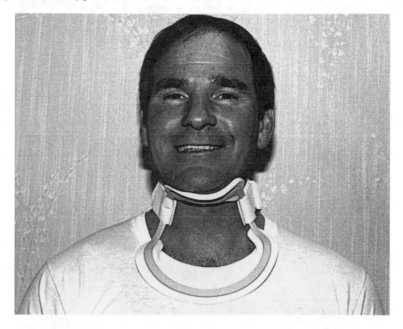

Figure 8-14. The Executive collar is made of molded plastic. Its great advantages are that it is lightweight, cool, and allows attachment of a ventilator.

Patient Lift Slings

A variety of sling designs can be ordered with a patient lift. The most versatile sling for home use with the "Transaid" lift is the "309 sling" (Figure 8-16). It has a commode hole opening for toileting and personal hygiene. The front of the hole is enclosed by two separate (right and left) leg pieces that can be crossed under the legs or woven in a figure eight, or can individually enclose each leg.

The greatest advantage of this sling is that it can be easily placed under a patient in the seated position without raising their buttocks. This is accomplished by spreading the right and left leg enclosures fully open and then sliding the back portion of the sling between the patient's back and the chair. The back piece is pulled down toward the buttocks as far as possible. The right and left leg pieces can then be tucked under the respective leg of the patient and crossed to the other side of the patient's body for attachment to the suspension chains or webs.

The advantage of enclosing each leg independently in its respective leg piece, rather than crossing under the legs to form an open sling, is that the two legs are held in an abducted position to allow for easy perineal care. The open sling style of attachment maintains the legs in a more modest position. Some patients, particularly those with excess trunk extensor tone, tend to slide out of the open sling because their legs are not enclosed. The method of enclosing the legs in a

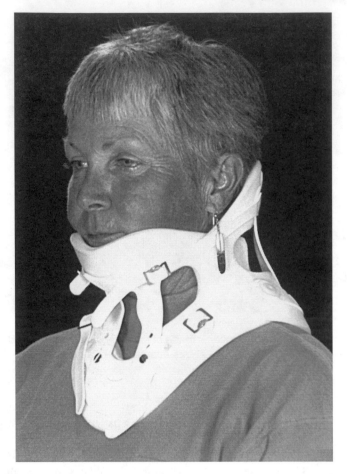

Figure 8-15. The Malibu collar is a cooler collar that provides firm, yet comfortable control of the head. The chin cup can be trimmed to allow for more chin movement and less restriction of cervical rotation.

figure eight is generally recommended for control of agitated patients or patients with neurological disorders characterized by athetoid or choreiform movements.

Wheelchairs

Manual Wheelchairs

There are special considerations that must be made before ordering a manual wheelchair for the ALS patient. While a patient is still ambulatory at a limited

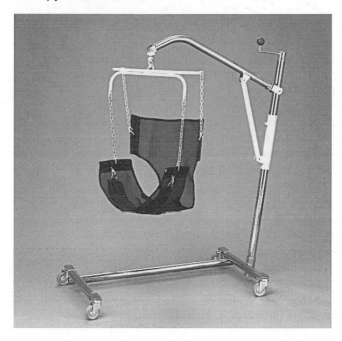

Figure 8-16. The "Transaid" lift with the 309 sling. This lift has a low profile base for ease of clearance under furniture. The 309 sling can be attached in a variety of ways to allow for greater patient safety and easier perineal care.

community level, they may benefit from the use of a wheelchair on a part-time basis. The appropriate wheelchair would be lightweight and portable so that their families could easily transport them. The physical therapist may sense a dilemma when realizing that the patient's insurance coverage should be used for a chair that will serve well when serious loss of trunk and neck strength necessitates use of a more expensive, bulky wheelchair. The best resolution of this dilemma is to arrange for rental of a lightweight chair until motor loss progresses to the point where a recliner chair is required. At that time, a more thorough assessment can be performed before ordering the final wheelchair.

Choosing a wheelchair requires a careful assessment of the individual's specific functional needs, home and work environment, and the need for future attachments. Many options are available to solve specific functional problems. There is no one model, however, that suits the needs of all patients. The options should be carefully selected to match the needs of the individual patient, remembering that each option adds to the bulk, complexity, and cost of the chair.

It is best to use input from the entire rehabilitaton team to select the final options for the wheelchair. The wheelchair specialist from the DME vendor can advise the team on the model that contains all desired features and can be modified for future attachments.

The occupational therapist can recommend attachments that facilitate hand use, prevent upper extremity dysfunction, and maximize self-care skills. They provide input on attachment of mobile arm supports (MAS) and must assure that the backrest upholstery allows for attachment of the MAS brackets. They also may recommend slanted armrests to decrease dependent hand edema. A lap tray may also be recommended to facilitate writing, feeding, or provide support for a personal computer.

The speech pathologist may provide input on desired positions of the trunk and neck to facilitate swallowing. Supplementing the reclining wheelchair with lumbar, neck, and head supports can prevent body positions that foster aspiration. The speech pathologist may recommend a small communication device that can be mounted on the chair and is accessible for the patient's use.

A reclining wheelchair with a headrest is nearly essential for the more involved ALS patient. Detachable armrests and legrests should be considered for the ALS patient to facilitate transfers and transportation of the chair. Adjustable height armrests allow for support of weakened shoulders to prevent subluxation.

Desk arms allow the patient to scoot up under ordinary tables. These arms can be reattached in reverse position to allow the patient to push to standing for transfer. Wraparound arms help narrow the overall width of the wheelchair, thus allowing for easy passage through narrow doorways, but they cannot be reattached in reverse position. Elevating legrests helps avoid dependent edema in the feet and ankles. Lowered seat heights allow the patient to use his feet for propulsion but make it harder to come to standing from the lowered seat. One should ascertain whether the patient will or will not accept a ventilator in the future. If ventilator use is a definite possibility, the chair must be able to accommodate attachment of a ventilator tray. Some fancy recliners have a pneumatic assist for the backrest, which precludes attachment of the ventilator tray.

One must also order an appropriate wheelchair cushion, lumbar support, and safety belt to assure skin integrity, proper trunk alignment, and trunk stability during transport. Elaborate seating systems may be indicated for those who lead an active life but have severe trunk and neck weakness. Wheelchair cushions come in a variety of shapes and thicknesses. Certain cushions are shaped to tilt the pelvis posteriorly in the chair and thus prevent the buttocks from sliding out of the seat. Other cushions emphasize flotation of the body weight above the seat in order to maximally protect the skin from breakdown. These cushions are very comfortable but are difficult to transfer from because of the instability of the surface.

The most efficient way to order a wheelchair is to have access to a wheelchair showroom where the patient can try a variety of chair and cushion models to see which combination provides the best comfort and function. Encouraging the patients to actively participate in the laborious task of choosing a wheelchair has the benefit of easing acceptance of this assistive device by allowing them a measure of control in its selection.

Motorized Wheelchairs

Consideration of an electric wheelchair should be made when the patient is unable to independently propel a manual wheelchair and needs a means of independent mobility in order to continue work or school or to remain in the home without hiring a caregiver. The purchase of an electric wheelchair is a large expenditure, and justification for its use frequently hinges on its contribution toward maintaining independence in self-care or continuation of a productive life-style.

The first consideration to be made is if the wheelchair needs to be transportable by the family. If so, the family has two options: (1) Purchase of a van and subsequent modification to allow for disabled accessibility, and installation of a proper restraint system to tie down the wheelchair and stabilize the patient. This option allows for consideration of most electric wheelchair models; (2) Purchase of a power unit attachment for converting a manual chair to power drive. This type of power wheelchair can be disassembled into multiple parts and can be placed in most medium to large car trunks.

The high cost of purchasing and converting a van for wheelchair use is prohibitive for many patients. They should be encouraged to investigate all financial resources for which they may be eligible, such as the Veterans Administration, the Department of Rehabilitation in the state of their residence, and grants from their place of employment, in order to subsidize purchase of the necessary equipment. A medical social worker can assist in exploring these resources. Private insurance usually aids the purchase of a power wheelchair when proper medical justification is provided, but it seldom assists in the purchase of a transport van.

Power Packs

Power units that attach to the rear of a wheelchair allow most patients the use of a power wheelchair and provide the possibility of transport in a standard automobile. This is advantageous for people who cannot afford a van, have limited access to or cannot afford to utilize disabled accessible transport services, and need to be transported on a regular basis.

The disadvantages of the power pack should be presented to the families so that an intelligent decision can be reached. Disassembly and reassembly of the wheelchair and power pack require some mechanical skills and about ten minutes. The wheelchair and batteries are heavy to lift into the car. The indirect drive does not provide the torque of most electric wheelchairs and thus cannot ascend as steep an incline. Moisture on the drive wheels can cause loss of the drive capability until the wheels are dry. Some recliner wheelchairs cannot use the power pack because the weight of the unit tips the chair over backwards. The angle of recline of the wheelchair backrest cannot be varied unless the entire drive unit is removed, reattached, and realigned. The unit attaches to the backrest and if the backrest is moved the drive wheels no longer contact the rear wheels of the chair and the drive function is inactivated.

The manual wheelchair chosen for the power unit needs to have a sturdy frame to accept the weight of the unit. The metal frame of the wheelchair backrest must be accessible for bracket attachment of the power pack. The wheelchair must be balanced so that tipping does not occur with use of the power pack. Treaded rear wheels provide better traction for the drive wheels of the power pack. Concurrent use of a ventilator may be impossible due to problems in balancing the wheelchair and restrictions for attachment of the units to the rear of the wheelchair.

Power Wheelchairs

Power wheelchairs seem to gain in complexity and option availability beyond the capability of the average physical therapist to remain informed. Maintaining a close relationship with an equipment vendor knowledgeable about these products serves to keep both the therapist and the patient current with product availability and informed of the performance records of various wheelchairs.

The most important general concept in ordering an electric wheelchair for an ALS patient is to order the wheelchair that will accommodate the patient's declining ability to function. Loss of trunk and neck strength require the use of a reclining backrest. Patients whose ability to remain independent at work is a condition of their continued employment may need to have a power recliner attached to the power wheelchair. This allows them to vary the back angle independently and can assist in pressure relief during prolonged sitting. The reclining back can also help to maintain a better position for chest expansion and diaphragm excursion and thus ease respiratory embarrassment. Special reclining units that keep shearing forces on the back to a minimum are also available. These help to prevent skin breakdown in the susceptible patient. Elevating legrests should accompany the use of a reclining backrest. Some power recline units are capable of coordinating the legrests with the backrest automatically.

The type of drive interface to be used by the patient is entirely dependent on the preserved muscle groups that are capable of activating the drive controls. When several motor groups are preserved at the time of ordering, the therapist should attempt to predict which groups may maintain usable function the longest and have the drive system adapted for that muscle group. The most common drive systems are for hand or finger use, sip and puff, head-activated, chin control, eyebrow control, and foot control.

If it is predicted that an attendant may have to drive the chair at a future date when the patient loses the ability to activate the controls, an attendant drive control should be included when ordering the wheelchair. Justification of this control is that it is much more expensive to retrofit a wheelchair at a future date, and assuring the usefulness of this chair for all phases of the disease eliminates the necessity of purchasing a manual reclining wheelchair at a future date.

Seat belts or chest restraints are highly recommended because of the possibility of falling out of the power wheelchair during abrupt stops or turns. Specialized seating systems may be necessary to stabilize the trunk and pelvis for the active wheelchair user with poor trunk strength.

The necessity for all other wheelchair options should be evaluated before ordering, as described in the preceding section on selecting a manual wheelchair. If possible, the entire rehabilitation staff should confer on the final ordering of the wheelchair to assure that communication devices can be positioned for proper access; activities of daily living (ADL) are facilitated by the chair design; mobile arm supports can be attached if necessary; and the family and patient have the cognitive skills and motivation to make use of the wheelchair under consideration.

Follow-up visits should be scheduled with occupational therapy and PT to assure that the patient and family can operate the wheelchair and all its options and that independence in self-care and activities of daily living is maximized. Ideally, these visits should be performed in the patient's home environment or work setting.

Summary

Central to the goals of physical therapy intervention for the ALS patient is the provision of education. Sharing knowledge about the disease process and what may be expected to occur helps shed a calming light on the vast unknown that faces each ALS patient. Fear and anxiety can be constant companions of the patient and can interfere with ability to retain instructions for new self-care skills or paralyze with indecision over the acquisition of necessary medical equipment.

The patient must understand that gradual changes in functional level are expected to occur. When difficulties in mobility or self-care become apparent, the patient should know to request referral to occupational or PT and thus become a more effective member of one's own health care team. Independence in mobility and self-care are certainly important goals of the PT program. A more important and long-lasting goal is to enable the patient to be an initiator in the management of health care.

Education about the disease and knowledge of the resources available will help the patient to cope with ongoing functional losses. This empowers the patient by allowing him to plan for the future. When the patient can be a *director* of change rather than a *prisoner* of a changing body, the ultimate goal of maintaining dignity will have been accomplished.

References

1. Norris FH. Amyotrophic lateral sclerosis: The clinical disorder. In: Smith RA, ed. *Handbook of Amyotrophic Lateral Sclerosis*. New York: Dekker, 1992.

2. Kisner C, Colby LA. *Therapeutic Exercise Foundations and Techniques*. Philadelphia: F. A. Davis, 1985.
3. Bohannon RW. Results of resistance exercise on a patient with amyotrophic lateral sclerosis: a case report. *Physical Therapy* 1983, 63(6):965–8.
4. Preston W, et al. *Managing Amyotrophic Lateral Sclerosis, MALS Manual II, Managing Muscular Weakness*. Sherman Oaks, CA: ALS Association, 1986.
5. Appel V, et al. *ALS: Maintaining Mobility*. Houston: Muscular Dystrophy Association.

9

Environmental Adaptations

Patricia Casey, M.S., O.T.R./L.

Environmental adaptations for amyotrophic lateral sclerosis include those phys-ical, mechanical, or procedural changes needed to accomplish activities of daily living (ADL). Adaptation may demand use of assistive devices or medical equip-ment, proper placement of furniture, utensils, or tools, or a change in the method of operation, i.e., pushing or sliding an object instead of lifting or carrying it.

Several factors affect the ability to make adaptations to the physical changes that occur with progression of the disease. Persons with ALS and their caregivers may have different perceptions of immediate and long-term needs and the degree to which increasing physical limitations will affect their lives. They may be in different stages of the grieving process, denial and depression making any changes very difficult. They may have different learning and problem-solving capacities that limit resolutions. Finally, families have different life-styles as well as varying social and financial resources. All of these factors need to be considered when assessing environmental adaptations for short- and long-term needs.

Solutions should be presented without supplying "too much" information or "too many" alternatives. This avoids overwhelming families who already have been stunned by the very need for such information. The purpose of adapting the environment to the patient's abilities is to make continued function easier or at least possible for him and his caregiver. *A person changes the way he performs a task only if the change makes accomplishing the task easier, or if the way he is performing is not accomplishing the task at all.*

Progressive physical limitations necessitate using a variety of assistive devices

Table 9-1. Classification of Amyotrophic Lateral Sclerosis

Recommended Assistive Equipment and Devices

Lightweight manual wheelchairs
    Companion model; Everest and Jennings (E&J)
    Other models; E&J, Invacare, Quickie
Recliner with headrest supports and ventilator trays; E&J, Invacare, Quickie
Adult stroller; Pogon
Motorized carts with adjustable tillers, hydraulic seat options
Cushions and seating systems
    Gel or T-Foam cushions, Jay, Roho cushions
    High back seating (make sure a headrest bracket can be attached), lateral
      supports
Wheelchair ramps
Power seat lift recliner chair
Padded shower commode on casters with U-shaped cushion, push handles, foot-
    rests; Activeaid models MD 250I, 450R, 461
Bath tub seat and bench, bathtub lift, bathtub attachment with separating sling or
    bath sling; Hoyer, Transaid
Hand Devices; Fred Sammons catalog
Infant monitor; Fisher Price

(Table 9-1). Use of these appliances may require modifying time, space, and location for activities. It eventually becomes necessary for the caregiver to perform the activity (e.g., feed, wash, dress, and so on). Occupational therapy in the home as well as in the clinic allows for periodic reevaluation to assess changing family priorities, the need for additional information, and the readiness to adapt the environment to maintain or improve function.

Recommendations for environmental adaptations are presented according to physical limitation rather than stage of the disease, since individual patients may present with disability at any stage. Along with patient's and caregiver's needs, consideration of insurance, Medicare, public assistance, and private organization policies for assistive equipment and environmental adaptations must be made to maximize limited benefits.

Ambulation with Limited Endurance

Once ambulation is affected by weakness, decreased endurance, or fatigability, assistive equipment is required to provide support for continued function at work, in the home, in the community, or at leisure. Depending on the rate of progression of the disease, careful selection of specific wheelchair and seating systems are made for short- and long-term needs. Most patients with lower extremity weakness require a lightweight manual wheelchair that can be easily placed in the back seat or trunk of a car. The caregiver's ability to lift and transport a wheelchair must be considered when prescribing such equipment. A suitable lightweight gel or dense foam cushion is always needed for adequate trunk and pelvic support. An adult stroller may be more supportive than a wheelchair for patients with neck and shoulder weakness since it has a high back, a slightly reclined seat/back angle, and offers the advantage of easy portability. The recliner wheelchair is bulky and difficult to transport in a car, although it is useful for persons with neck and trunk weakness who remain at home or use a van with a lift.

Some patients, especially those who are working or socially active, are interested in using motorized carts. Rental or loan of such equipment is indicated if the rate of progression of the disease is slow to moderate. Sitting posture, shoulder and hand function, and hip strength must be assessed to assure proper seating support. An adjustable tiller control or a hydraulic seat may be necessary.

Depending on family needs and resources, information may be provided regarding wheelchair racks and lifts, as well as lifts for motorized carts and power wheelchairs for cars and vans.

When fatigability is responsible for poor walking endurance, respiratory function may be at risk. Such patients may have already given some thought to ventilator-assisted lives and need guidance in selecting power recliner or manual wheelchairs with ventilator trays.

Once the decision is made that a wheelchair is required, easy entrance and exit from the house, car, and office must be considered. Portable wheelchair ramps provide the simplest means of negotiating one or two steps. Two motorcycle ramps are usually less expensive than a single wheelchair ramp. Wooden or metal ramps come in all shapes and sizes, depending on the configuration of front doors, walkways, shrubbery, and location of the house in relation to the sidewalk. Walkways along the side of the house allow space for a long ramp. A "Z"-shaped ramp is necessary when short front- or backyards do not provide length for a safe, long incline. A platform level with the door before the ramp begins is needed to rest the wheelchair safely while opening and closing the door. Ramp inclines of 1:12 but not more than 1.5:12 are safe and easy to climb. Hydraulic porch lifts may be the most economical and the only architectural choice for some homes. Local building ordinances must be taken into account.

Ambulation Requiring Assistance

Frequent falls occur when ankle weakness results in "drop foot" and weakness in the quadriceps causes the knees to "give out." Lightweight plastic ankle-foot orthoses (AFOs) with 5–10 degrees of plantar flexion can usually stabilize walking. Persons who wear braces and live in apartments or homes with stairs present problem-solving challenges. Standard orthoses usually decrease the ability to climb stairs. Articulating ankle joints may be considered when prescribing braces, but these preclude the floor reaction effect of the brace necessary for knee stability. Careful assessment is required by a physical therapist and an orthotist. If upper extremity weakness is severe, a walker with front casters can be helpful since it need not be lifted for smooth ambulation. A gait belt is often useful when assisted ambulation is necessary.

Trilevel, bilevel, and two-story homes with turning stairways are the most difficult challenges. Solutions depend on family resources. Stair lifts are an alternative solution for families unable or unwilling to move. Companies now rent stair lifts, which help in short- as well as long-term planning. A decision to move the patient to the most accessible level of the home with changes for toileting and bathing needs may be the most feasible solution in the long run. Finally, porch lifts have been installed inside homes to gain access to two levels with easy access to front and back doors, garages, and bathrooms.

Trunk and Hip Weakness

Initial difficulty rising from a seated to a standing position may simply require a firm 2″ or 3″ cushion added to the sitting surface. Sometimes sitting on a firm chair with supportive back and arms is needed. More often, purchase or rental of a powered seat lift recliner chair is required to provide independent change of position either to a standing, seated, or reclined position. In the bathroom, use of a plastic molded raised toilet seat is the simple solution with initial weakness. A padded shower commode with a U-shaped cushion on casters incorporates features required for problems of progressive weakness. It can be used over the toilet by the patient and easily removed by other family members. It provides a high seat and back support, removable armrests, a large opening for toilet hygiene, and can be used to transport the patient into the bathroom and shower when he can no longer ambulate. It can be placed at bedside for night use to avoid the inconvenience of donning braces and shoes.

Various bathtub seats, benches, lifts, and accessories are available to provide independent as well as assisted bathing. Selection depends on the bathroom layout and the willingness to make minor changes if expensive renovation is not feasible. A tiled floor with recessed drain allows access into a remodeled shower area using the shower commode. A standard shower stall with a 3″–4″ rim can be modified with a simple wood deck and removable ramp. Bathroom doors can be widened with inexpensive offset hinges. Commode chairs with casters usually clear doors as they measure 20–21 inches.

Early use of a full electric bed to facilitate safe standing and sitting can save energy and maintain independence. If space is adequate, a hospital bed frame (80″) without a headboard can be clamped to an extra long twin bed frame (80″) to form a king size bed, allowing spouses to continue sleeping together while providing power-operated assistance for positioning support. Some insurance companies will underwrite a queen or king size electric bed, but these usually do not raise to assist standing; other companies will cover only hospital beds.

Once weight bearing is not possible for standing and pivot transfer, a hydraulic lift is used for lifting in and out of bed, wheelchair, commode, seat lift, recliner chair, or car. A full size separating sling is easily placed under the patient and removed without lifting him. The extra long model provides head and neck support. One innovative person devised a ceiling lift using a garage door opener track and motor with attached bar and sling. Another family in a bilevel home installed an I beam and quarter-ton hoist on the ceiling. An attached swivel bar and sling enabled transport of the patient over the stairwell from top to ground level. The lower stairs were placed on rollers, and when rolled out of the way the wheelchair could be positioned directly below the hoist. This inexpensive renovation (under $2,000) allowed the family safe and easy access to both levels. It was considerably less expensive than installing an elevator or double stair lift. It also negated the need for the family to move to a one-level home.

Neck and Shoulder Weakness

Patients with mild to moderate weakness of the neck and shoulders may request a soft cervical collar or clavicle splint to provide mild support. A plastazote Philadelphia collar offers additional support without restricting neck muscles, but patients cannot eat, speak, or drive a car while wearing this collar. It also may not provide adequate head support while walking. The Oxford wire spring support collar allows some head motion for eating and speaking and gives lightweight support while walking. It also gives unrestricted neck support for ventilated patients. A sterno-occipital-mandibular immobilizer (SOMI) assures adequate head and neck control while walking or sitting. A simple sling should provide maximum support for flail upper extremities and minimize pressure on weak shoulder and neck muscles. Proper arm support while sitting can be managed with an adjustable overbed table and properly positioned pillows.

Upper Extremity Weakness

Weakness and atrophy in the shoulders and upper arms prevent placing the hand in a functional position, and weakness in the elbow, forearm, wrist, and hand limit use of the hand for manipulation of tools and utensils for self-care, work, or leisure activities. Intrinsic muscle weakness and atrophy affect grasp and prehension. Since many assistive devices are available for these symptomatic conditions, careful selection is required to promote function for as long as possible and reduce frustration for patient and caregiver as well.

Mobile arm supports (MAS) allow horizontal and vertical motion. Additional features can be attached to provide wrist support and allow for limited supination. Self-feeding and some grooming and personal care can be accomplished with the MAS once materials have been set up. It is possible to operate computer keyboards and communication devices using the MAS system.

Other useful devices for eating include lightweight wrist splints, utensil holders, foam or cork tubes for utensils, plastic or long-handled utensils, extra long straws, lightweight large-handled cups, plate guards, and suction holders or nonskid pads. Key holders, door knob extenders, light switch extension levers, lightweight reachers, self-opening scissors, and card holders assist with some usual daily activities. Button and zipper hooks, a long-handled sponge, a lightweight electric shaver, an adapted floss holder, a rechargeable electric toothbrush with rotary brush, and velcro fasteners help with hygiene, grooming, and dressing.

Communication aids include a rubber thumb, pencil grips, writing splints, Magic Slate, book holders, tilt-top overbed table, lap-style AbleTable, portable phone, speaker phone, use of TDD (telecommunication devices for the deaf) assistance through the phone company, infant monitor system, or small bell. Various augmentative electronic speech devices are used with patients who have adequate hand function to operate a keyboard, and single switch computer systems are available for those who do not.

Comfort in Bed

When patients spend more time in bed, comfort must be assured. Gel and foam mattresses with sheepskin padding are used by some patients. Contour neck pillows, foam boots, elbow pads, and blanket supports are sometimes helpful. An adequate communication system should be in place by this time whether it uses eyeblink, facial expressions, or a computer with speech synthesizer.

Conclusions

The purpose of all occupational therapy interventions is to maintain or improve the function of the patient with ALS. When this is no longer possible, the function and support of the caregiver becomes the main concern. Initially ALS forces a person to adapt himself to his environment. He changes the way he performs tasks in order to function as independently as possible. As weakness increases, however, the environment must be adapted to fit the patient's needs, to make function possible, if not easier. Each family has its priorities and each has its own style, format, and unique sense of timing. The occupational therapist intervenes in this dynamic process to help both patient and caregiver function as well as possible for as long as feasible.

Recommended Reading

ALS: Maintaining Mobility. New York: Muscular Dystrophy Association, 1987.

Caroscio J (ed.). *Amyotrophic Lateral Sclerosis: A Guide for Patient Care*. New York: Thieme Medical Publishers, 1986.

Foyder JE. *Family Caregivers Guide*. Cincinnati: Futuro Company, 1985.

Hamilton L. *Why Didn't Somebody Tell Me About These Things?* Shawnee Mission, KS: Intercollegiate Press, 1984.

Managing Amyotrophic Lateral Sclerosis: Managing Muscular Weakness. Woodland Hills, CA: ALS Association, 1985.

10

Long-Term In-Hospital Ventilatory Care for Patients with Amyotrophic Lateral Sclerosis

Hideaki Hayashi, M.D.

Introduction

Amyotrophic lateral sclerosis (ALS) is a chronic neurodegenerative disease that usually ends in respiratory failure and death. Although ventilatory support can sustain life beyond respiratory failure, this option raises complex medical and ethical issues. In Tokyo Metropolitan Neurological Hospital (TMNH), about half the patients with ALS who develop respiratory failure receive long-term ventilatory support and are cared for within the hospital. We have thus had the opportunity to follow closely the course of ALS beyond respiratory failure in a controlled environment.

In Japan, most patients have full medical insurance, paid for by either corporate or government programs. The insurance, however, would not cover the private room and the special caregiver that are required for patients on respirators. Family members of the principal insured may have less coverage depending on the type of the insurance. The decision to place ALS patients on ventilators after respiratory failure, however, has been affected by several other factors. Until recently, physicians did not tell patients of their diagnosis or prognosis. Even if family members learned the nature of the disease or treatment, they were not likely to share this information with the patient. Thus, many patients were placed on ventilators without knowing the implications. This practice is rapidly changing, but it is still very prevalent.

Since 1985, patients at TMNH have been notified of their diagnosis and prognosis before respiratory support was instituted (1). Moreover, we have taken an aggressive, positive approach in managing ALS patients. Home care options in Japan are limited, in part because the Japanese home is small and the burden on the family is correspondingly greater than in the United States. As a result, ALS patients are usually hospitalized and have greater access to the care needed for ventilation support. At TMNH, a metropolitan municipal hospital that is specifically designed to care for patients with neurological diseases, cost is at least not a major factor in the decision to provide ventilator care. These, then, are the major reasons why our patients are placed on ventilators at the time of respiratory failure more often than at any other hospital in Japan.

Ventilator Support of ALS Patients in Japan

Table 10-1 shows survival rates of ALS patients treated in Japan with and without mechanical ventilation. The data are based on a 1982 report by the Ministry of Health and Welfare of Japan, "Prognosis of Motor Neuron Disease in Japan," a survey that summarized the fate of 768 patients who died of ALS (2), and from our observations of 87 ALS patients treated at TMNH between July 1980 and May 1992.

Our results at TMNH contrast greatly with those contained in the 1982 Ministry report. Our experience indicated that ventilatory support could extend the lives

Table 10-1. Survival Rates for ALS Patients Treated in Japan With and Without Ventilator Support

Source (N)	Ventilator-Dependent N (% of all ALS patients with ventilator)	1-year Survival on Ventilator N (% of ALS patients with ventilator)	5-year Survival	
			Natural N (% of all patients without ventilator)	With N (% of all patients with ventilator)
Report[a] (472)	63 (13[b])	5 (8)	104 (13)	—
THNM[c] (87)	49 (56)	39 (80)	16 (18)	22 (26)

[a] Number represents responses to a survey of 768 cases in the Ministry report [2]. Only 472 patients (or their families) responded to the survey on the use of ventilator support.
[b] The percentage is based on 472 patients who responded to the survey on use of ventilator.
[c] Followed at TMNH between 1980 and 1992.

of ALS patients in respiratory failure and that the course of ALS beyond respiratory failure must now be considered.

In this chapter, I present our observations of ALS patients after respiratory failure. I describe the physiological deterioration caused by the disease after respiratory failure and discuss several quality of life and treatment issues raised by the option of long-term ventilator support. Our observations confirm that respiratory failure is only one of the neurological impairments of ALS (1,3–5).

Somatic Motor Function After Respiratory Failure

ALS involves all efferent motor functions concerned with movement and posture, including somatic motor and limbic functions (3). Somatic motor functions in ALS after respiratory failure can be put into four categories:

1. Extremity and axial functions (extremity and body movements of skeletal muscles).
2. Cranial motor functions (pontobulbar cranial functions: speaking and swallowing), excluding ocular function.
3. Respiratory muscle functions.
4. External ocular motor functions (eye movement).

Which somatic motor functions are involved first, and how rapidly the involvement progresses, varies for each patient. However, ontogenetically newer motor functions, such as fine motor control of the distal muscles and speech, appear to be involved earlier, whereas older ones, such as mass motor control of the proximal muscles and the external ocular muscles, seem to be involved later (3–5).

The onset of initial impairment and complete paralysis in the extremities, pontobulbar cranial functions, and external ocular motor functions in forty-nine ventilator-dependent ALS patients with respect to the time of respiratory failure are plotted in Figure 10-1. The duration from the time of diagnosis to the time of complete paralysis is shown in Figure 10-2. Complete paralysis is defined here as the absence of voluntary movement in the extremities, articulate speech (anarthria), the ability to swallow (aphagia), voluntary eye movements, and spontaneous respiration during sleep.

Impairment of extremity motor function was detected in all forty-nine patients before respiratory failure, but complete paralysis occurred in only twenty-two of the forty-nine (45 percent). Even after respiratory failure, the preserved motor function allowed patients to communicate. In fact, of the nineteen patients who survived on respirators for more than five years, nine were still able to use their extremities for communication. The onset of complete paralysis in the extremities appears to be more gradual than in the other categories.

The onset of complete paralysis of the bulbar cranial functions and respiratory

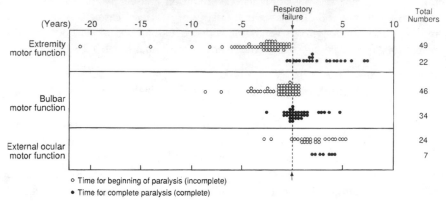

Figure 10-1.   Onset time of motor impairment and paralysis in 49 ALS patients.

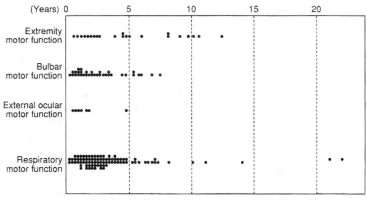

Figure 10-2. Time between diagnosis of ALS and complete paralysis of motor function in 87 patients.

functions was correlated in the majority of patients (Figure 10-2); that is, the complete paralysis of the one function followed the paralysis of the other function (5).

While external ocular motor function usually became impaired after respiratory failure, complete external ophthalmoplegia was not always the last of the four motor function categories to appear (5). ALS patients often die of respiratory failure before ophthalmoplegia can develop, which has resulted in underestimating the incidence of ophthalmoplegia and in interpreting it as a "negative sign" of ALS symptomatology.

Of thirty-nine patients who were ventilator-dependent for more than one year, complete paralysis occurred in one of the four function categories in twenty-five patients at least six months before ventilator care was begun. Of these twenty-five patients, twenty-one lost respiratory function completely, and four lost bulbar motor functions completely. Unexpectedly, after respiratory failure, more than half the ventilator-dependent patients (twenty-one of thirty-nine) retained some function in the other three categories. Although cases of respiratory failure without paralysis of other motor functions have been reported (6), this phenomenon was not widely recognized until the TMNH data were published (5).

Limbic Motor Function After Respiratory Failure

Forced crying and laughing are pseudobulbar signs of ALS. These synkineses are concerned with the expressive manifestations of innate emotive patterns; that is, laughing and crying are thought to be related to expressions of phylogenetically lower order facio-respiratory synergy, such as grunting and snarling, that might be related to yawning, sneezing, and coughing and have had social communication as an integrated autonomic component (7). These synkineses have also been discussed as facio-vocal (8) and facio-respiratory (9) functional motor units because emotional expressions are closely related to facial expression, vocalizations, and respiration. Motor function related to forced emotional expression can be included in limbic (emotional) motor functions as distinct from somatic motor functions. The limbic motor function might determine the level of neuronal functioning, which in turn might determine the emotional state of the individual (10).

Forced emotional expressions are triggered by subtle afferent stimuli, including emotional feeling, and involve facial contractions that are stronger and longer than voluntary facial contractions. Even when voluntary facial contractions become impossible, distinct facial contractions can be provoked by strong emotions. These findings suggest that the voluntary facial contractions mediated by the somatic motor function might be affected in ALS before the forced emotional expression mediated by the limbic motor function.

The efferent motor system of this forced emotional synkinesis is probably organized along the descending limbic-diencephalic connections and bulbar effector pathways at the level of the rostral midbrain (7). Forced emotional expression thus may be caused by impairments in the limbic system and related regions. On the other hand, subtle voluntary facial contractions were observed in some patients even after paralysis of emotional expression. This observation may be explained by the same mechanism that explains the faint voluntary movements of the extremities that sometimes remain after paralysis of somatic motor function (5). In fact, almost all of our ALS patients with forced emotional expressions do not report the expected accompanying emotional feelings.

We recently reported neuropsychological findings on personality and social behavior in ALS patients (11). Among thirty ventilator-dependent patients, nineteen sometimes expressed excessive irritability and social inappropriateness. In nine of these patients, the behavior was episodic. In the remaining ten patients, the behavior was probably triggered by subtle changes in daily routines; we refer to this circumstance as "disinhibition of emotional motor expression." This behavior pattern was also observed in patients with motor neuron disease with dementia, as described by Yuasa (12). Among these ten patients with disinhibition of emotional motor expression, forced emotional expression was detected in seven, spastic gaze fixation in eight, apraxia of the eyelids closing in seven, and supranuclear ocular limitation in all ten.

At TMNH, we examined four ALS patients with dementia (12) to determine if the dementia was related to the disinhibition of emotional motor expression (11). The two conditions had the following psychological characteristics in common:

1. The inability to shift from one stimulus to another (a type of perseveration).
2. The compulsive clinging to familiar situations and resistance to change.
3. The inability to discriminate himself or herself from others.
4. Excessive orderliness and an inability to think abstractly.
5. A psychologically labile state of busying themselves with activities intended to create stability.

These psychological characteristics in patients with ALS seem to be caused by the early impairment of the ontogenetically newer cortical function, namely, the abstract domain, leaving an older concrete thinking still intact (13). Motor neuron disease with dementia and ALS with clinical features of disinhibition of emotional motor expression share the findings that the limbic motor system is involved in both situations. This involvement is neuropathologically (14) and neuroradiologically demonstrated (15). Such evidence suggests that dementia occurring in motor neuron disease is caused by limbic motor involvement in ALS.

Patient Care and Family Support

The bulbar and respiratory motor functions lost in ALS patients can be treated symptomatically with nasopharyngeal feeding tubes or gastrostomy tube feeding and mechanical ventilation. We must realize that ALS patients may not die of ALS itself; that they must be cared for as patients not with a terminal illness but with a progressive, intractable, disabling disease. The issue now is how to activate the remaining motor functions and how to foster what the Japanese call *ikigai* —"something to live for" (1).

To cope with the impairments of advanced ALS, patients and their families must learn about the course of the disease and develop a strong degree of trust and confidence in their physician. Communication between patients, caregivers, and health care providers must be fostered.

Physical Problems

The physical problems of advanced ALS consist of neurological impairments related to ALS itself and the medical complications of ALS (Table 10-2).

Table 10-2. Manifestations Seen in ALS

I. Neurological Problems
  A. Extremity Motor Function (activity daily living [ADL] disturbance)
  B. Pontobulbar Motor Function
    1. Phonation and articulation (communication disturbance)
    2. Mastication and deglutition (swallowing disturbance)
  C. Respiratory Motor Function (respiratory failure)
  D. External Ocular Motor Function (communication disturbance)
  E. Limbic (Emotional) Motor Function (disinhibition of emotional motor expression, forced emotional expression)
II. Medical Problems
  A. Respiratory Disturbances: Pneumonia; Pneumothorax; Troubles with respirators
  B. Cardiovascular Disturbances: Changes of blood pressure in respirator setting or during sleep
  C. Gastrointestinal Disturbances: Sialorrhea; Aerophagia; Decreased peristaltic movements; Ileus (coarctation of upper mesencephalic artery); Perforation or penetration (gastric or duodenal ulcer); Postprandial diabetes
  D. Otological Disturbances: Serous otitis media, dizziness, or vertigo due to rapid changes of neck or body
  E. Vesicular Disturbances: Urinary retention, unusually frequent micturition
  F. Dermatological Disturbances: Pigmentation of dorsal skin of finger joints
  G. Sensory Disturbances: Abnormal sensation in oral cavity, photophobia, pains in various parts of body; muscle cramps
III. Social Problems
IV. Psychological Problems

Neurological Impairments

Our goal in treating physically impaired patients is not only to ameliorate each somatic limitation of the activities of daily living but also to enrich the quality of life through valuing the sanctity of life.

In general, when impairments in phonation and articulation prevent normal oral communication, we consider the use of communication devices. However, more importantly, the level of trust between patient and caregivers must be established. Before using any communication devices, "mental communication" between patients and their spouses (or caregivers) must be fostered. Without such trust, open communication about ALS and its effects does not happen, leaving the patient with a feeling of isolation and leading to a loss of hope.

From a practical standpoint, "somatic communication" (communication by movements and gestures when speech is impossible) can be classified into visual and nonvisual modes. We often use a transparent board bearing characters as a visual communication aid. Patients point to the characters on the board so that the caregiver can identify characters from the opposite side of the patient.

In nonvisual communication, a nurse-call is the fundamental need. The type of movements and signals to be used are selected by patients, and they vary from patient to patient. The important aspect is that the patient feels free to choose the specific signals and to define the specific meanings. Complete ophthalmoplegia is rare in ALS, and ocular movements themselves have been used for communication when other options have not been available (1).

At TMNH we encountered two specific problems in using ocular movements for communication. Ocular dyspraxia (uncoordinated volitional eye movements) occurred in six of our eighty-seven patients. These patients occasionally could not move their eyes or keep their gaze stable when attempting to fix a word on a word board, although none had complete paralysis of oculomotor function. All these patients had spasmodic gaze fixation, and all except one had supranuclear limitation, apraxia of the eyelids closing, and forced emotional expression. In these situations, with only their eye movements for communication, patients could select only a few words.

A more serious condition occurs when complete paralysis of all somatic motor functions results in a "total locked-in state" (TLS). It would be incorrect to assume that only patients on mechanical ventilation succumb to TLS. Patients may develop TLS before respiratory failure (16,17), and ophthalmoplegia occurs more frequently after respiratory failure than does TLS. Thus, TLS is not a new manifestation of ALS, but it is not widely recognized. It has become more noticeable since ventilatory support has been implemented after respiratory failure. Its incidence is not affected by the duration of ventilatory support.

Seven of our eighty-seven patients developed TLS. In six of these patients, ALS was characterized by a rapid onset, and complete external ophthalmoplegia occurred last (3). The seventh patient had a slower onset of ALS, and ophthalmoplegia did not occur last (5). In one patient, six years after the onset of TLS, electroencephalography revealed a slow alpha rhythm. After four more years, alpha suppression was no longer apparent on EEG. Patients with TLS do not appear to be brain dead; they simply, and tragically, cannot move. The three living patients with TLS have been well cared for by family members, who share the daily responsibilities with TMNH nurses. Family members believe that any inconveniences to them are insignificant compared to the lives and well-being of these patients.

Because respiratory failure is no longer a fatal characteristic in ALS, the possibility of ventilatory support should be explained to the patient and family early in the course of the disease. The possibility of complete ventilator dependency and complete reliance on nonverbal communication should be made clear. Although our patients had been informed of these possibilities well before respiratory failure occurred (18), none recognized the full impact of their situation until some time after ventilatory support had begun. Patients who elect to live with respirators require a great deal of psychological support and assistance in making decisions about their living circumstances from then on.

In treating ALS patients after respiratory failure, we must know, in addition to forced emotional expression, the occurrence of disinhibition of emotional motor expression, as defined previously. It is important to provide additional emotional support in these patients. Furthermore, because of afferent functional compensations for selectively impaired efferent motor functions in ALS, patients sometimes become hypersensitive to visual, cochlear, superficial, and visceral stimuli, again requiring special care to patients' surroundings.

Medical Problems

The medical problems in ALS are often caused by accidents resulting from motor restrictions or inexperience in living with a disabling condition. However, the medical problems may be caused by ALS itself, so we must pay careful attention to what patients say. For example, after respiratory failure patients often reported disturbances in hearing. On examination, they were found to have serous otitis media resulting from the paralysis of the tensor vili palatine muscle (2). Other examples include acute abdomen of coarctation of upper mesencephalic artery and postprandial diabetes caused by the decrease in total muscle volume. Patients do not often report pain, although they do report rare objective sensory disturbances, itching, and photophobia. Dryness or abnormal sensations in the mouth are more frequent than previously thought.

The medical problems in ALS can be fatal. Of forty-nine ventilator-dependent ALS patients (with and without tube feeding), twenty-five are now dead, twelve from intractable infections of the respiratory tract, six from sudden death during sleep, two from myocardial infarction, one from renal failure, one from a perforated stomach ulcer, and three from accidental death. Although respiratory infection was the most common cause of death, sudden death during sleep was the cause in six deaths. All these patients received continuous nocturnal ventilatory support, making sleep apnea an unlikely cause of death. Fluctuations in blood pressure, however, were detected in two of the six patients who died during sleep and in two who died from pneumonia. Physical disorders, such as pneumonia or heart insufficiency, apparently triggered instability in blood pressure. Recently, continuous twenty-four-hour recordings of blood pressure in an ALS patient confirmed that sudden death was preceded by significant depression in blood pressure during sleep and frequent paroxysmal elevation of blood pressure during arousal, probably as a result of pneumonia (Shimizu et al., personal communication).

Considering that the autonomic nervous system is not the primary target of ALS, blood pressure instability might be related to supranuclear efferent motor functions. Given that these fluctuating changes in blood pressure were observed in seven of ten patients with disinhibition of emotional motor expression, and that the disinhibition of emotional motor expression was verified in two patients who suddenly died during sleep, limbic motor functions might be involved in autonomic instability. According to Holstege (10), limbic motor functions might be setting the level of sensitivity for neurons high enough to be easily excited by some emotional stimuli. In some patients, the disturbance of limbic motor functions might precipitate a change in blood pressure and lead to cardiac arrest. If so, heart monitors might be used during sleep until the patient's general condition stabilizes.

Social Problems

Many caregivers continue to think of ALS as a disease that ends in death from respiratory failure within three or four years after diagnosis; that it, is a disease of "no cause, no cure, and no hope." With the institution of ventilatory support, ALS patients now live beyond respiratory failure, and their psychological and social needs must be addressed.

Psychological Problems

A major psychological issue is the anxiety about ALS itself. Family members may also experience this anxiety, and their needs must also be met. The difficulty is the highly individual nature of each patient and his or her circumstances and disease progression. In general, candid communication about the disease and its potential course, discussion of patients' and families' emotional reactions, and support in identifying and choosing treatment options provide a foundation for dealing with these problems.

Conclusions

Charcot (19) once said confidently, " . . . the verdict we will give a patient tomorrow will not be the same we must give this patient today." His enthusiasm was not shared for long, however, and the "no cause, no cure, no hope" stigma has haunted ALS for the past one hundred years, just as it did for tuberculosis and cancer (20). Despite this stigma, there is hope. From their personal experience of treating more than one thousand ALS patients, Norris et al. (21) and Smith (22) believe that "Indeed, ALS has no cure, but patients could be living longer and have more satisfactory lives due to symptomatic treatment. No one wants to hear that their circumstances are hopeless and that there is nothing to be done."

At TMNH, physical and medical problems in those living beyond respiratory failure were carefully assessed. As discussed in this chapter, respiratory failure is only one of the manifestations of ALS. However, in the current social and cultural climate, a majority of patients with ALS hold the "no cause, no cure, no hope" stigma of ALS; that is, respiratory failure in ALS is synonymous with the termination of the disease. I hope that our medical experiences with ALS patients on ventilators will cultivate a better understanding of the disease and break down the ALS stigma.

Acknowledgments

I thank all the patients and their relatives, the staff nurses and physicians at Tokyo Metropolitan Neurological Hospital, and particularly the members of the ALS project team, Drs. Shuuichi Kato, Akirhiro Kawada, and Toshio Shimizu, for their contributions to this chapter. I am also grateful to Mr. Tom Lang of the Department of Scientific Publications, The Cleveland Clinic Foundation, for his help with the manuscript.

References

1. Hayashi H. The clinical features and rehabilitation of advanced ALS. In: Tsubaki T, Yase Y, eds. *Amyotrophic Lateral Sclerosis*. New York: Excerpta Medica,1988.
2. Yase Y, Uebayashi Y, Tanaka H, et al. Prognosis study of motor neuron disease in Japan. The Committee of Intractable Degenerative CNS Diseases. Ministry of Health and Welfare of Japan (Chairman: Y. Toyokura). 1982.
3. Hayashi H, Kato S. Total manifestations in amyotrophic lateral sclerosis. ALS in the totally locked-in state. *J Neurol Sci* 1989, 93:19–35.
4. Hayashi H, Kato S, Kawada A, et al. Amyotrophic lateral sclerosis: Oculomotor function in patients in respirators. *Neurology* 1987, 37:1431–1432.
5. Hayashi H, Kato S, Kawada A. Amyotrophic lateral sclerosis patients living beyond respiratory failure. *J Neurol Sci* 1991, 105:73–78.

6. Hill R, Martin J, Hakim A. Acute respiratory failure in motor neuron disease. *Arch Neurol* 1982, 40:30–32.
7. Brown JW. Physiology and phylogenesis of emotional expression. *Brain Research* 1967, 5:1–14.
8. Kelly AH, Beaton LE, Magoun HW. A midbrain mechanism for facio-vocal activity. *J Neurophysiol* 1946, 9:181–189.
9. Wilson SAK. Some problems in neurology. II. Pathological laughing and crying. *J Neurol Psychopath* 1924, 4:299–333.
10. Holstege G, Descending motor pathways and spinal motor system: Limbic and nonlimbic components. In: Holstege G, ed. *Role of the Forebrain in Sensation and Behavior*. New York: Oxford, 1991.
11. Hayashi H, Kato S, Kawada A, Shimizu T. Significance of disinhibition of emotional motor expression in ALS. *Clin Neurol* 1992, 32:1412.
12. Yuasa R. Amyotrophic lateral sclerosis with dementia. *Clin Neurol* 1970, 10:569–577.
13. Goldstein K. *Human Nature in the Light of Psychopathology*. New York: Schocken Books, 1963.
14. Nakano I, Iwatsubo T, Hashizume Y, Mizutani T. Amyotrophic lateral sclerosis with dementia—lesions in the apical cortex and some deeper structures of the temporal lobes. *Neuropathol* 1992, 12:69–77.
15. Kato S, Hayashi H, Yagishita A. Involvement of the frontotemporal lobe and limbic system in amyotrophic lateral sclerosis: As assessed by serial computed tomography and magnetic resonance imaging. *J Neurol Sci* 1993, 116:52–58.
16. Harvey DG, Torack RM, Rosenbaum HE. Amyotrophic lateral sclerosis with ophthalmoplegia. A clinicopathological study. *Arch Neurol* 1979, 36:615–617.
17. Cohen B, Caroscio J. Eye movements in amyotrophic lateral sclerosis. *J Neural Transmission* 1983, 19:305–315.
18. Sivak ED, Gibson T, Hanson MR. Long-term management of respiratory failure in amyotrophic lateral sclerosis. *Ann Neurol* 1982, 12:18–23.
19. Goetz CG. Charcot's disease: Amyotrophic lateral sclerosis: A case of glosso-labial laryngeal paralysis. In: Goetz CG, ed. *Charcot the Clinician: The Tuesday Lessons*. New York: Raven Press, 1987.
20. Sontag S. *llness as Metaphor*. New York: Farrar, Straus & Giroux, 1978.
21. Norris FH, Smith RA, Denys EH. Motor neurone disease: Toward better care. *Br Med J* 1985, 291:259–262.
22. Smith RA. On behalf of the patient. *Adv Exp Med Bio* 1987, 209:319–322.

11

Respiratory Management and Home Mechanical Ventilation in Amyotrophic Lateral Sclerosis

Edward Anthony Oppenheimer, M.D.

Respiratory management in amyotrophic lateral sclerosis is essential to both comprehensive care and critical choices. Pulmonary consultation should be arranged soon after the diagnosis is made and then should continue as part of multidisciplinary support.

ALS almost always progresses to respiratory failure. This is the major cause of death directly related to ALS. Weakness of the muscles used for breathing and cough, as well as aspiration associated with bulbar involvement, results in pulmonary infection, sepsis, and respiratory failure. When respiratory failure and infection are prevented or treated, people with ALS can usually continue to live for additional years unless other medical problems occur. High priority must be given to reviewing the treatment options in advance and to informed decision making. Complex medical and ethical issues are involved.

Respiratory involvement in ALS often appears after quadriplegia, dysarthria, and swallowing problems, but it can occur earlier in the progression of ALS. Occasionally it occurs when there is considerable limb function, or when speech and swallowing are still good. The higher the functional level at the onset of respiratory failure, the more likely that a person may want to use a ventilator and continue living. Medical care can usually prevent death from respiratory complications unless this is not desired by the patient.

Survival and quality of life (QL) data indicate that long-term home mechanical ventilation (HMV) can be a successful option. Figure 11-1 shows survival data from the Kaiser Permanente HMV program in California, which started in 1985.

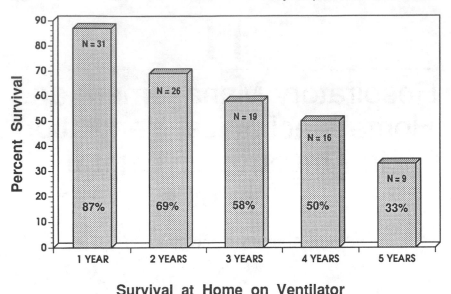

Survival at Home on Ventilator

Figure 11-1. ALS survival after hospital discharge on home mechanical ventilation (HMV). Data from the Kaiser Permanente Medical Care Program in California: 1985 to 1992. Percent surviving, of those discharged home one to five years ago. N: number of patients discharged home one to five years ago, respectively.

Patients and their families, as well as health care professionals, should understand HMV in order to make an informed choice before respiratory failure occurs. Clinical and physiological indications for mechanical ventilation in ALS are part of a broader context that is the basis for decision making. In the past, health care professionals have frequently either had a ''pessimistic nontreatment'' approach to ALS or have ''done everything'' as part of emergency and intensive care. A more reasonable approach involves early multidisciplinary individual and family evaluation, appropriate identification of those who might best benefit from HMV, and then physician counseling with a shared decision-making process. A multidisciplinary professional team is usually involved and should be assumed whenever ''physician'' is indicated in the discussion that follows; this includes psychosocial, rehabilitation, respiratory care, home health, and nursing professional staff as well as the personal physician and consultants.

Progression, Survival, and Pathophysiology

There is great variability in the pattern of progression of ALS. The time course of muscle weakness is usually linear (1); only occasionally does a plateau occur

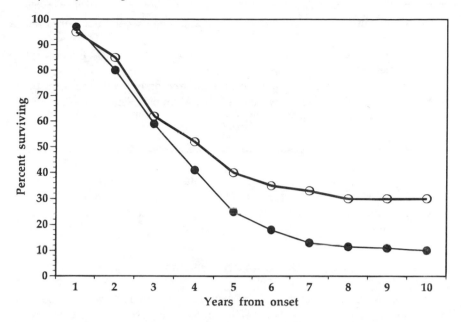

Figure 11-2. ALS survival data: ●: Mulder and Howard (6) [1976]: 100 ALS patients, Neurology Department, Mayo Clinic; ○: Caroscio (9) [1986]: 397 ALS patients, Neurology Department, Mount Sinai Medical Center, New York.

(2). In the past, the expected duration of life after onset of ALS was often stated as about two to four years, frequently limited by pneumonia and respiratory failure (3,4). In the past, 50 percent died during the first three to four years, but at least 25 percent lived five years or longer, with slow progression over many years (1, 5–7) (Figure 11-2). Longer survival for ten to fifteen years or more does occur (2,8–13). Some have little or no bulbar involvement, allowing speech, eating, and swallowing to continue. The rate of progression of ALS is not related to the presence or absence of bulbar involvement (1). In young patients ALS often progresses more slowly. Professor Stephen Hawking exemplifies slow progression of ALS, starting at age twenty-one, for more than twenty years, without persisting respiratory failure. Occasionally early involvement of respiratory muscle function occurs in ALS, when there is otherwise a high level of function and minimal need for assistance with activities of daily living (ADLs)(14–17). (See Patient 1, "Clinical Vignettes" at the end of the chapter.)

Impaired respiratory function in ALS is a result of:

1. Muscular weakness due to motor neuron disease and undernutrition.
   A. Weak inspiratory muscles: principally the diaphragm, plus the sternocleidomastoid, scalene, and internal intercostal muscles.

B. Weak cough due to weakness in abdominal and external intercostal muscles.
C. Weak gag reflex for upper airway protection due to paresis of the pharynx (18,19).
2. Reduction in pulmonary compliance due to monotonous ventilation at low tidal volumes; retention of secretions and aspiration; intercurrent lower respiratory infection; and discoordination of ventilatory efforts (20).

In ALS, unlike the myopathies, clinical respiratory failure often occurs over a short period of time, even a few days (21,22), especially when associated with aspiration or respiratory infection. A more gradual onset over weeks to months is less common. However, careful clinical and physiological monitoring can identify when respiratory weakness is present, track its progression, and forewarn when danger is imminent.

Signs and Symptoms

Dyspnea is frequent, but more often there may be few respiratory symptoms as respiratory muscle weakness develops gradually. Dyspnea with exertion or when lying supine suggests respiratory muscle weakness. Difficulty with talking, eating, and swallowing, indicating bulbar involvement, is often associated with respiratory problems. Cough and phlegm may reflect swallowing or feeding problems with aspiration, or pulmonary infection. Cough may be weak and clearing secretions difficult. Cough may be productive of clear mucous or food; purulent secretions suggest infection. Fatigue, hypersomnolence, mood disorders, and morning headaches may occur, often related to decreased ventilatory reserve, hypoxemia, and nighttime hypercapnia. There may be a need to sleep elevated or sitting up because of diaphragm weakness. Tachycardia or palpitation may occur with hypoxemia. Fever, tachypnea, tachycardia, and arrhythmias are warning signs of infection or respiratory failure (Table 11-1).

The patient should be examined both upright and lying flat while observing the respiratory rate, as well as chest and abdominal movement with breathing.

Table 11-1. Warning Signs and Symptoms

- Exertional dyspnea or orthopnea.
- Poor cough and aspiration.
- Basilar rhonchi and crackles.
- Tachypnea and tachycardia.
- Fever and purulent phlegm.
- Abdominal paradox or respiratory alternans.

Abnormalities may be most evident when lying flat because a weak diaphragm, the major muscle of respiration, is at disadvantage in this position. As respiratory muscle function becomes weaker, the effectiveness of both ventilation and cough is reduced. Physical examination by an experienced physician may detect abnormal signs before carbon dioxide (CO_2) retention and respiratory failure occur (23, 24). Increased respiratory rate and dyssynchronous movements of rib cage and abdomen, "respiratory alternans," are a sign of respiratory muscle fatigue, and may indicate impending respiratory failure. "Abdominal paradox" may occur. Normally during inspiration the inspiratory muscles enlarge the rib cage coincident with the descent of the diaphragm, which enlarges abdominal girth. Paradoxical inward inspiratory motion of the abdomen (or rib cage) is a sign of severe weakness of the diaphragm (or of the intercostal muscles). Percussion may identify decreased excursion of the diaphragm. On auscultation there may be coarse breath sounds or inspiratory crackles, particularly at the lung bases due to poor bronchial clearance, patchy atelectasis, aspiration, or infection. These findings may be masked by shallow breathing and inability to take a deep inspiration. Upper extremity weakness may be associated with expiratory muscle weakness and poor cough. The clinician should also note emotional responses, quality of speech, nutritional status, pedal edema, and signs of other problems, such as cor pulmonale.

Pulmonary Function and Other Tests

Pulmonary function testing (PFT) should be done soon after ALS is diagnosed for initial baseline assessment. Other respiratory problems amenable to treatment may be identified, such as asthma or chronic obstructive pulmonary disease (COPD). Initial PFT should at least include: spirometry with vital capacity (VC), air flow measurement, flow volume loop, maximum voluntary ventilation (MVV), and maximal static pressure measurements. In ALS progression of inspiratory muscle weakness, strength, and endurance, results in decreasing VC, MVV, and maximal static inspiratory pressure (P_{Imax}) (10,25–28). Maximal static expiratory pressure (P_{Emax}) measures expiratory muscle force, necessary for effective cough. Maximal static pressures (P_{Emax} and P_{Imax}), sometimes called maximal inspiratory and expiratory force (MIF and MEF), are more sensitive than reduction in VC, MVV, or arterial blood gas (ABG) abnormality; they measure muscle force, but not endurance. Many patients with considerable respiratory muscle weakness have a normal VC but a decreased P_{Emax} and P_{Imax}. ABG abnormality may not occur until maximal static pressures have decreased to less than 30 percent predicted (24). Respiratory muscle weakness is aggravated by aspiration, atelectasis, pneumonia, and undernutrition. Breathing at low tidal volumes, with a poor ability to sigh, may further compromise lung function, with resulting microatelectasis and decreased compliance. VC and MVV may decrease by as much as 50 percent of predicted without being noticed by the patient or physician (25). PFT values may decline gradually over one to two years or may at any point start falling more quickly over a few months or even days. Careful PFT studies in ALS have shown the variable patterns of gradual and sometimes sudden decline (25, 29). Clinical symptoms and ABG abnormalities may lag and not give much advance warning before respiratory failure and critical illness occurs.

When the VC decreases to one half of normal, careful frequent monitoring and follow-up is needed. People with ALS are at risk of respiratory complications and death when the VC is reduced to one-third of normal or less (20). As the respiratory abnormalities progress, there is a high risk of sudden life-threatening respiratory failure due to a small aspiration, some mucus plugs, a relatively minor respiratory illness, or even without any clear additional event. Patients with bulbar involvement and aspiration may have a decreased PaO_2, without alveolar hypoventilation. A stable elevated $PaCO_2$ while awake is not common in ALS. If $PaCO_2$ becomes elevated, the PaO_2 falls reciprocally. This often progresses quickly with respiratory acidosis to a life-threatening critical event. Additional studies that can be useful include comparison of pulmonary function and ABG measurements both upright and lying flat to allow earlier identification of progressing respiratory muscle weakness, because the work load of the diaphragm is greater when lying flat. Noninvasive sleep studies may show significant abnormality of PaO_2 and $PaCO_2$ before these are evident while awake and forewarn that respiratory failure is developing. Small portable transcutaneous monitoring devices that enable overnight home monitoring, similar to Holter monitoring units, are becoming available; they retain eight to twelve hours of data that can be printed for review.

The most useful PFT parameters to monitor regularly are: VC, MVV, and the maximal static pressures. The ABG values should be obtained when the latter values are low or if there is clinical concern. Simple inexpensive devices that can be used for home VC monitoring are available. When VC or the maximal static pressures are approaching 40 percent to 30 percent of normal, there is a high risk of sudden life-threatening respiratory failure (Table 11-2).

Chest radiographs are important for initial evaluation to identify other medical problems and for clinical assessment when there is suspicion of infection or aspiration. Regular office visits allow continued comprehensive medical evalua-

Table 11-2. Physiologic Indicators of
Impending Respiratory Failure

- VC and MVV ≤ 30% of predicted.
- $P_{Emax} \leq +30$ cm H_2O.
- $P_{Imax} \leq -30$ cm H_2O.
- Hypoxemia, mild hypercapnea, and acidosis.

tion as well as the opportunity for doctor, patient, and family members to become comfortable discussing care and planning.

Decision-Making Issues

Medical management of ALS varies. At this time, the majority of patients and their doctors do not support prolonging life after the onset of respiratory failure (30,31). This may in part reflect the generally pessimistic nontreatment approach that has characterized some ALS care in the past. Many doctors feel that prolonging life with a ventilator simply prolongs an unacceptable condition of living, results in increased suffering for the patient, and places an unnecessary burden on the family and other caregivers and on their resources. Frequently there is minimal physician involvement in ongoing care, resulting in a feeling of abandonment and hopelessness by patient and family. Also, some physicians have been reluctant to convey the truth about the diagnosis to the patient because of the poor prognosis (32,33). This may deprive people of the opportunity to become informed and properly plan their care. Some ALS patients decide to oppose even temporary respiratory support because of denial, or because they are severely incapacitated by ALS or other disabilities. For others, there is a reluctance to be a care burden to their family; or they may wish to avoid advanced ALS; or they identify the lack of available resources to assist with long-term care. Therefore, many ALS patients, with the assistance of their families, avoid hospitalization when respiratory failure occurs and refuse cardiopulmonary resuscitation and intubation. They choose to die at this point. Many may have little medical assistance or medication to ensure comfort during this difficult terminal experience. Patient autonomy is stressed together with the right to limit or refuse various "invasive" therapeutic interventions such as respiratory or nutritional support (34,35).

Considerable experience now favors a more positive engaged approach to medical management for people with ALS and emphasizes effective symptomatic and supportive care (9,36–39). In addition to physicians experienced with pulmonary rehabilitation and long-term ventilator assistance, voluntary charitable organizations (e.g., the ALS Association in the United States and the Motor Neurone Disease Association in England) and many people with ALS have contributed to a positive approach to living with the disease (37,40–45). Many now consider that death due to respiratory failure in ALS may be "premature" and represent therapeutic failure. The physician should advise the patient after careful assessment, should be able to distinguish what should be done from what can be done, and should be sensitive to patient and family preferences.

The decision whether to use a ventilator is often difficult and is highly individual. Long-term ventilator assistance is elected in advance by only a small minority

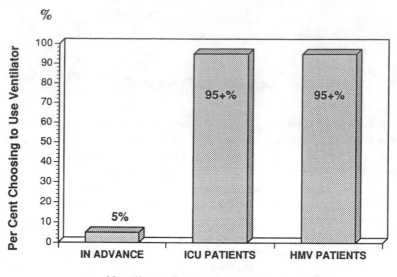

Ventilator Decision-making in ALS

Figure 11-3. Ventilator decision-making in ALS: electing, withholding or withdrawing. Percent choosing to use mechanical ventilation: A. electively in advance; B. when stable in the ICU after emergency intubation; C. after being on HMV. HMV: home mechanical ventilation. ICU: intensive care unit. Data from the Kaiser Permanente Medical Care Program in California, and Moss *et al.* (30).

of people with ALS (Figure 11-3) (30). However, patient autonomy and decision making may be a sham unless people who need help are provided considerable support in the form of knowledge about care options and support in accessing those options and managing their long-term care. People with ALS who are most likely to electively choose HMV in advance (Table 11-3) are those:

Table 11-3. Characteristics That Favor Home Mechanical Ventilation

- Patient is highly motivated and engaged in living.
- ALS is progressing slowly.
- Patient is able to communicate and do some ADLs.
- Patient and family understand the options.
- Family is able to and wants to participate in HMV.
- Resources for equipment and caregivers are available.
- Experienced multidisciplinary team supports HMV.

1. With gradually progressing disease that has allowed incremental accommodation;
2. With onset of respiratory failure when they still have some independent function and good ability to communicate;
3. Who still enjoy and are actively engaged in life; and
4. Who have good resource support available (see Patient 2, p. 158).

Essential resources needed for HMV include experienced professionals, assistance from family or friends, and a home care program that can provide care coordination plus both the needed equipment and additional caregiver assistance. Informed patient and family participation in decision making is essential (31, 46–52). Peer relationships and counseling are advocated. We encourage interested patients and their families to meet other patients who have experience with different options including HMV. In the future there may be increasing demand for resources to support long-term home care including HMV, when desired by the patient and family.

Most people with ALS retain normal cognitive capacity for planning and for participation in decision making. They should clarify their preferences for medical care with their family in consultation with their physician. The use of advance directives to record this should include designating a "proxy" decision maker. We encourage use of the Durable Power of Attorney for Health Care or other legally recognized form. Many people are reluctant to complete these forms. Physician notes in the medical record, or any written record by the patient or family, can be very useful documentation of advance directives. People should be told that they can change their mind (and directives) at any time. Although most people's wishes concerning ventilator care remain stable, they should be periodically reevaluated regarding their wishes (31). A competent adult (see Patient 3, p. 158) can stop any treatment, including mechanical ventilation, if it becomes burdensome and is consistently not desired (in the absence of an acute reactive depression) (35,53–55). I strongly encourage people with ALS, who decide to use HMV, to identify limits beyond which point mechanical ventilation and other treatment should not be continued (e.g., permanent coma or the complete inability to communicate in any way). Frank discussion is needed, as well as advice by the physician.

Because of the great burden of HMV and long-term home care on family caregivers, family members should participate in decision making as well as the patient (30,51,52,56–59). They also need special psychosocial support (60, 61). Family caregivers should carefully evaluate the impact that HMV will have on their lives and review this with other HMV families before they decide to take on this commitment (47,48,50,62). HMV can go on for many years (Patient 1); it is not a short-term decision. They need permission to make an independent choice. Even when this is done carefully, feelings of entrapment and resentment by family members may become major issues. In our experience and other studies, even though they identify the burden, stress, and unmet needs, most families say that the prolongation of life with HMV is worthwhile and state that they would make the same decision again (30).

General Aspects of Respiratory Care

Clinical evaluation of the ALS patient should identify any other medical condition that might contribute to respiratory problems. For example, asthma, COPD, and congestive heart failure are common and are amenable to specific therapy. Risk factors, such as cigarette smoking, secondhand smoke, dusts and fumes, and exposure to people with acute viral respiratory illness, should be identified and avoided. Pneumovax immunization and yearly influenza immunizations are advised. Careful attention to swallowing and feeding is important so as to initiate aggressive management when needed to avoid aspiration and weight loss. Bronchitis with purulent sputum or any evidence of lower respiratory tract infection should be evaluated, including chest radiographs, and treated to improve bronchial clearance of secretions, plus prompt antibiotic therapy. Patients with chronic cough should have medication and instructions available at home so that antibiotic treatment can be started when indicated without delay. In a few cases, there may be value in teaching postural drainage and percussion (or use of a mechanical percussor device) to help clear secretions.

Using an incentive spirometer at home may help prevent patchy atelectasis, as well as provide daily monitoring. Simple VC measuring devices are available for more reliable home monitoring. Maximal static pressures could be monitored at home, but these instruments are more expensive and not as frequently available.

Sometimes excessive saliva (sialorrhea) can be a problem and may respond to medications such as amitriptyline HCl (Elavil®), nortriptyline HCl (Pamelor®), trihexyphenidyl HCl (Artane®), or clonidine HCl (Catapres®). Codeine and antihistamine cough preparations should be avoided if they aggravate bronchial clearance of secretions. Simple glycerol guaiacolate cough preparations are safe to use. Beta-adrenergic bronchodilator medication can be tried if needed to help clear secretions; these are available in metered dose inhalers, tablets, or liquid preparations. Sedative, antianxiety, and sleep medications should be used only after considering their potential for decreasing ventilatory performance. Oxygen may be used at home to treat hypoxemia. The indication for home oxygen is a persisting $PaO_2 \leq 55$ mmHg, or $SaO_2 \leq 88\%$ by either ABG or oximetry (63). The home oxygen flow rate via nasal prongs is adjusted to achieve an oxygen saturation of 92–95 percent.

If a patient decides in advance to avoid intubation or ventilator support after appropriate counseling (see Patient 4), then the family should plan what to do in an emergency and what medication to give to relieve respiratory distress. The physician must continue to stay involved to provide support and symptomatic care (9,37,42,43,64). Hospice care, available in many communities, can be very helpful. Contingency planning helps to avoid a panic request for emergency medical services (EMS) that are not desired by the patient. Some communities now have a form that can be completed in advance, and will be honored by EMS and emergency room staff, to limit emergency care to comfort measures. Without planning and good communication, some family members may be reluctant to limit care when a crisis occurs. Morphine sulfate in liquid form or as a sublingual tablet, used every two to four hours at a sufficient dose to relieve distress, is an excellent medication for relieving respiratory distress when ventilator assistance is not desired. Sedative, antianxiety, and sleep medications should also be used without hesitation when prolonging life is not desired (55).

Short-Term Mechanical Ventilation

Acute respiratory failure may occur associated with pneumonia or other causes before a person is permanently unable to sustain breathing. Medical care should try to reverse the acute underlying causes and provide rehabilitation to restore the highest level of independent function (62,65,66). Temporary ventilator support can be given using noninvasive ventilation or by endotracheal intubation. The method chosen should reflect the experience of the medical center to achieve the safest and most effective care. If the patient is conscious and able to cooperate and cough effectively, then a useful noninvasive approach may be mouth intermittent positive pressure ventilation, nasal intermittent positive pressure ventilation (NIPPV), exsufflation (''pneumobelt''), tank negative pressure ventilator, or chest cuirass. The most common emergency method is ventilation by endotracheal intubation. This is particularly important when the mental status is poor, aspiration is a problem, and cough is not effective. Some people with ALS can recover from acute respiratory failure and regain fully independent breathing for a considerable period of time; this may happen repeatedly before it is necessary to consider long-term mechanical ventilation. Alternatively, there may be a period of time when mechanical ventilation is needed for only part of the twenty-four hours, such as during sleep, allowing considerable ''free time'' off the ventilator during the day. The hospital staff need to understand the difficulty the patient may have feeling secure off the ventilator; considerable patience and continual encouragement are needed when physiologic parameters (e.g., VC, ABGs, P_{Emax} and P_{Imax}) suggest that weaning to unassisted ventilation should be possible (66). Transition to unassisted ventilation (''weaning'') is more likely to be successful if ventilator support is set to a tidal volume of 350 to 500 ml, rather than the high tidal volume techniques often used in the intensive care unit (ICU).

Tracheostomy

Elective tracheostomy should be considered when there are considerable problems with aspiration of upper airways secretions or feedings. If breathing and cough are still strong, some aspiration can be managed without tracheostomy. Early percutaneous endoscopic gastrostomy should be considered if swallowing and feeding problems with aspiration do not respond to noninvasive management or if weight loss is occurring. The tracheostomy provides an avenue for suctioning when cough is ineffective, but it creates additional secretions itself and requires extra care. Tracheostomy has been the most common method in the United States for administering long-term mechanical ventilation. However, if bulbar problems with swallowing and aspiration are minimal, noninvasive alternative methods of mechanical ventilation should be considered first (2,67,68) (see Patient 5).

Tracheostomy is often thought of as the first step to a commitment to permanent long-term ventilator support. Thus it requires considerable discussion and careful informed consent, realizing that this may evoke concerns about many other issues. Although tracheostomy can be life-saving, it requires some adjustment and skill to allow verbal communication and swallowing to be reestablished (if they were functional prior to tracheostomy). A tracheostomy with an inflated cuff prevents verbal communication. A deflated cuff or cuffless tracheostomy can often be used, even with a ventilator (69), despite bulbar problems, to allow speech and decrease the risk of tracheal mucosal injury. The use of a speaking valve, such as the Passy-Muir™ valve (Irvine, California), is often helpful with a fully deflated cuff or a cuffless tracheostomy tube. Assistance from a speech-language pathologist experienced with ALS may be of assistance to reestablish effective verbal communication or augmentative communication. Specially designed tracheostomy tubes are available to enable talking or for better comfort (70). During the first year the stoma usually requires regular ENT physician follow-up evaluations, to make needed changes and to treat granulations or other problems. Besides important cosmetic concerns, tracheostomy has many potential problems, so it should not be used unless necessary. The potential problems include an avenue for infection, drying of secretions, tracheal mucosal injury, tracheoesophageal fistula, pneumothorax, subcutaneous or mediastinal emphysema, hemorrhage, tracheal stenosis or tracheomalacia, and accidental decannulation or upper airway obstruction (71). With careful training, the patient and caregivers become competent in tracheostomy/stoma care and proper ''clean'' suctioning techniques for home care so as to minimize (but not eliminate) complications. After about two to three months, the stoma matures sufficiently to allow family members to learn how to do regular or emergency changes of the tracheostomy tube. Some people are hesitant to learn this, but with continued teaching and encouragement competency can usually be accomplished over several months; this improves the safety and independence of home care. If there are purulent secretions, the tracheostomy tube will need to be changed every two to three weeks. When the stoma is stable and there are minimal clear secretions, then tracheostomy tube changes may be needed only every six to eight weeks, or even less often.

Long-Term Mechanical Ventilation

Drinker and Shaw demonstrated in 1929 that a mechanical ventilator, the iron lung, could prolong life in respiratory failure due to neuromuscular disease (72). Home care for ventilator-dependent people with poliomyelitis resulted in increasing experience since the 1950s and has expanded greatly in the last twenty years (56). Published experience is most enthusiastic about results for those with stable neuromuscular disease and kyphoscoliosis (73–76). Although there has been considerable experience with HMV for ALS, many physicians are ambivalent due to the prognosis and progressive nature of ALS, the high level of dependence that increases home care requirements, and quality of life (QL) concerns.

The goals of long-term ventilator assistance include (75,77) relieving respiratory symptoms and distress; ensuring satisfactory ventilation; prolonging life; reducing morbidity; allowing the respiratory muscles to rest in order to enable some time off the ventilator; good quality and safety of ventilator care; and enhancing the QL, with the greatest independence in the least restrictive environment. These goals can be achieved with ALS. There is little data regarding respiratory muscle rest in ALS (78–80).

Usually respirator support for ALS has been nonelective, instituted as an emergency measure, often without clear advance decision making about the desirability and feasibility of long-term mechanical ventilation (11,12,30,37). People with ALS and their families often avoid making a decision or are not ready to do so. They may have received little experienced help from physicians. Often respiratory failure and sepsis develop suddenly, with survival due to hospital intensive care. Most people with ALS who use long-term mechanical ventilation are ICU survivors of acute respiratory failure, unable to be weaned. By temperament they are not "quitters" and usually decide to continue ventilator support rather than withdraw the ventilator. Alternatives for people who cannot be weaned successfully (e g , institutional care) usually favor HMV, although for some HMV should neither be considered nor offered (74). A few ALS patients decide to withdraw ventilator support (31), particularly people who have all along strongly desired to avoid using a ventilator and those without the needed resources for HMV (Patient 3).

In contrast, only about 5 percent of people with ALS decide in advance that they would want to use a ventilator when respiratory failure occurs (30). Denial may play a part, as may a reluctance to lose independence and become "ventilator dependent" and the desire to avoid becoming a burden to others. Possibly most people with ALS who use mechanical ventilation would not, had they had the opportunity to properly review their options and make their choice before the onset of respiratory failure. Information and assistance from other people with ALS who use HMV (peer counseling) can be helpful. Those who choose electively to use ventilator assistance are almost always able to arrange continuing care at home (42), particularly if resources support HMV. Otherwise many can become "hospital trapped" for lack of resources.

For most people with ALS, sixteen to twenty-four hours per day of ventilator support are needed initially, or frequently within the first year. A minority at first need only eight to ten hours or fewer daily. Additionally, people with ALS generally become quadriplegic and require assistance with all ADLs (bathing, eating, dressing, toileting, grooming) and instrumental ADLs (cooking, cleaning, laundry, shopping), with minimal or no independence of daily function. At some point many need gastrostomy feeding, a communication augmentation device, plus considerable special equipment at home and for transportation. This typically results in high home care costs and greater burden for the caregivers. As respiratory muscle weakness progresses, most ALS patients tolerate little time off the ventilator after the first year at home. A few retain the ability to have some hours of "free time" off the ventilator each day for several years. In France, among twenty-four ALS patients using HMV, there was only a 24 percent one-year survival (81). However, data from the Kaiser Permanente HMV program in California, which provides up to sixteen hours per day of paid caregiver assistance to the families, found 84 percent one-year survival based on thirty-one patients and 58 percent three-year survival based on nineteen patients (Figure 11-1). The addition of caregiver assistance to the family may explain the longer survival. Long-term survival for disabled people with ALS on HMV is very resource-dependent. With considerable resources and good care at home, people with ALS can survive many years after they require ventilator assistance. ALS does not itself cause death directly. Complications such as respiratory failure, pneumonia, and malnutrition can usually be treated successfully.

The patient and family must decide how long to continue full care. How long is worthwhile? For example, should full care and ventilator support continue if communication becomes extremely limited or impossible or if permanent coma occurs? These questions are not easy to address initially and are often avoided. Most of our ALS patients on HMV do not set any limits unless strongly advised by their physician. The physician needs to suggest a reasonable plan. Then with this clear advice and counseling and time to reflect, the patient should make a decision. Decision making becomes more and more difficult when communication barriers increase, particularly if a totally locked-in state occurs (Patient 6, p. 159). With long-term ventilator support, muscle weakness can progress in some cases to total paralysis (82–85), sparing only sensory and cognitive function.

For many, life continues to be sufficiently satisfying on HMV. Often health care professionals evaluate the QL of someone who is severely disabled as unacceptable. However, such patients report that they are satisfied with their QL (30, 31,43,86), that it is better at home than long-term hospital care, and that the quality of care (QC) is as good or better than hospital care (11, 87). They have adjusted to HMV and compare it to the consequences of withdrawing ventilator support. Family members' QL may be more burdened by HMV than that of the patient (47–49, 59).

Most people with ALS on HMV report that they are satisfied and would want to make the same decision again (11,30,43). They indicate that it would be worthwhile even if it provided only a relatively short period of prolonged life at home, perhaps even as little as a month. When decision making is carefully assisted by an experienced health care team and resources are available to support home care, almost all ALS patients who cannot be weaned after intensive care are able to continue their care at home (11,42). This can be accomplished by experienced professionals at community hospitals with a program of regional support (11,76,88,89), as well as by special university and rehabilitation medical centers (74,90–92). Medical centers just beginning their experience with HMV might benefit from working closely with established HMV programs to review experience and share policies and procedures. Although HMV can be very expensive, there is generally a cost advantage to HMV compared to acute hospital care (11,74,76,93,94). More restrictive hospital bed utilization policies and economic pressures encourage discharge to home care. In some cases, due to the high cost of nursing care in the home (compared to the use of aides or personal attendants), the cost of care at home may not be cost-effective (95). This is particularly likely if more than fourteen to sixteen hours per day of nurse caregivers are used.

Extensive experience and consensus is now available to guide high quality hospital assessment and preparation for HMV and coordinated home care (9,12,37,43,50,56,59,65,74–77,79,81,89,96–110). In addition to repeated discussion and training, we use an informed consent form for HMV, as well as other forms to clarify the roles, expectations, and responsibilities for each party in the home care process and to document caregiver training and demonstrated competency.

Indications for Home Mechanical Ventilation for Patients with ALS

Basic Issues

As many of the characteristics that favor HMV as possible should be present (Table 11-3). Additionally, the patient and family need good interpersonal skills and adaptability. Careful psychosocial evaluation of the patient and family should confirm that there is nothing to contraindicate HMV and should identify any support needed (58,59,61,111). Decision making, planning, and preparation for home care must be carefully and successfully completed (74,75,77,98). Reasonable clinical and physiological stability is needed for home care. The limits of care desired as ALS progresses should be defined in advance.

Physiological Indications

1. Progressive hypercapnia and respiratory acidosis that cannot be controlled without ventilator assistance and do not improve with short-term ventilator management.

2. Marginal ventilatory reserve: VC decreased to 30 percent of predicted or less; MVV decreased to 30 percent of predicted or less; P_{Imax} of -30 cm. H_2O or less. These values are guidelines. Clinical judgment is needed for each patient. It is best to provide support earlier rather than too late.

Clinical Indications

1. Respiratory failure necessitating acute ventilator support: acute hypercapnic ventilatory failure. Most ALS patients require continuous use of ventilator assistance after their initial hospitalization with respiratory failure. However, some have large reversible components and slow progression that may allow weaning and independent autonomous ventilation, or ventilator assistance only 6–12 hours per day.

2. Inability to be weaned off ventilator support, despite optimal medical, respiratory, and rehabilitation management (66,105), including special attention to nutrition (poorly nourished patients have significant impairment of muscle strength and endurance, and without any intrinsic neuromuscular disease can have 60 percent decrease in P_{Imax} and P_{Emax} (112)) and management of infection and aspiration.

3. Repeated episodes of respiratory failure; increasing symptoms of shortness of breath with minimal exertion; and physiologic indicators (Table 11-2)

4. Impending respiratory collapse: symptoms of shortness of breath and borderline physiological status that cannot be improved. When HMV is desired, it is important to recognize progressive respiratory muscle weakness and to intervene before life-threatening complications arise. Clinical judgment is required to decide when to intervene with mechanical ventilation because of imminent respiratory crisis.

5. Elective HMV has been advocated as a way to prepare a patient and family, as well as to provide hands-on experience for decision making (29,78,79,80). Noninvasive mechanical ventilation may be used at home as a trial (Patient 5).

Types of Home Mechanical Ventilation

Noninvasive ventilation (NIV) should be considered when there is little or no bulbar involvement. It is easier to accomplish when there is effective cough and the ability to breathe independently for at least an hour or more at a time; when the patient can do some ADLs with minimal assistance; and when the ALS and respiratory muscle weakness are only slowly progressive (2,24,29,67,106,108, 113–115). There are many alternative methods for NIV (116,117), including nasal or mouth positive pressure, cuirass, pneumobelt, and rocking bed. The best choice will depend on the clinical findings and will change as ALS progresses. NIV has also been advocated as a reasonable option when there is a desire to avoid entrapment or a commitment to long-term HMV as ALS progresses or when resources are limited. NIV may be more acceptable than tracheostomy to many patients. It may be safer, easier, and more cost-effective (67,69,93,96). NIV more easily allows nonprofessional assistance with care (93). However, in the United States clinical experience at this time indicates that only a minority of ALS patients who require a mechanical ventilator are good candidates for NIV. This may be due to bulbar involvement, or that the ability to be off ventilator support is less than an hour at a time. More people may be able to use NIV when mechanical ventilation is started electively on a trial basis earlier in the progression of ALS.

Tracheostomy positive pressure ventilation (TPPV) should be used when there are significant problems related to bulbar involvement (bronchial clearance of secretions, dysphagia, aspiration), ineffective cough, or when there have been unsatisfactory results with NIV. TPPV is usually preferable when the patient cannot sustain independent ventilation for at least an hour or more at a time. This should be reserved for those people who are appropriate candidates for long-term mechanical ventilation (see previously) and where the necessary resources for HMV are available.

Excellent small portable ventilators, portable oxygen, and suctioning equipment are available for use at home and in the community (70,116,117). Internal and external battery support allows travel worldwide. When properly maintained, the equipment is quite reliable. A backup ventilator system is advised for people who cannot tolerate at least an hour off the ventilator. The pulmonary physician and respiratory care practitioner experienced in HMV, with participation from the patient, should advise which ventilator would be best and the settings. Whenever possible, a cuffless or deflated cuff tracheostomy tube should be used (69). Usually the delivered tidal volume needs to be greater than the exhaled volume, due to variable air leak around the tracheostomy tube to allow speech and prevent tracheal damage. Volume controlled mechanical ventilation is commonly used; this can be modified to pressure controlled ventilation to improve reliability and compensate for the varying air leak (118). The assist/control mode (or controlled rate mode) is often used. The rate should be adjusted to equal the patient's usual respiratory rate so that there is no effort required to cycle the ventilator. A humidification device is used, or a moisture exchanger that avoids liquid in the ventilator tubing may be preferable for part of the day. Many people on HMV have strong preferences about their ventilator settings; whenever possible, these should be respected. Often people with neuromuscular disease prefer to be hyperventilated to a low $PaCO_2$ and feel uncomfortable if settings are changed to achieve a normal $PaCO_2$. People with ALS frequently do not need supplemental oxygen except when infection, aspiration, or an additional pulmonary disease is present. When the patient is clinically stable, only occasional measurements of ABG and oximetry are needed. Overnight oximetry monitoring may be useful at times (118); this can now be done using a portable oximeter in the home, with eight-hour memory capacity. Regular technical equipment checks and preventive maintenance are essential. Empirical use of antibiotics for clinical signs of infection usually works well. Occasionally medical center evaluation, and sometimes hospitalization, is required if empirical therapy is not successful.

Barriers to Home Care Using Mechanical Ventilation

Numerous obstacles may thwart HMV (77,103). The most common include psychological problems involving the patient or family; economic and resource limitations; lack of sufficient caregiver support; lack of support needed for family caregivers to counterbalance their burden and stress; lack of an experienced and coordinated hospital and home care program; and lack of availability of communication augmentation devices. Other factors that are often absent, but are needed for success, include opportunities to network with others (peers); social activities out of the home; a positive attitude by health care professionals and agency administrative staff; and special transportation needs.

The health and social services provided by many communities are often inadequate to support home care for ventilator-assisted people. Public and private health care programs frequently do not include comprehensive long-term home care benefits nor benefits to cover both the medical and the overlapping social assistance needed. Charitable organizations have limited resources.

HMV home care can be costly (30,74,76,79,93,95,119–123) (Figure 11-4). The following cost data reflect our 1991 HMV experience in California.

1. Necessary equipment may cost $20–35 per day when rented, but less if purchased. The rental cost should include emergency respiratory care services, teaching for caregivers, and equipment maintenance.

2. Paid caregivers, to supplement family members, are the most expensive part of home care for people with ALS, usually for eight to sixteen hours per day in the home while family members work or sleep. Personal attendant care costs about $8 to $10 per hour. Licensed vocational (practical) nurse (LVN) care costs about $25 per hour when obtained through an agency. There is no data to indicate that quality of care is better when nurses are used. The continuity of care, the patient's locus of control, and cost-effectiveness may be better with personal attendant caregivers (93,103,104). Medical care programs are commonly required to use licensed nurses, who are often in short supply; this results in more expensive home care. Personal attendants or aides are commonly employed by individuals, families, schools, or with social service agency funds.

3. Supplies, medications, and special feedings add to the daily costs and may not be covered by home care programs.

4. Professional care coordination and home visits by professional staff may add 5 to 10 percent or greater additional cost. Few people have the personal means to pay for this ''catastrophic'' level of home care themselves. The cost of health care has been increasing dramatically during the last twenty years. There

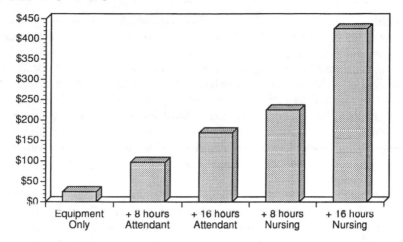

Selected Costs of Home Mechanical Ventilation per Day

Figure 11-4. Cost of home mechanical ventilation, depending on resources used: A. equipment only; B. equipment plus 8 hours attendant care; C. equipment plus 16 hours attendant care; D. equipment plus 8 hours nursing care; E. equipment plus 16 hours of nursing care. Costs include home health agency care coordination and some supplies. Data from the Kaiser Permanente Medical Care Program in California: 1985 to 1991.

may be very limited monies available for very expensive care that benefits only a small number of technology-dependent people (124). The physician in clinical practice should be an advocate for resources for appropriate care in the best interest of the patient and family. The need for wise public policy regarding resource allocation and prioritization in health care is increasing.

Advances in the delivery and organization of intensive home care may result in high quality home care at a lower cost in the future. The alternative of remaining in a hospital or subacute institutional setting is unattractive to most ventilator-assisted people. HMV can be cost-effective compared to acute hospital costs and allow beds to be available for people who need acute hospital care. Residential or congregate living facilities for people with ALS using ventilator support might be an alternative to HMV, but are not usually available.

Clinical Vignettes

The brief vignettes that follow illustrate some of the clinical issues discussed. They are from medical records of our clinical experience working with people with ALS.

Patient 1. J.M. had gradual onset in 1974 of ALS at age forty-seven. Respiratory problems occurred early. Tracheostomy was elected after several episodes of acute respiratory failure, ICU care, and complete weaning. HMV started in 1975, initially eight hours per day. Two years later he was completely quadriplegic and required the ventilator twenty-four hours per day. During seventeen years of HMV, he has required fewer than four days of hospital care per year. He continues to enjoy his life. He has no bulbar involvement and is able to eat and speak. The burdens of HMV are at times overwhelming for his wife. Equipment, some supplies, sixteen hours per day of LVN care, and home health visits with care coordination provided by the home care program cost $438 per day. Medicare covers some additional costs.

Patient 2. I.T. developed ALS in 1985 at age fifty with gradual limb muscle weakness. He and his wife decided in advance to use HMV when respiratory failure occurred. In November 1990, he was still able to ambulate and had only minimal bulbar involvement. Speech was clear. Respiratory muscle weakness became severe with poor cough. He was electively admitted to the hospital for tracheostomy and preparation for HMV. He was able to tolerate only short periods of time off the ventilator. After discharge home, he resumed his usual work schedule. Almost complete quadriplegia and gradual loss of the ability to speak developed over the following two years. He produces and directs educational films and videotapes. With some remaining strength in one foot, he is able to control his video console and editing equipment using specially adapted ball track technology. In 1992 a computer-assisted communication system was selected that uses an infrared switch activated with eye blinks, and a voice synthesizer. With sixteen hours per day LVN assistance, he works ten hours most days and moves about the community in his wheelchair and specially adapted van. Facial muscle function continues normally, as well as the ability to eat and swallow if done carefully. He is medically stable on HMV and enthusiastic. His wife continues her professional career while supporting him in every way possible. They recently completed an educational video for people facing the ventilator decision: ''It's Your Choice'' (Valona Productions, 14621 Titus Street, Suite 108, Van Nuys, CA 91402).

Patient 3. J.D. had onset of ALS in 1990 at age forty-seven. She was divorced and lived alone. Progressive muscle weakness was followed by unexpected pneumonia, emergency care with intubation, mechanical ventilation, and tracheostomy. Unable to be weaned, she tolerated only short periods off the ventilator. HMV was arranged with sixteen hours of LVN nursing care following careful planning and caregiver preparation. Her ex-husband returned to assist her, but quickly found that her care required more than he had anticipated. Unable to cope, he left after one week. She was rehospitalized, unable to find any friend or family member to help with home care. After extensive review of the remaining options with the hospital staff and her minister, she decided that life in a hospital or nursing home would not be acceptable. She requested to withdraw ventilator care. This persistent decision was reviewed by psychiatry, social services, and the hospital Bioethics Committee. After four months of ventilator support, it was withdrawn. Symptom-relieving medication was given and she died.

Patient 4. C.C. had onset of ALS in 1991 at age fifty-four, with rapid progression of limb weakness and bulbar involvement. After nine months, gastrostomy was needed and reluctantly accepted. Speech became difficult to understand, and respiratory muscle weakness became severe. Her children encouraged her to consider HMV; resources were available. She decided on hospice care instead. Symptomatic medication was used to relieve distress as respiratory failure progressed. She died at home with her family ten months after the initial symptoms appeared.

Patient 5. A.H. had gradual onset of ALS in 1991 at age forty-six. Respiratory muscle weakness began a year later, together with some lower extremity weakness. Not sure about long-term HMV, he used a nasal mask for NIPPV for nine months at home, initially eight hours at night, but this gradually increased to almost twenty-four hours daily. Unable to work, he lost health care coverage and qualified for public assistance. He and his family decided to continue HMV. Cough became ineffective. He was admitted to the county hospital for elective tracheostomy and was later discharged home on the Medi-Cal (Medicaid) In-Home Medical Care Services (IHMCS) waiver program, which provides equipment and up to sixteen hours of LVN nursing care per day in lieu of continued acute hospital care. He and his family continue to be satisfied with HMV.

Patient 6. T.L. developed ALS in 1985 at age forty-five with bulbar involvement and then increasing limb weakness. Denial was a major problem. Speech and swallowing problems became severe. After eighteen months he was admitted to the hospital with sepsis, bibasilar pneumonia, and respiratory failure. He responded to ICU care, which included gastrostomy and tracheostomy, but was unable to be weaned. He and his wife decided on HMV, with successful preparation and discharge to home care in 1987. Bulbar involvement progressed and speech was not possible. Despite complete quadriplegia, he was able to take out-of-town trips with his wife and LVN and goes out of the home several times a week. He used augmentative communication methods, including a computer-assisted system, up to 1990. He repeatedly indicated that he wants full medical care without limitations. Muscle weakness progressed so that no voluntary control remains, including all facial and oculomotor muscles. His cognitive and sensory functions are normal, but he is in a totally locked-in state. There are occasional periods of crying, related to severe discomfort without any ability to immediately identify the cause. Otherwise he is continued medically stable on HMV, with a very devoted wife and children.

Conclusion

HMV can be a successful option for people with ALS. It should be reserved for selected, highly motivated patients and families who can arrange the considerable resources, preparation, and caregiver support needed. Physician counseling and advance planning should be started soon after ALS is diagnosed. Every person with ALS needs continuing physician support and respiratory care no matter which option is selected.

References

1. Appel V, Stewart SS, Smith G, Appel SH. A rating scale for amyotrophic lateral sclerosis: description and preliminary experience. *Ann Neurol* 1987, 22: 328–333.
2. Alba A, Pilkington LA, Kaplan E, Baum J, Schultheiss M, Rugieri A, Lee MHM. Long term pulmonary care in amyotrophic lateral sclerosis. *Resp Ther* 1976, 11/12: 49–105.
3. Kurtzke JF. Epidemiology of amyotrophic lateral sclerosis, In: L.P. Rowland, ed. *Human Motor Neuron Diseases*. New York: Raven, 1982.
4. Kristensen O, Melgaard B. Motor neuron disease: prognosis and epidemiology. *Acta Neurol Scand* 1977, 56: 288–308.
5. Mortara P, Chio A, Rosso MG, Leone M, Schiffer D. Motor neuron disease in the provence of Turin, Italy, 1966–1980. *J Neurol Sci* 1984, 66: 165–173.
6. Mulder DW, Howard FM. Patient resistance and prognosis in amyotrophic lateral sclerosis. *Mayo Clin Proc* 1976, 51: 537–541.
7. Granieri E, Carreras M, Tola R, Paolino E, Tralli G, Eleopra R, Serra G. Motor neuron disease in the province of Ferrara, Italy, in 1964–1982. *Neurology* 1988, 38: 1604–8.
8. Iwata M. Clinico-pathological studies of long survival ALS cases maintained by active life-support measures. *Adv Exp Med Biol* 1987, 209: 223–225.
9. Caroscio JT. *Amyotrophic Lateral Sclerosis. A Guide to Patient Care*. New York: Thieme Medical Publishers, 1986.
10. Nakano I, Hirano A. A clinicopathological study of two cases of sporadic amyotrophic lateral sclerosis with long survival. *Neurol Med* (Tokyo) 1981, 15: 45–53.
11. Oppenheimer EA, Baldwin-Myers A, Tanquary P. Ventilator use by patients with amyotrophic lateral sclerosis. In: 3rd International Conference on Pulmonary Rehabilitation and Home Ventilation, 1991, Denver, Colorado, 49.
12. Oppenheimer EA. Amyotrophic lateral sclerosis: home mechanical ventilation. *Eur Respir Rev* 1992, 2:323–329.
13. Roger J, Pache D. A propos des formes lentes de la sclérose latérale amyotrophique. Bilan clinique d'un case de S.L.A. évoluant depuis douze ans. *Rev Neurol* (Paris) 1959, 100: 234–238.
14. Fromm GB, Wisdom PJ, Block AJ. Amyotrophic lateral sclerosis presenting with respiratory failure. *Chest* 1977, 71: 612–614.
15. Hill R, Martin J, Hakim A. Acute respiratory failure in motor neuron disease. *Arch Neurol* 1983, 40: 30–32.
16. Meyrignac C, Poirier J, Degos JD. Amyotrophic lateral sclerosis presenting with respiratory insufficiency as the primary complaint. *Eur Neurol* 1985, 24: 115–120.
17. Sivak ED, Streib EW. Management of hypoventilation in motor neuron disease presenting with respiratory insufficiency. *Ann Neurol* 1980, 7: 188–191.
18. Braun SR. Respiratory system in amyotrophic lateral sclerosis. *Neurol Clinics* 1987, 5: 9–31.

19. Kreitzer SM, Saunders NA, Tyler HR, Ingram Jr. RH. Respiratory muscle function in amyotrophic lateral sclerosis. *Chest* 1978, 73: 266–267.
20. Miller A. Pulmonary function and respiratory failure in neuromuscular disorders with reference to amyotrophic lateral sclerosis, In: J.T. Caroscio, ed. *Amyotrophic Lateral Sclerosis. A Guide to Patient Care.* New York: Thieme Medical Publishers, 1986.
21. Munsat TL, Andres PL, Finison L, Conlon T, Thibodeau L. The natural history of motor neuron loss in amyotrophic lateral sclerosis. *Neurology* 1988, 38: 409–413.
22. Munsat TL. Adult motor neuron diseases. In: L.P. Rowland, ed. *Merritt's Textbook of Neurology.* Philadelphia: Lea & Febiger, 1989.
23. Cohen CA, Zagelbaum G, Gross D, Roussos C, Macklem PT. Clinical manifestations of inspiratory muscle fatigue. *Am J Med* 1982, 73: 308–16.
24. Rosen MJ. Respiratory failure in amyotrophic lateral sclerosis. In: J.T. Caroscio, ed. *Amyotrophic Lateral Sclerosis. A Guide to Patient Care.* New York: Thieme Medical Publishers, 1986.
25. Fallat RJ, Jewitt B, Bass M, et al. Spirometry in amyotrophic lateral sclerosis. *Arch Neurol* 1979, 36: 74–80.
26. Griggs RC, Donohoe KM, Utell MJ, Goldblatt D, Moxley R. Evaluation of pulmonary function in neuromuscular disease. *Arch Neurol* 1981, 38: 9–12.
27. Hyatt RE, Black LF. Maximal static respiratory pressures in generalized neuromuscular disease. *Am Rev Resp Dis* 1971, 103: 641–650.
28. Poloni M, Mento SA, Mascherpa C, Ceroni M. Value of spirometric investigations in amyotrophic lateral sclerosis. *Ital J Neurol Sci* 1983, 4: 39–46.
29. Fallat RJ, Norris FH, Holden D, Kandal K, Roggero PC. Respiratory monitoring and treatment: objective treatments using non-invasive measurements. *Adv Exp Med Biol* 1987, 209: 191–200.
30. Moss AH, Casey P, Stocking CB, Roos RP, Brooks BR, Siegler M. Home ventilation for amyotrophic lateral sclerosis patients: outcomes, costs, and patient, family and physician attitudes. *Neurol* 1993, 43:438–443.
31. Silverstein MD, Stocking CB, Antel JP, Beckwith J, Roos RP, Siegler M. Amyotrophic lateral sclerosis and life-sustaining therapy: patient's desires for information, participation in decision making, and life sustaining therapy. *Mayo Clin Proc* 1991, 66: 906–913.
32. Carey JS. Motor neurone disease: A challenge to medical ethics. *J Roy Soc Med* 1986, 79: 216–220.
33. Carus R. Motor neurone disease: A demeaning illness. *Brit Med J* 1980, 280: 455–456.
34. Malcolm AH. *This Far and No More, A True Story.* New York: Times Books, Random House, Inc., 1987.
35. Herr SS, Bostrom BA, Barton RS. No place to go: refusal of life-sustaining treatment by competent persons with physical disability. *Issues in Law & Medicine* 1992, 8: 3–36.
36. Mulder DW. *The Diagnosis and Treatment of Amyotrophic Lateral Sclerosis.* Boston: Houghton Mifflin, 1980, 367.
37. Preston W, Donohue KM, Eyck LGT, Goldblatt D. Managing Amyotrophic Lateral Sclerosis Manual III: Managing Breathing Problems. Sherman Oaks, CA: The ALS Association, 1986.
38. Rabin R. *Six Parts Love: A Family's Battle with Lou Gehrig's Disease (ALS).* New York: Charles Scribner's Sons, 1985, 224.

39. Tandan R, Bradley WG. Amyotrophic lateral sclerosis: Part 1. Clinical features, pathology, and ethical issues in management. *Ann Neurol* 1985, 18: 271–280.
40. Chenevert BJ. *Taking Hopelessness Out of Helplessness*, 2nd ed. Southfield, MI: MetroStaff Home Health Care, 1989.
41. Hamilton L. *Why Didn't Somebody Tell Me About These Things?* Shawnee Mission, KS: Inter-Collegiate Press, 1984, 139.
42. Norris FH, Smith RA, Denys EH. Motor neurone disease: towards better care. *Brit Med J* 1985, 291: 259–262.
43. Norris FH, Holden D, Kandal K, Stanley E. Home nursing care by families for severely paralyzed ALS patients. *Adv Exp Med Biol* 1987, 209: 231–238.
44. Hawking S (ed.). *Stephen Hawking's A Brief History of Time: A Reader's Companion*. New York: Bantam Books, 1992, 194.
45. White M, Gribbin J. *Stephen Hawking: A Life in Science*. New York: Dutton, 1992, 304.
46. Goldblatt D, Greenlaw J. Starting and stopping the ventilator for patients with amyotrophic lateral sclerosis. *Neurol Clin* 1989, 7: 789–806.
47. Agich GJ. Reassessing autonomy in long-term care. *Hastings Center Report* 1990, 20: 12–17.
48. Collopy B, Dubler N, Zuckerman C. The ethics of home care: autonomy and accommodation. *Hastings Center Report* 1990, 20: 1–16.
49. Callahan D. Families as caregivers: the limits of morality. *Arch Phys Med Rehab* 1988, 69: 323–328.
50. Colbert AP, Schock NC. Respirator use in progressive neuromuscular diseases. *Arch Phys Med Rehab* 1985, 66: 760–762.
51. Gilgoff IS, Prentice WS, Baydur A. Patient and family participation in the management of respiratory failure in Duchenne's muscular dystrophy. *Chest* 1989, 95: 519–524.
52. Nelson JL. Taking familes seriously. *Hastings Center Report* 1992, 22: 6–12.
53. American Thoracic Society Bioethics Task Force. Withholding and withdrawing life-sustaining therapy. *Ann Int Med* 1991, 115: 478–485.
54. Bone RC, Rackow EC, Weg JG, Panel AC. Ethical and moral guidelines for the initiation, continuation, and withdrawal of intensive care. *Chest* 1990, 97: 949–958.
55. Wilson WC, Smedira NG, Fink C, McDowell JA, Luce JM. Ordering and administration of sedatives and analgesics during the withholding and withdrawal of life support from critically ill patients. *JAMA* 1992, 267: 949–953.
56. Fischer DA. Long-term management of the ventilator-dependent patient: levels of disability and resocialization. *Eur Respir J* 1989, 2: 651s–654s.
57. Jecker NS. The role of intimate others in medical decision making. *Gerontology* 1990, 30: 65–71.
58. Sharp JW, Sivak ED. The role of social work in contemporary home care planning. *Cleve Clin Q* 1985, 52: 355–358.
59. Thomas VM, Ellison K, Howell EV, Winters K. Caring for the person receiving ventilatory support at home: care givers' needs and involvement. *Heart & Lung* 1992, 21: 180–6.
60. Clark K. Psychosocial aspects of prolonged ventilator dependency. *Respir Care* 1986, 31: 329–333.
61. Gale J, O'Shanick GJ. Psychiatric aspects of respirator treatment and pulmonary intensive care. *Adv Psychosom Med* 1985, 14: 93–108.

62. Caplan AL, Callahan D, Haas J. Ethics & Policy: issues in rehabilitation medicine. *Hastings Center Report* 1987, 17: 1–20.
63. O'Donohue WJ . Prescribing home oxygen therapy: what the primary care physician needs to know. *Arch Int Med* 1992, 152: 746–748.
64. Smith RA, Norris FH. Symptomatic care of patients with amyotrophic lateral sclerosis. *JAMA* 1975, 234: 715–717.
65. Prentice WS, Wilms D, Harrison LB. Outpatient management of ventilator-dependent patients. In: J.E. Hodgkin, ed. *Pulmonary Rehabilitation: Guidelines to Success.* Boston: Butterworth Publishers, 1984.
66. Tobin MJ. Weaning from mechanical Ventilation. In: D.H. Simmons, ed. *Current Pulmonology.* Chicago: Year Book Medical Publishers, 1990.
67. Bach JR, Alba A, Mosher R, Delaubier A. Intermittent positive pressure ventilation via nasal access in the management of respiratory insufficiency. *Chest* 1987, 92: 168–170.
68. Branthwaite M. Assisted ventilation. 6-Non-invasive and domiciliary ventilation: positive pressure techniques. *Thorax* 1991, 46: 208–211.
69. Bach JR, Alba AS. Tracheostomy ventilation. A study of efficacy with deflated cuffs and cuffless tubes. *Chest* 1990, 97: 679–683.
70. McPherson SP. *Respiratory Home Care Equipment.* Dubuque: Kendall Hunt Publishing, 1988,182.
71. Stauffer JL, Silverstri RC. Update: Complications of endotracheal intubation, tracheostomy, and artificial airways. In: D.J. Pearson, ed. *Respiratory Intensive Care.* Dallas: Daedalus, 1986.
72. Drinker P, Shaw LA. Apparatus for prolonged administration of artificial respiration: I, design for adults and children. *J Clin Invest* 1929, 7: 229–247.
73. Fischer DA, Prentice WS. Feasibility of home care for certain respiratory-dependent restrictive or obstructive lung disease patients. *Chest* 1982, 82: 739–743.
74. Make BJ, Gilmartin ME. Mechanical ventilation in the home. *Crit Care Clin* 1990, 6: 785–796.
75. O'Donohue WJ , Giovannoni RM, Goldberg AI, Keens TG, Make BJ, Plummer AL, Prentice WS. Long term mechanical ventilation. Guidelines for management in the home and at alternate community sites. *Chest* 1986, 90: 1S–37S.
76. Robert D, Gerard M, Leger P, et al. Long-term IPPV at home of patients with end stage chronic respiratory insufficiency. *Chest* 1982, 82: 258–259.
77. Plummer AL, O'Donohue WJ, Petty TL. Consensus conference on problems in home mechanical ventilation. *Am Rev Resp Dis* 1989, 140: 555–560.
78. Stoller JK. Physiologic rationale for resting the ventilatory muscles. *Respir Care* 1991, 36: 290–296.
79. Splaingard ML, Frates RJ, Jefferson LS, Rosen CL, Harrison GM. Home negative pressure ventilation: report of 20 years of experience in patients with neuromuscular disease. *Arch Phys Med Rehab* 1985, 66: 239–42.
80. Goldstein RS, Avendano MA. Long-term mechanical ventilation as elective therapy: clinical status and future prospects. *Resp Care* 1991, 36: 297–304.
81. Salamand J, Robert D, Leger P, Langevin B, Barraud J. Definitive mechanical ventilation via tracheostomy in end stage amyotrophic lateral sclerosis. In: 3rd International Conference on Pulmonary Rehabilitation and Home Ventilation, 1991, Denver, Colorado, 50.

82. Hayashi H, Kato S. Total manifestations of amyotrophic lateral sclerosis. ALS in the totally locked-in state. *J Neurol Sci* 1989, 93: 19–35.
83. Hayashi H, Kato S, Kawada T, Tsubaki T. Amyotrophic lateral sclerosis: oculomotor function in patients in respirators. [Published erratum appears in *Neurology* 1987, 37(10):1606] *Neurology* 1987, 37: 1431–2.
84. Hayashi H, Kato S, Kawada A. Amyotrophic lateral sclerosis patients living beyond respiratory failure. *J Neurol Sci* 1991, 105: 73–8.
85. Mizutani T, Aki M, Shiozawa R, et al. Development of ophthalmoplegia in amyotrophic lateral sclerosis during long-term use of respirators. *J Neurol Sci* 1990, 99: 311–319.
86. Bach J, Gombas G. Quality of life perceptions of ventilator-assisted individuals. *IVUN News* 1990, 4: 1.
87. Smith RA. On behalf of the patient. *Adv in Exp Med and Biol* 1987, 209: 319–322.
88. Goldberg AI. The regional approach to home care for life supported persons. *Chest* 1984, 86: 345–346.
89. Robert D, Gérard M, Leger P, et al. La ventilation méchanique a domicile définitive par trachéostomie de l'insuffisant respiratoire chronique. *Rev Fr Mal Resp* 1983, 11: 923–936.
90. Daras M, Spiro AJ, Swerlow M. Respiratory failure in amyotrophic lateral sclerosis. *N Y State J Med* 1984, 84: 570–572.
91. Sivak ED, Cordasco EM, Gibson WT. Pulmonary mechanical ventilation at home: a reasonable and less expensive alternative. *Resp Care* 1983, 28: 42–49.
92. Sivak ED, Gibson WT, Hanson MR. Long-term management of respiratory failure in amyotrophic lateral sclerosis. *Ann Neurol* 1982, 12: 18–23.
93. Bach JR, Intintola P, Alba AS, Holland IE. The ventilator-assisted individual. Cost analysis of institutionalization vs rehabilitation and in-home management. *Chest* 1992, 101: 26–30.
94. Wagner DR. Economics of prolonged mechanical ventilation. *Am Rev Resp Dis* 1989, 140: S14-S18.
95. Indihar FJ. Cost comparison of care for chronic ventilator patients [letter]. *Chest* 1991, 99: 260.
96. Branthwaite MA. Home mechanical ventilation. *Eur Respir J* 1990, 3: 743–745.
97. Gilmartin M, Make B. Home care of the ventilator-dependent person. *Resp Care* 1983, 28: 1490–1497.
98. Gilmartin ME. Long-term mechanical ventilation: Patient selection and discharge planning. *Respir Care* 1991, 36: 205–216.
99. Goldberg AI. Home care for life-supported persons in England: the responaut program. *Chest* 1984, 86: 910–914.
100. Goldberg AI, Faure EAM. Home care for life supported persons in France: the regional association. *Rehab Lit* 1986, 47: 60–64, 103.
101. Goldberg AI. Home care for life supported persons—Is a national approach the answer? *Chest* 1986, 90: 744–748.
102. Goldberg AI. Home care for life supported persons: the French system of quality control, technology assessment, and cost containment. *Publ Hlth Reprts* 1989, 104: 329–336.
103. Goldberg AI. Mechanical ventilation and respiratory care in the home in the 1990's: some personal observations. *Resp Care* 1990, 35: 247–259.

104. Goldberg AI, Alba AS, Oppenheimer EA, Roberts E. Caring for mechanically venti-
     lated patients at home. *Chest* 1990, 98: 1543.
105. Indihar FJ. A 10-year report of patients in a prolonged respiratory care unit. *Minn
     Med* 1991, 74: 23–7.
106. Leger P, Bedicam JM, Cornette A, Degat OR, Robert D, Polu JM, Jeannin L. Long
     term follow up of severe chronic respiratory insufficiency patients (n = 373) treated
     by home nocturnal non-invasive nasal IPPV. *Amer Rev Resp Dis* 1991, 143: A73.
107. Make BJ, Gilmartin ME. Care of ventilator-assisted individuals in the home and
     alternative community sites. In: G.G. Burton, J.E. Hodgkin, and J.J. Ward, eds.
     Respiratory Care: A Guide to Clinical Practice. Philadelphia: J.B.Lippincott Com-
     pany, 1991.
108. Sawicka EH, Loh L, Branthwaite MA. Domiciliary ventilatory support: an analysis
     of outcome. *Thorax* 1988, 43: 31–35.
109. Sivak ED. Long-term management of the ventilator-dependent patient: preparation
     for home care. *Cleve Clin Q* 1985, 52: 307–314.
110. Thompson CL, Richmond M. Teaching home care for ventilator-dependent patients:
     the patients' perception. *Heart & Lung* 1990, 19: 79–83.
111. Iwata M. Severity stages of ALS and the psychological management. *Adv Exp Med
     Biol* 1987, 209:
112. Arora NS, Rochester DF. Respiratory muscle strength and maximum voluntary venti-
     lation in undernourished patients. *Am Rev Resp Dis* 1982, 126: 5–8.
113. Braun SR, Sufit RL, Giovannoni R, O'Connor M, Peters H. Intermittent negative
     pressure ventilation in the treatment of respiratory failure in progressive neuromuscu-
     lar disease. *Neurol* 1987, 37: 1874–1875.
114. Ellis ER, Bye PTP, Bruderer JW, Sullivan CE. Treatment of respiratory failure during
     sleep in patients with neuromuscular disease, positive pressure ventilation through
     a nose mask. *Am Rev Resp Dis* 1987, 135: 148–152.
115. Strumpf DA, Millman RP, Hill NS. The management of chronic hypoventilation.
     Chest 1990, 98: 474–480.
116. Bach JR, Beltrame F. Alternative approaches to home mechanical ventilation. In:
     Rothkopf MM, Askanazi J, eds. *Intensive Homecare*. Baltimore: Williams & Wilkins,
     1992.
117. Marino WD, Kvetan V. Home positive pressure ventilatory support. In: Rothkopf
     MM, Askanazi J, eds. *Intensive Homecare*. Baltimore: Williams & Wilkins, 1992.
118. Gilgoff IS, Peng R, Keens TG. Hypoventilation and apnea in children during mechan-
     ically assisted ventilation. *Chest* 1992, 101: 1500–1506.
119. Eddy DM. Clinical decision making: from theory to practice. The individual vs
     society. Resolving the conflict. *JAMA* 1991, 265: 2399–401.
120. Eddy DM. Clinical decision making: from theory to practice. The individual vs
     society. Is there a conflict? *JAMA* 1991, 265: 1449–50.
121. Eddy DM. What care is 'essential'? What services are 'basic'? *JAMA* 1991, 265:
     786–8.
122. Motwani JK, Herring GM. Home care for ventilator-dependent persons: a cost-
     effective, humane public policy. *Health and Social Work* 1988, 13: 20–24.
123. Rosen RL, Bone RC. Economics of mechanical ventilation. *Clin Chest Med* 1988,
     9: 163–169.
124. Eddy DM. Clinical decision making: from theory to practice. Connecting value and
     costs. Whom do we ask, and what do we ask them? *JAMA* 1990, 264: 1737–9.

12

Life Support: Realities and Dilemmas

Mark B. Bromberg, M.D., Ph.D.

Amyotrophic lateral sclerosis type of motor neuron disease is a neurodegenerative disorder characterized by slowly progressive weakness that ultimately involves muscles of respiration and leads to respiratory failure. The slow rate of progression provides time for patients to reflect on their mortality and gives them the opportunity to make decisions regarding their death. Although death is a consequence of living, it is the one universal experience for which there is no sage advisor available for consultation. Because of the very personal issue of mortality, questions about respiratory failure and support are uncomfortable topics, not only for the patient and family but also for health care providers. Accordingly, management of respiratory failure is the greatest challenge for patients and all involved in their care. This chapter is derived from a panel presentation and discussion that addressed both practical issues of respiratory failure and life support and the difficult decisions that affect all participants involved with ALS.

In this chapter, the term *ALS* is used to include all progressive forms of motor neuron disease that lead to respiratory failure. Respiratory failure is defined here as the point at which full-time respiratory support is required. Although some ALS patients may benefit temporarily from noninvasive and part-time ventilatory assistance, the progressive nature of the disorder ultimately makes full-time support necessary (1). With the goal of treating artificial ventilation as a handicap and not a reason for institutional confinement, this chapter focuses on full-time artificial ventilation for ALS patients as managed in the home.

The "reality" in ALS is the predictable progression to respiratory failure, and the accompanying "dilemma" is whether to support respiration artificially or to discontinue support at a later time. Intertwined with the principal reality of failure and dilemma of support are a number of other realities and associated dilemmas. A primary role of health care providers is to give full information to the patient and family about respiratory failure and artificial support. It is during the dissemination of information that these less obvious issues in ALS become apparent. One goal is to guide the patient and family through the decision process, maintaining patient autonomy.

This chapter is divided into two sections. The first section discusses the various realities of respiratory failure and artificial support. Early symptoms of respiratory failure must be recognized in order for the patient and family to make decisions in a timely and comfortable manner. Although patients with ALS learn from a variety of sources that the disease is progressive and that death is most frequently from respiratory failure, they rarely fully understand the mechanism, time course, and physical events that occur with respiratory failure and death. Specific information may be reassuring and may resolve some dilemmas.

The second section discusses the dilemmas of making choices and carrying them out. Feelings about continuing life in the face of respiratory failure will be unique for each patient and will affect their choices. Influential factors include personality, emotional state, life experiences, and met and unmet goals. Artificial ventilation also poses a dilemma for clinicians, whose manner of presentation of information is based on their personal philosophy and experience. The ability of the clinician to remain neutral may be one of the most important factors in helping ALS patients to make choices, but this is often difficult. There is also a dilemma for home care providers, who usually are family members. Artificial ventilation increases the responsibilities and decreases the freedom of home care providers, and the attitudes and feelings of these individuals must be considered. The cost of artificial ventilation in the home is formidable and can pose a financial dilemma. Finally, the decision to discontinue artificial respiratory support as the disease progresses may be the ultimate dilemma for the patient, family, and clinician.

The Realities of Respiratory Failure

This section concerns the recognition and consequences of respiratory failure. Although detailed presentations of respiratory physiology and failure and measurement of pulmonary function are presented in other chapters from the pulmonary point of view (Chapters 10, 11), this chapter focuses on disease progression from the perspective of neurology, and brief descriptions of respiratory physiology, failure, and measurement are included where helpful.

Muscles of Respiration

The muscles of respiration are skeletal muscles. The diaphragm is the major muscle of inspiration, and the external intercostal muscles are secondary or accessory muscles of respiration. Muscles of respiration, like limb and bulbar muscles, are innervated by lower motor neurons and are at risk to degenerate and die during the progression of ALS. The lower motor neuron cell bodies for the diaphragm are in the upper portion of the cervical spinal cord, segments C_3 through C_5, and reach the muscle via the phrenic nerve. Lower motor neurons to neck and shoulder muscles, which include some of the accessory muscles of respiration, originate from the same cervical region. There is evidence for local spread of lower motor neuron death in the spinal cord (2), and muscles sharing the same segmental distribution usually become weak with the diaphragm. Thus weakness of neck flexion and extension, shoulder abduction, elbow flexion, and lower cervical-upper thoracic paraspinal muscles (reflected in stooped posture) predict involvement of respiratory muscles (2,3).

Death of motor neurons innervating a muscle is usually not detected clinically as weakness until 40–50 percent of the motor neurons have died (4). This delay in recognition is due to collateral reinnervation, the growth of new nerve terminal branches in muscle from the surviving nerves in an attempt to reinnervate denervated muscle fiber. When only a few motor neurons have died, collateral reinnervation can adequately compensate, and weakness is not appreciated. However, when strength is measured quantitatively with a dynamometer, mild weakness can be detected (5). As more motor neurons die, the limits of collateral reinnervation are reached and exceeded, and weakness becomes apparent. Weakness occurs earlier in rapidly progressive forms of ALS because muscle fibers are denervated at a faster rate than they can be reinnervated. Although collateral reinnervation is an important compensatory process, once it begins to fail, the clinical manifestations of respiratory failure may progress rapidly.

Respiratory Muscle Fatigue and Failure

Respiratory failure initially appears as muscular fatigue, defined as the inability to continue to generate the required level of muscle force (6). Diaphragm fatigue is related to several factors. The first and most important is reduced strength of the diaphragm because of loss of lower motor neurons in the spinal cord. There will be an inability to increase minute ventilation when required. Another factor is failure of nerve transmission across the neuromuscular junction to activate muscle, because reinnervated neuromuscular junctions are less efficient at transmission (7,8). Both factors frequently appear as acute shortness of breath when the work of breathing increases, such as during bathing and dressing. A third factor is metabolic and includes several components. In poor nutritional states, muscle energy stores may be low (6). With fever or infection, increased metabolic and work demands on the diaphragm reduce the threshold for fatigue (9). Increased carbon dioxide from hypoventilation can reduce diaphragm contractility, which in turn increases fatigue, and thus contributes to a positive feedback state (10).

The work of breathing is increased during recumbency. In the upright position, the chest wall and abdomen move outward together during inspiration, and the diaphragm expends little energy as it flattens and displaces abdominal organs (11). In the supine position, the diaphragm must work harder to displace organs and move the abdomen and may fatigue if weak. As the diaphragm fatigues, accessory muscles of inspiration become active. With further fatigue, the weak diaphragm begins to passively follow the outward movement of the chest wall. This produces a paradoxical pattern of movement, with the rib cage moving outward while the abdomen moves inward (12,13). Routine pulmonary function tests, usually conducted with the patient in a sitting position, may not be markedly abnormal, but values may fall by half in the supine position (14,15).

Symptoms of Respiratory Muscle Failure

The consequence of respiratory muscle weakness is hypoventilation. Hypoventilation impairs both the renewal of oxygen in the blood, leading to hypoxemia, and the removal of carbon dioxide from the blood, leading to hypercapnia. The initial symptoms of respiratory failure in ALS patients are more often related to hypercapnia than to hypoxemia (13). Other factors that can increase the production of carbon dioxide, and may be present in individual patients, are superimposed infection with fever and poor gas exchange from underlying lung disease such as emphysema (10).

The slow progression of muscle weakness in ALS means that early symptoms and signs of respiratory failure frequently appear transiently as fatigue. Early symptoms of fatigue may occur only during exertion. Initially, this may be a subjective sensation of inadequate respiration felt by the patient and not associated with tachypnea, but later there is a clear increase in breathing effort. With disease progression, even the exertion of bathing and dressing brings on respiratory fatigue. Because patients may unconsciously adjust their activity to reduce fatigue, early symptoms must be actively sought by specific questions.

Early fatigue and failure of the diaphragm and intercostal muscles may become noticeable at bedtime and during sleep. A progression of respiratory failure might start with respiratory discomfort and inability to lie prone or supine. With further denervation of the diaphragm, respiratory fatigue and failure occur when lying in the lateral decubitus position. At a later period, sleeping with the head of the bed at ever steeper angles will be necessary, until sleeping sitting up is the only comfortable position (16).

The slow progression also means that symptoms will predominate and laboratory findings will be minimal. In patients with abnormal pulmonary function tests, symptoms of "exertional shortness of breath," "disturbed sleep," "excessive day time drowsiness," "inattentiveness during the day," and nocturnal or morning "headaches" (17,18,19) are more common than specific blood gas abnormalities, such as low arterial oxygen and high carbon dioxide tensions (20,21).

Sleep Disturbances

During sleep, a number of physiologic changes occur that may affect ALS patients. These include changes in body position of which the patient is unaware, but which result in diaphragm fatigue and reduced activation of accessory muscles of respiration during REM sleep (22). Sleep studies indicate that in most ALS patients the overall quality of sleep is similar to that measured in normal subjects of similar age (23,24). Arousals and mild disorders of breathing occur, but are infrequently associated with clinically significant hypoxemia ($pO_2 < 80$ mmHg) (23,24). An occasional patient will have profound nocturnal hypoventilation and hypoxia (18,25). These patients respond affirmatively when asked about "difficulty sleeping" or being "sleepy during the daytime" (23). A polysomnogram should be performed to demonstrate significant nocturnal hypoxemia, for these patients may respond dramatically to noninvasive ventilatory assistance.

Measurement of Progression

Weakness in ALS is progressive, both in the degree of weakness within muscles and in the distribution among muscles in the body. Weakness of muscles of respiration progressing to respiratory failure is the end point of the disease for patients who choose not to have artificial ventilation and is the leading cause of death in ALS patients (26). Patients and family often ask about the rate of progression of weakness, the amount of time before muscles of respiration become involved, and when a decision about artificial ventilation must be made. These are emotionally charged questions for the patient to ask and difficult for the clinician to answer because the rate of progression for an individual patient cannot be accurately predicted.

Longitudinal studies show a broad range of survival times. Survival curves are skewed, and although the median survival time is approximately four years (27), some patients die within months of symptom onset, while others with slowly progressive forms of motor neuron disease live for one or more decades (28, 29). Most studies show shorter survival times when the onset of symptoms is later in life (26,27,28,30,31) and longer times in patients with the less common forms of motor neuron disease of primary lateral sclerosis and progressive muscular atrophy (27). It is uncertain whether patients with the progressive bulbar palsy form of motor neuron disease progress more rapidly than patients with initial limb involvement. Although a number of studies indicate a more rapid progression for bulbar patients (26,30,31), other studies report no differences (27). Alternatively, the shorter survival time for these patients may be accounted for by an older age at symptom onset (32). These epidemiological studies point out the difficulties in using survival data to give meaningful answers about progression to individual patients.

Attempts to accurately predict survival in individual patients are based on measurement of limb muscle strength by dynamometry, and respiratory muscle strength by pulmonary function tests (5), or by composite scores that include performance in activities of daily living (27,28). Quantitative dynamometry and pulmonary function testing yield interval data values, while the 0 to 5 Medical Research Council (MRC) manual muscle testing scale is nonlinear. Serial studies show highly linear rates of loss of strength over time when values from a group of ALS patients are averaged (33,34). However, these linear rates are derived from patients during the active phase of their disease, and patients with early symptoms and normal strength, or those at a late stage with minimal change in strength, are not included (34). When patients are considered individually, variability in deterioration rates are found (34,35). The rate of progression may rarely increase during the terminal phase of the disease (28). The variability in strength and function points out how unreliable measurements of progression can be in individual patients.

The most important question for the ALS patient is, "When will muscles of respiration become involved?" It is unusual for these muscles to be the initial symptomatic group (17,28,36,37). More commonly, the onset of respiratory muscle weakness is delayed compared to limb muscles, and it is not uncommon for patients to have paralyzed lower extremities but unchanged respiratory function.

Pulmonary function tests are the most common method of assessing respiratory muscle strength. Full or formal testing, as performed in a pulmonary physiology laboratory, provides maximal amounts of data, but serial testing to follow a patient's course by this comprehensive format is impractical in terms of scheduling, patient effort, and expense. Simplified or "bedside" pulmonary function testing can be performed in the clinic as a practical alternative with respect to these factors and provides useful information for prediction and management of respiratory failure.

When first tested, pulmonary function in ALS patients may be unexpectedly abnormal, and values less than 50 percent of predicted are not uncommon (20). As diaphragm weakness progresses, pulmonary function test values decline linearly, and forced vital capacity is a reliable measure to follow (38). Although respiratory impairment usually develops insidiously, terminal failure in ALS patients usually occurs acutely and unexpectedly (39). It is prudent to initiate discussion about respiratory failure and artificial ventilation when values fall below 50 percent of predicted. Forced vital capacity values of less than 25 percent of predicted may be tolerated by patients (Bromberg, unpublished observations), but the suddenness of respiratory failure makes a frank discussion at these values imperative.

Respiratory Failure

Without artificial ventilation, the most common penultimate physiologic event preceding death from respiratory failure is hypercapnia leading to impaired consciousness (40). The ultimate cause of death is likely from hypoxemia and cardiac dysrhythmia (27). Although patients often assume that choking and gasping will occur, death occurs peacefully for most, often during sleep. Aspiration may be more likely in patients with a poor cough and coexistent bulbar dysfunction, but postmortem examinations show that aspiration leading to bronchopneumonia is a factor in less than half of cases (27). During the terminal phase, if patients become anxious and restless, use of sedatives and narcotic analgesics are effective in making death comfortable (41).

Artificial Ventilation

A question frequently raised by patients is, ''What is it like being on artificial ventilation?'' (42). Being placed on artificial ventilation produces psychological stress, the severity of which depends on the individual patient's perceptions of the situation and its meaning (43). Descriptions by patients on permanent artificial ventilation, although personal experiences, are informative. Initially, there may be panic with intubation and mechanical inflation (44). Because some respiratory muscle function is present, there is usually a period of adjustment during which the natural rhythm of respiration fights with the artificial pattern of mechanical ventilation (45). There is apprehension that mechanical ventilatory failure might occur and a question of whether it will be attended to in time. When initially hospitalized for intubation and ventilation, the alarm soundings from other patients' ventilators potentiate this apprehension (46). Speech, if possible before intubation, is not possible during the first few weeks after intubation. Dependency on a machine and inability to communicate easily raise strong feelings of isolation and frustration (44).

There are also physical discomforts. Supported ventilation remains permanently ''artificial,'' and the ventilator cannot provide sighs, gasps, or sneezes, which have been described as part of the ''respiratory vocabulary'' (43). The necessary tracheal suctioning brings relief of respiratory discomfort, but it is an uncomfortable procedure at best and agonizing in unskilled hands (44). Suctioning may be infrequent, but under certain circumstances may be so frequent as to preclude other activities (45). When patients on artificial ventilation require assistance in changing body position, they may not be able to communicate their discomfort and may become dependent on a time schedule. The perception of time under these circumstances may become altered, and reasonable time schedules can appear unbearably long to the patient (46).

After the initial fears and tribulations of artificial ventilation are dealt with, there is a different type of adjustment period in which a patient begins to reestablish self-worth, regain control, and think about and make decisions concerning the future (45). At this time, the reality of all that is involved with artificial ventilation becomes apparent. This transition has been described as ''getting on with life'' (45). Factors include adjustments in life-style and physical living arrangements in the home, reestablishing vocational and avocational interests, and integrating them with the interests and activities of the rest of the family. The transition phase must be an active and continuous process, because more adjustments become necessary with the passage of time as strength and function continue to decline.

The Dilemmas of Respiratory Failure

The Choice of Artificial Ventilation

The principal dilemmas for an ALS patient are whether to start artificial ventilation and whether to stop it if it proves unsatisfactory. The proportion of patients who are on artificial ventilation, by choice or by chance, is not known accurately, nor is the number who die naturally or after intentional disconnection. Estimates from a regional survey in the midwestern United States suggest that up to 8 percent of ALS patients are placed on artificial ventilation (47). Although artificial ventilation prevents death from respiratory muscle failure, patients are at risk for dying from other medical causes. Some patients choose to terminate artificial ventilation. Correcting for these factors, the estimated point prevalence of ALS patients on artificial ventilation is closer to 5 percent (47).

Prospective data are not available to determine how many patients actively choose no ventilation and die a natural death, how many die a natural death without having made a choice, and how many are forced into a decision by a medical emergency. Data from patients on artificial ventilation indicate that while most were informed about the dilemma, only a minority chose it in advance (47,48). The majority make the choice, or their families do, under emergency conditions.

Dissemination of Information on Respiratory Failure and Support

The failure of the majority of patients to make decisions may be a result of insufficient information about respiratory failure and artificial support, or presentation of the information at the wrong stage of the illness. There is a certain volume and content of information that a patient and family can process and use in making decisions. The extreme manner of information presentation, in which all facts about the progression of ALS and ultimate respiratory failure are given at the time of diagnosis, will be unsuccessful. Most ALS patients state that they desire as much information as possible (42), but early in the course of the disease, respiratory failure is a frightening idea and may not be perceived by the patient as a real possibility (49). Although half of the patients are satisfied with their level of understanding, a third want more, including information on the progression of failure and use of ventilators (42). It is necessary to repeat information on respiratory failure at intervals as weakness progresses, with greater focus when respiratory symptoms appear. Even though a discussion of artificial ventilation by the clinician may evoke sadness and anxiety, a detailed description of the symptoms and signs of respiratory failure, experiences on artificial ventilation, and the manner of death from respiratory failure is often satisfying and may be reassuring to patients as they consider their options.

The request by patients for full information presents a dilemma for clinicians in the manner of their presentations and discussions with the patient and family. Clinicians have personal thoughts and feelings about artificial ventilation that are based on their background and their clinical experiences. These feelings may come through in their description of life on a ventilator and the logistics of the personnel and financial support required. ALS patients may also directly ask the clinician for advice. In a survey of ALS center clinical directors, there was a seven-fold and statistically significant difference in the percentage of patients on artificial support among the five centers. The survey questions revealed an association between clinicians' personal feelings about artificial ventilation and the likelihood that one of their patients will choose it (47).

ALS patients have difficulty discussing their feelings about artificial ventilation and only half are able to do so, most commonly with their spouse. Although these feelings are expressed less often with their physician, patients generally feel comfortable and in control during these discussions. Despite the fact that a majority of patients seen in an ALS center receive information about respiratory failure and support and half of them discuss these issues, 30 percent prefer to leave care and treatment decisions to their physicians (42). It is not clear if the physicians are aware of this preference.

Patient Decision Making

It is important that a patient be encouraged to make a decision in a timely fashion. An approach used in our Motor Neuron Disease Clinic is to discuss decisions about artificial ventilation in terms of a neutral document, the Durable Power of Attorney for Health Care. We invoke the argument that every person of legal adult age should consider their medical management, make their thoughts known, and entrust them in such a document.

Reaching a decision about artificial ventilation is difficult, and patients should be given permission to change their minds as their experience with ALS grows and circumstances change. The emphasis in our clinic is to keep the control of decisions with the patient at all times. We also stress that there are no "right" or "wrong" decisions regarding artificial ventilation. Patient control is especially important in family situations where some members are opposed to the patient's wishes.

Patient Indecision

When a patient abdicates the decision about artificial ventilation, either by active transfer or by passive indecision, the clinician is faced with the dilemma.

One clinician's approach is to classify symptomatic treatment in ALS as either "ordinary" or "extraordinary." Positive pressure artificial ventilation is considered an example of extraordinary treatment. Under these definitions, a passive "no decision" can be interpreted as a decision against the extraordinary therapy of artificial ventilation (19).

Termination of Artificial Ventilation by the Patient

ALS patients on artificial ventilation may lead very productive lives at home and in their professional arenas (45). The majority of ALS patients on artificial ventilation, whether placed on it by choice or by circumstances, report overall satisfaction at being alive under these conditions (47,48). From individual patient histories, it is likely that ambulation and in particular the ability to communicate are important factors in feeling satisfied (50). It is clear that with artificial ventilation the natural course of ALS is altered, and patients can live long enough to experience unanticipated disabilities (51). What is not clear is the lowest level of function associated with a satisfactory quality of life for artificially ventilated patients. Some patients consider terminating artificial ventilation when weakness progresses to a certain level, when communication is no longer possible, or when some goal in life is met (19,52,53). In this context of failing function, the most difficult dilemma for a patient may be when to request that artificial ventilation be stopped. In one survey, 17 percent of patients chose to withdraw from artificial ventilation, but the reasons were not given (47). In another, only one of nineteen patients requested withdrawal from artificial ventilation when home care could not be continued (48). Goldblatt argues eloquently that the clinician and other health and home care providers must stand by the patient to advocate life, but also to respect the patient's "liberty to die" (49). The majority of physicians who have had experience with ALS patients reveal that they would honor a request by a patient to discontinue artificial ventilation (52).

Termination of Artificial Ventilation by the Family

Termination of artificial ventilation when weakness has progressed to preclude communication and the patient's wishes are not known can be a dilemma for the family. This situation is also likely to be a dilemma for the patient. With artificial ventilation, ALS can progress so that essentially all lower motor neurons die, including those responsible for voluntary eye movements and rectal sphincter muscle control (54). This precludes any expressive communication, but patients are likely to retain sensory function and consciousness (55; Bromberg, unpublished observation). In a review of "locked-in" ALS patients, EEG recordings showed only mild disturbances of background activity, and in some there was alpha wave reactivity (54). The repertoire of sensations expressed by communicative ALS patients includes pain from pressure and immobility that may be prominent when muscle and fat masses are lost (50), visceral pain from constipation, and discomfort from heat, cold, and pruritis. Although locked-in ALS patients cannot communicate their experiences, reports from physically dependent patients temporarily on a ventilator indicate the frequent occurrence of psychotic symptoms under these conditions (56). Relief is most likely to be inadequate when these discomforts cannot be communicated, and the concept of a totally locked-in state takes on horrifying prospects (52).

The Home Caregiver

Home caregivers are a group of individuals with their own set of dilemmas, but are often overlooked in the dissemination of information on artificial ventilation to ALS patients. This chapter focuses on long-term artificial ventilation support in the home, which gives the ALS patient the psychological benefits of being independent of institutional support (1). However, uninterrupted patient attention is required, and the burden rests mostly on the spouse. The great majority of home caregivers are women (90 percent), although the male to female ratio in ALS is approximately 1.5 to 1 (47).

The task of home care must be divided. The average daily time spent by the family for patient care is nine hours, with the balance from outside personnel, for a total average daily involvement of 3.5 persons per patient (47). Relief from some of these burdens by hiring outside personnel is not without stress. Stressors include finding and interviewing candidates, assessing their level of competency, and the reliability of their attendance. Qualifications alone are not sufficient, for experienced personnel may be burnt out from previous work with patients on ventilators. Caring for ALS patients in whom weakness and disability will progress may be especially trying for personnel who only have experience caring for patients with stable disabilities or who eventually improve their level of function.

The impact of home ventilatory care on the family, especially on the spouse, is tremendous, but is largely hidden from discussion. With the trend toward families assuming more of the burden of long-term patient care, questions about the psychological, ethical, and moral limits of their obligation have been considered (57). Half of the home caregivers consider the time commitment to be a major burden (47). The initial enthusiasm frequently wanes, and anger and resentment are common. Anger may be directed toward the patient. Previously established patterns of coping are often used, and family conflicts may become channeled through the patient (50,58). Anger can also be directed back to the caregiver. The anger, in turn, often generates guilt, and home caregivers frequently suffer in silence (57). As a consequence, many experience ill health (47).

After living with these difficulties, most caregivers surveyed were happy that their ALS patient chose artificial ventilation (47). This finding may reflect in part the complex and ambivalent nature of feelings toward the patient. Their experience with artificial ventilation did affect them, however, and only half would choose artificial ventilation if they themselves developed ALS (47).

Financial Burden

The dilemma of financing artificial ventilation is formidable. It is less costly to care for patients in the home than in hospitals (58). The monthly home costs vary widely, from $407 to $35,000 (47,58,59). In one survey, the mean and median monthly costs were $12,771 and $7,250 respectively, and the average yearly cost was $153,252 (47). The major factor affecting cost is the need for hiring outside personnel. The major financial concern for the family is the amount of insurance coverage. Eighty-three percent of the monthly costs listed were covered by insurance, with more than half of the families receiving full coverage. When incomplete, coverage was usually denied for outside personnel, and the uncovered monthly expenses ranged from $100 to $7,200 (47). These data suggest that if the financial profile shifts away from 100 percent insurance coverage, or if families are less well-to-do, the burden of home care shifts to the spouse.

Comments

Presentation of the full spectrum of dilemmas associated with respiratory failure shows them to be formidable in number and complexity. However, they are all manageable. Indeed, the ALS patient and family who chose artificial ventilation are satisfied with the choice (47). Such is the will and power of the human spirit to deal with and overcome obstacles.

The advantage of presenting the full spectrum of dilemmas is that it encourages discussion among patient, family, and health care workers. Problems must be identified before they can be investigated and solved. Particular problems, such as the psychological aspects of being an ALS patient and caring for an ALS patient, may be hidden, but are present nonetheless. Thus, a full presentation and open discussion is very important for the well-being of those who choose and those who refuse artificial ventilation.

Summary

The reality of respiratory failure in ALS profoundly affects the patient, the family, and the health care providers, and the dilemmas are shared by all. The opportunity to make decisions regarding the manner of one's death is a unique feature of this disorder. Although these decisions are frightening, they reflect a control over life, which becomes an important issue in light of the technological advances in medicine and should be considered the right of every person. In ALS, full information should be made available in a neutral manner by health care providers. Educational material about respiratory failure and artificial ventilation are available to assist in dissemination of information (60,61). Decisions by the patient should be encouraged and made informally to the family and formally in a document, such as a Durable Power of Attorney for Health Care. It is the obligation of the health care providers to honor these decisions.

The hope for all involved with ALS is that advances in understanding will lead to an effective therapy, and that these realities, dilemmas, and decisions will not be part of the disease in the future.

Acknowledgments

I would like to thank Dr. A. Moss for making available a prepublication copy of his manuscript, D. Forshew, R.N., for her indefatigable efforts in the Motor Neuron Disease Clinic and review of the manuscript, the ALS patients from whom I have learned much, Drs. M. Aldrich and J. Bromberg for review of the manuscript, and D. Scott for assistance in preparing the manuscript. Supported in part by grants from the Muscular Dystrophy Association, the FDA (FD-R-000512-01), and the NIH (MO1-RR00042).

References

1. Sivak ED, Gipson WT, Hanson MR. Long-term management of respiratory failure in amyotrophic lateral sclerosis. *Ann Neurol* 1982;12:18–23.
2. Brooks BR, DePaul R, DeTan Y, Sanjar M, Sufit RL, Robbins J. Motor neuron disease. In: Porter RJ and Schoenberg BS, eds. *Controlled Clinical Trials in Neurological Disease*. Norwell: Kluwer Academic, 1990.
3. Kreitzer SM, Saunders NA, Tyler HR, Ingram, RH. Respiratory muscle function in amyotrophic lateral sclerosis. *Am Rev Respir Dis* 1978, 117:437–447.
4. Beasley WC. Quantitative muscle testing: principles and applications to research and clinical services. *Arch Phys Med Rehab* 1961, 42:398–425.
5. Andres PL, Hedlund W, Finison L, Conlon T, Felmus M, Munsat TL. Quantitative motor assessment in amyotrophic lateral sclerosis. *Neurology* 1986, 36:937–941.
6. Roussos C, Macklem PT. The respiratory muscles. *N Engl J Med* 1982, 307:786–797.
7. Denys EH, Norris FH. Amyotrophic lateral sclerosis—impairment of neuromuscular transmission. *Arch Neurol* 1979, 36:202–205.
8. Bernstein LP, Antel JP. Motor neuron disease: decremental responses to repetitive nerve stimulation. *Neurology* 1981, 31:202–204.
9. Braun SR, Sufit RL, Giovannoni R, O'Connor M, Peters H. Intermittent negative pressure ventilation in the treatment of respiratory failure in progressive neuromuscular disease. *Neurology* 1987, 37:1874–1875.
10. Weinberger SE, Schwartzstein RM, Weiss JW. Hypercapnia. *N Engl J Med* 1989, 321:1223–1231.
11. Gothe B, Bruce EN, Goldman MD. Influence of sleep state on respiratory muscle function. In: Saunders NA, Sullivan CE, eds. *Sleep and Breathing*. New York: Marcel Dekker, 1984.

12. Cohen CA, Zagelbaum G, Gross D, Roussos C, Macklem PT. Clinical manifestations of inspiratory muscle fatigue. *Am J Med* 1982, 73:308–316.
13. Rosen MJ. Respiratory failure in amyotrophic lateral sclerosis. In: Caroscio JT, ed. *Amyotrophic Lateral Sclerosis*. New York: Thieme Medical, 1986.
14. Newsome-Davis J, Goldman M, Loh L, Casson M. Diaphragm function and alveolar hypoventilation. *Q J Med* 1976, 45:87–100.
15. Serisier DE, Mastaglia FL, Gibson GJ. Respiratory muscle function and ventilatory control—I in patients with motor neurone disease—II in patients with myotonic dystrophy. *Q J Med* 1982, 202:205–226.
16. Sivak ED, Streib EW. Management of hypoventilation in motor neuron disease presenting with respiratory insufficiency. *Ann Neurol* 1980, 7:188–191.
17. Hill R, Martin J, Hakim A. Acute respiratory failure in motor neuron disease. *Arch Neurol* 1983, 40:30–32.
18. Al-Shaikh B, Kinnear W, Higenbottam TW, Smith HS, Shneerson JM, Wilkinson I. Motor neurone disease presenting as respiratory failure. *Br Med J* 1986, 292: 1325–1326.
19. Goldblatt D. Decisions about life support in amyotrophic lateral sclerosis. *Semin Neurol* 1984, 4:104–110.
20. Fallat RJ, Jewitt B, Bass M, Kamm B, Norris F. Spirometry in amyotrophic lateral sclerosis. *Arch Neurol* 1979, 36:74–80.
21. Gay PC, Patel AM, Viggiano RW, Hubmayr RD. Nocturnal nasal ventilation for treatment of patients with hypercapnic respiratory failure. *Mayo Clin Proc* 1991, 66: 695–703.
22. Kreiger J. Breathing during sleep in normal subjects. In: Kryger MH, Roth T, Dement WC. *Principles and Practice of Sleep Medicine*. Philadelphia: Saunders, 1989.
23. Gay PC, Westbrook PR, Daube JR, Litchy WJ, Windebank AJ, Iverson R. Effects of alterations in pulmonary function and sleep variables on survival in patients with amyotrophic lateral sclerosis. *Mayo Clin Proc* 1991, 66:686–694.
24. Minz M, Autret A, Laffont F, Beillevaire T, Cathala HP, Castaigne P. A study on sleep in amyotrophic lateral sclerosis. *Biomedicine* 1979, 30:40–46.
25. Carre PC, Didier AP, Tiberge YM, Arbus LJ, Leophonte PT. Amyotrophic lateral sclerosis presenting with sleep hypopnea syndrome. *Chest* 1988, 93:1309–1312.
26. Boman K, Meurman T. Prognosis of amyotrophic lateral sclerosis. *Acta Neurol Scand* 1967, 43:489–498.
27. Caroscio JT, Mulvihill MN, Sterling R, Abrams B. Amyotrophic lateral sclerosis—its natural history. *Neurol Clin* 1987, 5:1–8.
28. Jablecki CK, Berry C, Leach J. Survival prediction in amyotrophic lateral sclerosis. *Muscle Nerve* 1989, 12:833–841.
29. Mulder DW, Howard FM. Patient resistance and prognosis in amyotrophic lateral sclerosis. *Mayo Clin Proc* 1976, 51:537–541.
30. Jokelainen M. Amyotrophic lateral sclerosis in Finland. *Acta Neurol Scand* 1977, 56: 194–204.
31. Rosen AD. Amyotrophic lateral sclerosis—clinical features and prognosis. *Arch Neurol* 1978, 35:638–642.
32. Daube JR. Electrophysiologic studies in the diagnosis and prognosis of motor neuron diseases. *Neurol Clin* 1985, 3:473–493.

33. Andres PL, Finison LJ, Conlon T, Thibodeau LM, Munsat TL. Use of composite scores (megascores) to measure deficit in amyotrophic lateral sclerosis. *Neurology* 1988, 38:405–408.
34. Munsat TL, Andres PL, Finison, Conlon T, Thibodeau L. The natural history of motoneuron loss in amyotrophic lateral sclerosis. *Neurology* 1988, 38:409–413.
35. Nau KL, Bromberg MB, Katch VL, Forshew DA. Progressive strength loss in patients with amyotrophic lateral sclerosis. *Med Sci Sports Exerc* 1992, 24:S73.
36. Fromm GB, Wisdom PJ, Block AJ. Amyotrophic lateral sclerosis presenting with respiratory failure. *Chest* 1977, 71:612–614.
37. Daras M, Spiro AJ, Swerdlow M. Respiratory failure in amyotrophic lateral sclerosis. *N Y State J Med* 1984, 84:570–572.
38. Sufit RL, Brooks BR. Longitudinal changes of pulmonary functions (PFT) in amyotrophic lateral sclerosis (ALS): a pilot study for natural history and clinical trials. *Neurology* 1990, 40:315.
39. Bradley WG. Respirator support in amyotrophic lateral sclerosis. *Ann Neurol* 1983, 13:466.
40. Desmedt M, Clement J, Schepers R, Van de Woestijne KP. Respiratory failure: correlation between encephalopathy, blood gases and blood ammonia. *Respiration* 1976, 33: 199–210.
41. Wilson WC, Smedira NG, Fink C, McDowell JA, Luce JM. Ordering and administration of sedatives and analgesics during the withholding and withdrawal of life support from critically ill patients. *JAMA* 1992, 267:949–953.
42. Silverstein MD, Stocking CB, Antel JP, Beckwith J, Roos RP, Siegler M. Amyotrophic lateral sclerosis and life-sustaining therapy: patients' desires for information, participation in decision making, and life-sustaining therapy. *Mayo Clin Proc* 1991, 66: 906–913.
43. Gale J, O'Shanick GJ. Psychiatric aspects of respirator treatment and pulmonary intensive care. *Adv Psychosom Med* 1985, 14:93–108.
44. Castillo A, Egan H. How it feels to be a ventilator patient. *Respir Care* 1974, 19: 289–293.
45. Charles RA. Coping with life on a portable ventilator. *Home Health Nrs* 1985, 3: 27–30.
46. Parker MM, Schubert W, Shelhamer JH, Parrillo JE. Perceptions of a critically ill patient experiencing therapeutic paralysis in an ICU. *Crit Care Med* 1984, 12:69–71.
47. Moss AH, Heidkamp PC, Stocking CB, Roos RP, Brooks BR, Siegler M. Home ventilation for amyotrophic lateral sclerosis patients: outcomes, costs, and patient, family and physician attitudes. *Neurology* 1993, 43:438–443.
48. Oppenheimer EA, Baldwin-Meyers A, Tanquary P. Ventilator use by patients with amyotrophic lateral sclerosis. *International Conference on Pulmonary Rehabilitation and Home Ventilation*. Denver, 1991, 49.
49. Goldblatt D. Caring for patients with amyotrophic lateral sclerosis. In: Smith RA, ed. *Handbook of Amyotrophic Lateral Sclerosis*. New York: Marcel Dekker, 1992.
50. Bregman AM. Living with amyotrophic lateral sclerosis: major concerns of patients and families. In: Charash LI, Wolf SG, Kutscher AH, Lovelace RE, Hale MS, eds. *Psychosocial Aspects of Muscular Dystrophy and Allied Diseases*. Springfield: CC Thomas, 1983.
51. Sivak ED, Cordasco EM, Gipson WT, Stelmak K. Clinical considerations in the

implementation of home care ventilation: observations in 24 patients. *Cleve Clin Q* 1983, 50:219–225.

52. Goldblatt D, Greenlaw J. Starting and stopping the ventilator for patients with amyotrophic lateral sclerosis. *Neurol Clin* 1989, 7:789–806.

53. Wilson JP. Why I pulled the plug on a competent patient. *Med Econ* 1990, 138–143.

54. Hayashi H, Kato S. Total manifestations of amyotrophic lateral sclerosis. *J Neurol Sci* 1989, 93:19–35.

55. Mizutani T, Aki M, Shiozawa R, et al. Development of ophthalmoplegia in amyotrophic lateral sclerosis during long-term use of respirators. *J Neurol Sci* 1990, 99: 311–319.

56. Viner ED. Life at the other end of the endotracheal tube: a physician's personal view of critical illness. *Prog Crit Care Med* 1985, 2:3–13.

57. Callahan D. Families as caregivers: the limits of morality. *Arch Phys Med Rehab* 1988, 69:323–328.

58. Sivak ED, Cordasco EM, Gipson WT. Pulmonary mechanical ventilation at home: a reasonable and less expensive altermative. *Respir Care* 1983, 28:42–49.

59. Lehner WE, Ballard IM, Figueroa WG, Woodruff DS. Home care utilizing a ventilator in a patient with amyotrophic lateral sclerosis. *J Fam Pract* 1980, 10:39–42.

60. MALS Manual III: *Managing Breathing Problems*. Order from: The ALS Association, 21021 Ventura Blvd., Suite 321, Woodland Hills, CA 91364, Phone: (818) 340-7500.

61. Video on Ventilator Decision: *It's Your Choice*. Order from: The ALS Association, 21021 Ventura Blvd., Suite 321, Woodland Hills, CA 91364, Phone: (818) 340-7500.

13

ALS Nursing Care Management: State of the Art

Barbara T. Beal Libby, R.N., M.N., P.H.N.

Neurologic nursing textbooks covering care of patients with ALS have improved dramatically in the last few years (1,2). Content is organized using the concept of nursing diagnoses. This relatively new method is helping nurses define and organize professional nursing practice in a logical sequence. In the future we should see generalist nurses graduating with basic concepts to understand ALS care.

This chapter does not cover nursing basics. Rather than attempt to be comprehensive, "state of the art" functions of specialist nurses described here illustrate current trends in nursing management of ALS.

For the nurse caring for a person dying of ALS, very little is available in journals on nursing care requirements. Case examples are provided here to illustrate this area of nursing expertise.

A discussion on "dying readiness" is included in this chapter in the section "Endstage Disease and Dying After Ventilator Disconnect." A pattern emerged from my experience with families facing the death of someone with ALS. Some of the people with ALS chose not to use life supports and to allow death by respiratory failure. Some chose to use the ventilator when breathing failed and later to discontinue it and let death ensue. Table 13-2 outlines the steps used in my private practice.

Current Trends in Nursing Management of ALS

Most people with ALS live at home and at some point must receive nursing help. The level of excellence of nursing management provided can determine the level of coping, comfort, and general health of the ALS person and the whole family.

Nursing care is almost always given in a combination of ways—by family, friends, and by part- or full-time hired help.

Hired personnel may be nurses. They are usually nursing attendants who do not hold any health care licenses. Some are skilled in ALS care, but many are not. Licensed practical or vocational nurses (LPNs, LVNs) and registered nurses (RNs) know basic nursing practice but may not be familiar with the special approaches required for people with ALS. Home health agencies can provide nursing supervision of home care given by others, but few people can afford agency fees. Therefore, the main source of guidance for the patient and family is the family caregiver who may know exactly what the person likes, but who may not know good nursing care. ALS clinics (contact the ALS Association and the Muscular Dystrophy Association for available ALS clinics) and ALS home care nursing consultants are relatively new and are playing an increasing role in guiding home care.

ALS Nursing Care Is "Different"

Many conditions involve motor weakness and paralysis. The unique feature in ALS is the experience of severe progressive motor loss. Because needs change quickly, one discovers that the care and planning provided one week may be inadequate the next week.

The major nursing problems in ALS stem from upper and lower neuron losses resulting in motor paralysis. Brainstem dysfunction results in gradual loss of swallowing, speech, and breathing. These meteoric losses create unique nursing care problems. Supporting this slow dying process is one of the most challenging areas in all of nursing care.

ALS usually happens to otherwise healthy and mentally normal people. Perhaps this explains why nursing consultants find that with relatively little guidance from them, patients and families cope very well with even devastating care problems.

Nursing Consultation

By definition, a consultant is one who helps the patient draw on his/her own resources and use them effectively. Most of us who call ourselves ALS nursing consultants do more than this. We also become educators, advocates for our clients, referral and liaison agents, equipment finders, and, occasionally, direct caregivers.

Nurses who have specialized in ALS care often find themselves in all these roles because the need for information and support is so great.

The issue of educational preparation of the nurse consultant is deliberately omitted here. At present, this is undefined. Nurses with a variety of backgrounds are functioning in the role.

Who are the clients? The consultant's clients may be the ALS person, the family, or the home care nurse.

Consultant Roles

Home Care Consultation

Success of a consultation depends on the accuracy of the nurse's assessment of the client's readiness to address his/her needs as well as how far advanced the symptoms are (3). Coping skills differ for everyone.

Based on professional nursing assessment, we can provide explanation of symptoms (4). We teach home care techniques. Life support options are described. We discuss hopes and fears and describe the dying process. We also discuss feasibility of the home setting for the care that is needed and available community services. We have learned that when people face life-threatening illnesses, they ask the same questions of many persons before they make a decision.

People use knowledge gained to cope with long-term planning as well as with the day-to-day nursing problems. Attempts to use unorthodox therapies that promise cure are often tried (see Chapter 5). Some are quite costly. The person may or may not tell the physician about these activities, but will often tell the nurse consultant. If the diagnosis seems in doubt, referrals for medical second opinions are provided. Many misconceptions can be cleared up.

Consultations with Home Care Nurses

Consultants hold care conferences at home care agencies and go on home visits with agency nurses in order to solve problems together.

Direct Care Giving

At times there is need for direct caregiving. One steps out of the consultant role and functions as a licensed caregiver. I prefer to provide any care with the primary caregiver present—family or nurse—so that the tasks performed can become part of the daily care given by others.

Telephone Consultations

Some chapters of the ALS Association sponsor telephone consultation programs as a free service to people with ALS, as well as to health professionals. Home health nurses phone the service for help with specific patients. For program protocol used in Orange County, California, see Table 13-1.

An open-ended free service could, of course, be subject to abuse by callers. Observation by experience is that ALS families simply do not misuse such a service. They call when, and only when, they need help. Even the occasional long calls are rewarding. Feedback from people who have received help is positive

Table 13-1. ALS Telephone Consultation Program Protocol (as developed for the Orange County Chapter of the ALS Association)

• Services Provided	Professional consultation for multiple complex issues faced by ALS patients and their families. The consultant assesses by phone and provides education about how to care for the individual in the home. Also evaluates and troubleshoots the special problems presented. A free service sponsored by the local ALSA chapter.
• Clients	ALS persons, families, caregivers (in the home, home health agencies, nursing homes, hospitals).
• The Consultant	An ALS nursing care specialist with a Master's degree in nursing.
• Fees	Paid by the chapter to the consultant by prearrangement.
• Telephone	A phone line located at the consultant's premises. Costs covered by fees to consultant.
• Hours	Set hours not used. Most people call during the work day, unless given permission to call other times.
• Record-keeping	Several methods tried. Control-o-fax* proved to be most satisfactory. This system includes a telephone log page and individual client data slips to record all incoming and outgoing calls. Lends itself to data retrieval, billing, and content analysis.
• Utilization Review	Periodic review of methods and records provided by a medical social worker familiar with the consultation process. Reports to the chapter board.
• Benefits of Program	Highly stressed anxious patients and caregivers can continue to function when receiving timely help, support, and education about problems faced. Consultant readily accessible. Highly cost-effective. Costs of program generally are covered by donations from clients who have benefitted. The program has aided in chapter development and fulfillment of patient service goals.
• Alternatives Available	Physician office visits, health professional home visits, emergency room and hospital stays, or no service available at all (except 911 emergency, which is almost never appropriate).
• Program Outcomes and Comments	Telephone time—approximately 10 hours/week, excluding overhead time used for problem solving. At times, the consultant serves as an advocate for services needed (placing referral calls for stressed-out clients). At present, a variety of "information only" phone services are available from many chapters. There is no national standardization for a telephone consultation protocol at present. Social workers serve effectively in this role for all but nursing care techniques.

* Control-o-fax, Box 778, Waterloo, Iowa 50704—1-800-344-7777.

on the whole. The following examples demonstrate how amazingly well people cope with disastrous problems when given a relatively small amount of professional guidance in a timely fashion. This means guidance when they need it, not when it is convenient for professional hours or appointments. Hospital admissions are avoided when problems can be prevented.

Ventilator Nurses Round Table

Ventilator care in the home is one of the areas where ongoing nursing education (beyond the required initial orientation to home equipment) is greatly needed. In Orange County, California, we developed a ventilator nurses round table that functioned under the sponsorship of the local chapter of the American Lung Association. A "round table" is a forum, not a support group. Expert approaches developed by these special nurses were shared with each other.

The impetus for starting the group was the expressed need of LVNs caring for "vent" persons at home. Although the round table was short-lived, the concept was good. With the right leadership and promotion, such groups could make a real difference in home ventilator care.

Professional Writing and Public Speaking

Another way the consultant can help the home care nurse is by professional writing and public speaking. We provide talks on specific ALS topics at local and national conferences as well as in-service instruction to home health agencies and nursing homes. Our ALSA chapter mailing list deliberately includes many home care nurses. We have excellent feedback from nursing care articles published in local ALS newsletters.

Third Party Reimbursement

Although nursing care is the greatest need of the person with advanced ALS, it is the one element that is generally uninsurable. Home visits by a professional nurse are usually covered only as long as they are necessary to teach the family to provide the care themselves. This offers little hope for exhausted caregivers and means that those without sufficient private means have to go without vital nursing expertise at the time when they need it most.

When private insurance companies know of the ALS nursing consultant's work, preauthorization is sometimes provided for home care consultations. At times, requests for consultant services come directly from the insurer. Consultation services need to be reimbursed by third party payers under an authorization category separate from visiting nurses since the services are generically different. Insurers who use the services of an ALS nursing consultant save costs of hospitalization for problems that can be solved at home. This practice must be encouraged by medical practitioners caring for an ALS population.

Sample Problems from Consultant Practice

Examples cited in this section are drawn from my private practice. They illustrate common nursing problems encountered in the home.

Constipation

''Bowel care'' is rather well known by most nurses. Elimination problems are primarily those resulting from inactivity. Combined with reduced fluid intake and loss of Valsalva action (abdominal straining against a closed glottis), constipation can and does become severe rapidly. It is not uncommon for constipation to precipitate costly hospitalizations and even death.

Example. Mr. S's wife called for a consultation for her husband who was quadriplegic from ALS and had chosen not to have any life supports. He was eating little and had had no bowel movement for over a week. There was no reported breathing problem. On consulting with the home care nurse, it was quickly apparent that constipation was not considered enough of a problem for the agency to authorize a nurse home visit. The statement repeatedly given was, ''He is just going to have to realize that he is dying and not to complain so much.''

On physical exam in the home, I found Mr. S. to be chair-ridden, severely dysphasic, dehydrated, with a beginning sacral pressure sore, shallow respirations, poor diaphragm excursion, poor secretion clearance, reduced muscle tone, and without a Valsalva action.

Nursing consultation in this case was followed by the provision of direct care. After manual bowel evacuation with Mr. S. lying on the floor in the bathroom (his only comfortable position), the problem cleared. The teaching provided was not lost on him or his wife, and in his remaining three months of life, constipation did not recur, despite the rapid downhill course of the disease.

Dying of ALS

Once people learn that their vital breathing and swallowing can weaken, they need to learn about life support options (5). Dying without life support for breathing is the ''natural'' way. Extending life with machines is an available option. Three main avenues of choice are:

1. The physician provides all care and decision making if/when the time comes that life support is needed.

2. The person lets events take their course and falls prey to whatever is available for his or her needs, usually at the time of a predictable emergency.
3. The person learns the options and makes realistic plans based on all information available. It is not easy to learn what is available, nor is it a palatable subject for anyone to have to investigate. The powerful protective mechanisms of denial keep people from addressing anxiety-provoking topics.

Although it seems to me that the third option (self-determination) is the best, this is not always so. Early planning with a client requires skill, sensitivity, and the right timing. When fear cannot be addressed successfully, a trusting patient-doctor relationship may dictate that the person rely solely on his physician for making life-and-death decisions.

Since Congress passed the Patient Self-Determination Act (6) in 1990, nearly all states have enacted advance directives such as the Durable Power of Attorney for Health Care (DPA/HC), which permits and legally supports self-determination regarding life support decisions (7). While an increasing number of physicians are addressing what can be called the "life care plan," the reality is still that the home care nurse is often required to initiate the plan. Agency nurses are not usually ready for this and can use the ALS consultant to help.

Some health care agencies support self-determinations (the DPA/HC) by developing policies for nursing care of the person wishing to avoid, or even discontinue, life supports. Without an agency policy, the home care nurse cannot be allowed to attend a person who wishes to discontinue the ventilator. Thus, the dying patient may be deprived of trusted assistance most needed at the time of death.

Communication Losses

Losing the ability to communicate, a most devastating happening, occurs with combined anarthria and total paralysis. Eventually only the most sophisticated communication devices can be used and even they end up on the closet floor. The alert, intuitive family caregiver or the nurse is often the only one left who can reliably understand what the person is trying to communicate.

Example. When I first met Sue, she had been homebound for five years. With vocal cord paralysis and quadriplegia, she could make her needs known by only a series of facial expressions, an alphabet board, and loud noises when she was distressed. Her mainstay was her father, who died the following year. Her mother, whose health was deteriorating, then provided all care with help from Sue's sister and a neighbor.

California state medical insurance does not cover communication devices. Through referral to the communication device program of the local ALSA chapter, Sue was provided with a computer communicator. For a while, she did the shopping lists and remembered her mother's medication times for her. Her mother had several health emergencies, and Sue could do nothing for her. Things went from bad to worse, and spoon-feeding became increasingly difficult. She weighed sixty pounds and began to develop pressure sores. Several ulcers were at Stage 4. The house was a mess. She had stopped using the computer because it was so hard to keep it set up and leave space for her other required care.

At this point, her mother requested another consultation visit. The choice seemed to be "where to die." Sue had avoided all discussion of this subject. I raised it, forcing the issue into the open. She was adamant in her refusal to go to the hospital or to accept the feeding tube. Systemic infection from pressure sores finally forced hospitalization, at which time Sue relented and accepted the feeding tube.

She survived the ordeal and went from the hospital to a nursing home, taking her computer with her. Within weeks, she became everyone's "pet" and the staff learned to communicate with her. Her sores healed and she gained weight. At present, Sue is glad to be alive, and it seems clear that the communication device is her link to survival and obtaining the loving care her spirit needs. She wrote me that the real reason she accepted the tube and nursing home placement was that she realized she was being selfish to hold out.

An Unusual Family Member Coping Problem

In the following case, referrals to community experts proved unnecessary.

Example. I knew Jean well. She and her brother had consulted with me when their mother, Laura, became disabled with ALS. They could not cope with their mother's childish, demanding nature, and both had left home years before. They expressed concern for their grandmother who, despite her own cardiac condition, was providing all the home care for Laura. They loved their Grannie and did everything they could to ease her burden, but avoided Laura and her petulant demands. About a month after Laura died, Jean called me in alarm. She was developing symptoms of ALS. Questioning revealed that her mother had placed a hex on her, saying "Wait 'til I die, and then see what you get."

At the end of the telephone consult—one of my longest calls—I offered to find Jean a referral for the help she so obviously needed. I immediately located help from one of our chapter medical advisers, who had received an Irish medical education that included exorcism. He offered help. Her response was, "Since our phone call, my symptoms have disappeared and I am fine now. I don't need any referrals." The only follow-up was with her grandmother, who said Jean was functioning well.

Dying Without Life Support

Example. In this case, there was no nursing agency involved. Mr. F. had ALS. His daughter, Kathy, worked nights as a nursing aide in a nursing home. Kathy called for a consultation. Her father had not been sleeping, was depressed, and had missed two ALS support group meetings, which was rather unlike him.

Physical examination showed use of the diaphragm, but no use of intercostal or accessory muscles for breathing, and he had shallow, fast respirations. He could no longer speak but could walk and use his hands.

An inarticulate man even when he could speak, he had no questions or demands—just the round-eyed look of a mute appeal for help. I framed questions for him and he nodded "yes," that while he did not want to hear the news, he needed to know what lay ahead. I knew from support group discussions that he had chosen no life support.

I described in some detail what respiratory failure is like, pointing out his symptoms to him and his family. I also described what life supports are like, what they cost, what laws prevail, giving information calmly, factually, and carefully neutral.

I was able to tell him that in my experience, I had never seen anyone strangle to death even though that is what he had been told was likely to happen. He said nothing. Kathy followed me out to the car, saying that nobody dared to speak thus to him and that she was grateful.

He slept soundly from that night on. Soon after, Kathy took leave from work to provide all his nursing care. On the day he died, she looked at him and said, "Today's the day, isn't it, Dad?" He nodded and smiled. She called relatives and friends to visit, and he died peacefully nine hours later.

Consultation with the Home Health Agency Nurse and the Family

At times, the consultation is more effective for the family than for the person with ALS.

Example. Chuck knew about ventilators and did not want one. He could suction himself through his open "trach" and refused all personal help. His wife, Brunella, brought piecework home from her factory job in order to care for Chuck herself.

He wanted to kill himself but did not have the strength to pull the trigger of his pistol. His anger turned onto his wife daily as he rejected her solicitous care. He could still swing at her with his arms and walk out of the house, creating constant worry for her, even though weapons were removed.

Joint consultation with the home health agency nurse was provided for this couple. The agency nurse had never before seen a person with ALS. During the initial visit, we were both pushed bodily out of the room by Chuck. Both Brunella and the home care nurse called me when problems became insuperable. The nurse and I supported her efforts to leave him free and not become panicked about the gun threats. She was to call one of us if she was desperate. She could not leave, even to attend the local support group, and Chuck refused professional counseling. One night he was admitted to the hospital and died the following day of pneumonia complications, all the while continuing his vigorous refusal of the ventilator and repeated requests for someone to please kill him. Before dying, he did indicate thanks to Brunella for her patience.

In this case, our services were more for the support of Brunella than for Chuck. We felt that his unresolved problems could have resulted in frequent hospitalizations if we had not been available to help her with the incredible stress.

Endstage Disease and Dying After Ventilator Disconnect

One case is detailed here of experience with people who discontinued ventilator support at home and died as a result (8–11). Many people prefer to die at home than in a hospital and could be granted their wishes if we, as home care personnel, were prepared.

The ventilator home care nurse must be prepared to help the person and the family with readiness-to-die issues. Using careful assessment and calling in qualified consultants as needed, the home care nurse can effectively initiate home assessment of the physical, emotional, and mental factors without costly hospitalization.

A pattern emerged from our clinical experiences and an outline of the process is shown in Table 13-2 as a guideline for home care agencies, physicians, and attorneys to follow and refine through further experience (11).

Although guidelines are fairly clear for weaning a person from the ventilator to independent breathing (a hospital procedure) (12,13), predictive indices have not been identified for people whose goal is to permit death to follow disconnect. I suggest the following definition for successful outcome of ventilator disconnect as ''a peaceful death within thirty minutes to twenty-four hours of the disconnect, providing all steps in the readiness process have been satisfactorily completed.''

Step 7 includes the trial disconnect. Temporary disconnects are routinely done by all caregivers for suctioning the airway, but not to assess tolerance off the ventilator. This is done by the physician at the time of the first home visit. It provides subjective feedback to the person and can reduce fears. Spontaneous breathing and apnea can be noted. Breathing and heart rate, exhaled volume, skin changes, and oxygen saturation, as well as emotional readiness, can be inexpensively assessed.

Compensated respiratory alkalosis, a typical condition for the long- term ventilator-dependent person, can confound the assessment due to temporary apnea following disconnect. This is due to CO_2 depletion and depression of the respiratory drive. Patient comfort may dictate terminating the trial disconnect before eucapnia resumes and hypoxic drives, if present, can override the apnea.

Despite these difficulties, trial disconnects have been successfully used with patients in my caseload and contributed significantly to patient comfort and trust. The actual disconnect is done as a second visit. The waiting time is very important and should not be truncated, since the family's comfort level also takes time to develop, regardless of their stated desires to ''get on with it'' once the decision has been made.

Table 13-2. Ventilator Disconnects at Home: A Ten-Step Process

1. Wish Identification	By the ALS person or the home caregiver, frequently the nurse, who contacts the consultant or physician.
2. Motivation Assessment	A delicate process—the accuracy depending on the person/family being well-informed and without outside influences that can color motivation. Open communication is mandatory. Step 2 takes several months.
3. Legal Consultation	DPA/HC is revalidated. Use of an attorney is encouraged, especially when communication is severely compromised by dysphasia and hand paralysis.
4. Plans Regarding Dialing 911	Depends on local paramedic laws and policies. In many areas, calling "911" results in mandatory resuscitation. Orange County, California, has pioneered a method whereby paramedics are not obliged to resuscitate dying people. (14)
5. "No Code" Orders	"Do not resuscitate (DNR)" orders must be in place if home health agencies are providing care. At present, many agencies have no policies. Hospice usually requires DNR orders. The patient must be involved in this step.
6. Contingency Planning for Respiratory Arrests	Includes written instructions posted by the telephone and all relevant phone numbers. Timing is very important. Plans can be set only after the person is comfortable with his/her decision.
7. First Physician Home Visit	Physician meets with the person, family, and staff. A trial disconnect is done by the physician and a date is set.
8. Prescriptions	Obtained by family (not the nurse) and made available for the home care personnel. (15) This step helps family readiness.
9. Discontinuing Ventilator Support Including Second Physician Home Visit	Anxiety-relieving medication is given as ordered about two hours ahead of physician arrival. Nursing consultant is present. Physician disconnects at the trach site.
10. Follow-Up	By the nursing consultant several weeks or months later to clarify any confusion and provide emotional support and maintain open communication. A most rewarding final step.

The whole process requires many months, as decision making requires time for clarification and reflection. For details, see Beal Libby "Discontinuing Ventilator Support at Home: Clinical Experience with ALS in Orange County, California" (11)

Without exception, the disconnects, done at the later visit, were without struggle and families were content with the outcome.

Example. Ken was paralyzed "up to the eyebrows"—almost literally. He had no dependable nonverbal communication left; even eye blink and eye gaze were not dependable. A keyboard communicator stood idle. Mary, the LVN, was the only one who could understand what he wanted. One day he indicated to Mary that he wanted to see me because he wished to disconnect his ventilator. At the consult visit, it was clear he was not ready. He only wanted help to send an application for a cure about which he had just heard from the night nurse. Afterwards I phoned his physician, who had never been involved in this type of care but said he would support our action by counseling with the children.

Three months later, Ken had a week of constant crying. No reason could be found, but Mary had a hunch. She said, "Ken, are you crying because you want to see Barbara again?" He immediately stopped crying and his eyes tracked her around the room. Their lawyer made a home visit to verify the DPA/HC and to revalidate Ken's intent. Ken was able to use a slight shoulder shrug to communicate reliably. The medical director of the local Muscular Dystrophy Association visited Ken twice, first to conduct a trial disconnect, and to set the date. The nursing agency allowed Mary to be in the kitchen, but not in the room. I administered the premedication. The physician arrived thirty minutes later and talked with Ken, his wife, and the three boys. The family opted to stand by in the kitchen with Mary. Ken took no breaths after the ventilator was disconnected and died fourteen minutes later. His family was supported by the nurse and their priest. Follow-up six months and one year later revealed that the experience had left no regrets for any of them, including the caregivers.

Summary and Comments

Many levels and types of nursing care are given people with ALS. Most caregivers occasionally need expert guidance. They also need hope and much emotional support. Such guidance from nursing experts is not accessible through many insurance plans.

Most home care generalist nurses have had little or no education about ALS in their basic programs. The improvement found in recent nursing textbooks, discussed in this chapter's beginning, should soon be reflected in an improvement in professional nursing care available in the home.

Nursing care of the person dying from ALS is different from the care of other dying people because of the nature of this progressive and fatal neuromuscular disorder.

Yet it is clear to us, as nursing consultants, that by conferring with people on the unique care required to get through a devastating disease such as ALS, we have saved the health care industry thousands of dollars. We have helped people cope and find peace in handling a disease for which there is no high tech solution and for whom hospital is not the appropriate place to receive long-term expert care.

References

1. Hickey JV. *The Clinical Practice of Neurological and Neurosurgical Nursing.* Philadelphia: Lippincott, 1992, pp. 634–640.
2. Smeltzer SC, Bare BG, eds. *Brunner and Suddarth's Textbook of Medical-Surgical Nursing,* 7th ed. Philadelphia: Lippincott, 1992, pp. 1720–1722.
3. Silverstein MD, Stocking CB, Antel JP, Beckwith J, Roos RP, Siegler M. Amyotrophic lateral sclerosis and life-sustaining therapy: Patients' desires for information, participation in decision making, and life-sustaining therapy. *Mayo Clin Proc* 1991,66: 906–913.
4. Krantz DS, Baum A, Wideman M. Assessment of preferences for self-treatment and information in health care. *J Pers Soc Psychol* 1980;39:977–990.
5. Strull WM, Lo B, Charles G. Do patients want to participate in medical decision making? *JAMA* 1984;252:2990–2994.
6. Omnibus Reconciliation Act 1990. Title IV. Section 4206. Congressional Record, October 26, 1990;12638.
7. Emanuel LL, Barry MJ, Stoeckle JD, Ettelson LM, Emanuel EJ. Advance directives for medical care—a case of greater use. *N Engl J Med* 1991;324:899.
8. American Thoracic Society. Withholding and withdrawing life-sustaining therapy. *Am Rev Respir Dis* 1991;144:726–731.
9. The Hastings Center. *Guidelines on the Termination of Life-Sustaining Treatment and the Care of the Dying.* Briarcliff Manor, NY: The Hastings Center, 1987.
10. Ruark JE, Raffin TA and the Stanford University Medical Center Committee on Ethics. Initiating and withdrawing life support. Principles and practice in adult medicine. *N Engl J Med* 1988;318:25–30.
11. Beal Libby BT. Discontinuing life support at home: Clinical experiences in Orange County, California. In: Colbert A, et al. The Ventilator: Psychosocial and Medical Aspects, Philadelphia: Charles Press Publishers (in press).
12. Yang KL, Tobin MJ. A prospective study of indices predicting the outcomes of trials of weaning from mechanical ventilation. *N Engl J Med* 1991;324:1445–1450.
13. Strickland JH Jr, Hasson JH. A computer-controlled ventilator weaning system. *Chest* 1991;100:1016–1019.
14. Jones L. O.C.'s terminally ill can soon halt medics' heroics. *Los Angeles Times* 1991; Sunday, July 14, A1–29.
15. Edwards BS, Ueno WM. Sedation before ventilator withdrawal. *J Clin Ethics* 1991; 9:118–122.

14

Successful Home Care

Mary Beth Parks, R.N.

Agency Nursing Care

A majority of ALS patients will require professional at-home nursing services at some point during the progression of this long-term catastrophic disease. Experience tells us that the quality of the nursing services received affect both the quality of life and the dignity of the patient.

ALS patients present unique and demanding challenges to the caregiver or health professional. Effectively dealing with ALS patients requires not only "generic" nursing skills to address the patient's physical needs but also specialized nursing skills in order to handle the patient's emotional and psychological concerns. Unfortunately, the highly specialized types of services needed by the patient are rarely obtained, so the bulk of home care service frequently falls to a relative, friend, or other caregiver who is neither licensed nor skilled in ALS care. Although the services of an LVN or RN experienced in general health care may be retained, the LVN or RN may not be trained in the special approaches required by the ALS patient. In some cases, insurance companies do not cover the expenses involved in ALS nursing services; home visits are covered only to the point whereby the patients have been sufficiently educated to take care of themselves. Since nursing care is one of the largest expenses involved in ALS cases, we find that those families without private funds tend to do without vital nursing needs at the very time they most need them.

Although many families manage to cope relatively well with the devastating

197

health care problems presented by ALS, those with sufficient financial resources will turn to a home health care agency for education and guidance. The need for information and support is great in ALS cases. Due to the unique progressive nature of the disease, it is soon discovered that the care and planning provided one week become inadequate for the same patient by the following week. Additionally, agency nurses often find themselves alternately cast into the roles of direct caregiver, grief counselor, problem-solver, educator, referral agent, and equipment-finder.

As the need for highly specialized ALS home care increases, newly formed ALS clinics and ALS consultants appear to be instrumental in providing guidance to agencies as well as to individual families. Agency nurses may dual-schedule the ALS consultant to accompany them on the initial home visit in order to reap the benefits of specialized advice in the areas of planning, counseling, problem-solving, and nursing assessment.

Nursing Assessment

Once an initial home visit has been scheduled, the consultant will counsel with the agency nurse, the patient, the patient's current caregivers, and physician. A nursing assessment will evaluate the extent of the patient's disability, the level of function, the equipment, and life-style adaptation.

Specifically, nursing assessment should focus on the major concerns that present the greatest amounts of difficulty to a patient suffering with ALS.

Neurological

For the typical ALS patient, there generally is no decline in rational thought processes; there is normal mentation throughout all stages of the illness. However, once bulbar dysfunction manifests itself, the patient's ability to speak, swallow, and eat may be severely impaired. For example, speech may become slurred, nasal, low in tone, or garbled. ALS patients often become frustrated trying to make their needs known. When speech is down to a whisper, an amplifier can be held or worn near the mouth, attached either to eyeglasses or on the front collar a of shirt or blouse. Many patients are still able to mouth the words distinctively enough to be understood by lipreading.

When there is no upper extremity difficulty and hands can be used, patients may write or point to alphabetic letters in order to make known their needs. The consultant may recommend the use of communication devices, such as light boards, magic doodles, Speak and Spell, Ouijas, and simple picture boards. The John Delserone board, in particular, works very well as it can be memorized easily, allowing the patient to communicate well enough to eliminate board use.

The consultant may suggest a computerized voice synthesizer or techniques to teach the patient to speak slowly and succinctly when upper extremity difficulty is present. Additionally, the consultant may instruct the patient in techniques for swallowing or advise medication or suctioning as means of managing hyper-salivation in patients affected by bulbar dysfunction.

Cardiopulmonary

The ALS patient may suffer impaired lung functioning caused by aspiration and weakening of the diaphragm muscles. If the consultant assesses lung problems at the time of the home visit, specific nursing techniques such as positioning, coupled with medication management, can be used. The patient who displays a mottled or cyanotic appearance may be displaying the effects of poor circulation due to inactivity. If the consultant determines that this is the problem, nursing measures to improve circulation will be recommended.

Abdominal

Constipation is one of the most common complaints among ALS patients. The malady is caused by immobility and poor nutrition. Often the patient is unable to manipulate food around in the mouth with the tongue. The consultant may coach the patient to take in a balanced diet that includes bulk in the form of vegetables and fruit. If the patient is on a liquid diet, warmed prune and apple juice, as well as over-the-counter remedies such as Metamucil and Fibercon, can be utilized as a method of alleviating the problem. Recommendations will be made to increase daily fluid intake to 2000–3000 cc and to engage in increased physical activity such as standing, changing positions, and exercising legs and arms frequently. In short, the consultant will counsel the patient to draw on his or her own resources to solve the problem.

Skin

The ALS patient should be kept mobile and should practice good skin care and general hygiene in order to avoid such skin maladies as the dryness, oiliness, and flaking associated with the disease. Since common problem areas target new hair growth, the consultant may suggest any of a variety of cremes, powders, and tar-based shampoos to treat scalp, underarm, pubic, and facial hair spots.

Fluids and Electrolytes

In regard to patient intake, a patient's weight maintenance is very important to sustain his or her quality of life. Weight maintenance is often very difficult to achieve. Because of muscle atrophy, which is natural in the course of ALS progression, the patient will lose weight. To further complicate issues, bulbar involvement creates the need to continually adjust the patient's diet. By modifying the consistency and texture of the foods and fluids, the risks of aspiration are decreased. When changes in consistency of foods become necessary, it is useful to think in terms of familiar foods. The five diets for swallowing problems are: steak consistency diet, pot roast consistency diet, meat loaf consistency diet, pudding consistency diet, and cream consistency diet (tube feedings). In whatever manner calories are obtained, the ambulatory patient will still require up to 2500 calories daily in order to maintain weight, the wheelchair- or bed-bound patient 1200–1500 calories.

The ALS patient who is consuming food five or more times daily, yet is still unable to maintain a stable weight or sufficient caloric intake, should be counseled in the pros and cons of using a nasopharyngeal or gastrostomy tube. The nasopharyngeal tube can be inserted quite easily, and the patient can avoid a surgical procedure. This tube, however, requires monthly replacement, and patients often complain about the annoyance of the tube as it hangs from the nose or the discomfort in the back of the throat.

The gastrostomy tube seems to be used more by most ALS patients. A percutaneous endoscopic gastrojejunostomy (PEG) can be inserted at the bedside under a local anesthesia . It is inserted with endoscopy and can be maintained for years. The contraindications for this tube are thoracic stomach, ventriculoperitoneal shunt, severe coagulopathy, active peptic ulcer disease, previous left upper quadrant surgery, oral and esophageal pathology, gastric retention, morbid obesity, or marked ascites. The patient can usually be discharged when the feedings are tolerated and bowel function is normal, usually a four- to seven-day process.

In regard to patient output, we find that bladder muscle functioning is usually not affected until the final stages of the disease. However, urinary complaints from ALS patients stem from their inability to get to a bathroom facility in time by themselves. With male patients who ambulate slowly, an easily accessible urinal is recommended.

Activity

ALS patients need to be counseled on the enormous benefits of remaining mobile. Aids such as ankle and weight supports, canes, walkers, and, eventually, wheelchairs may be suggested in order to keep the patient moving. Movement is of extreme importance as even exercising muscles that are no longer used will stave off contractures. If contractures can be prevented, the patient's ability to sit comfortably for long periods of time in a recliner or wheelchair will be greatly enhanced. Again, the consultant's role here is to underscore and reinforce the patient's commitment to maintain an active life-style for as long as possible.

Emotional

ALS patients report that it can be very disturbing and embarrassing when they become uncontrollably weepy, short-tempered, or "silly." The patient, as well as friends and family members, must be made aware of the fact that ALS can produce emotional roller coaster reactions; highs and lows are part of the disease and cannot be controlled by the patient. The consultant can inform and counsel the family concerning the types of medications that can help alleviate emotional instability in individual ALS cases.

Patients should be strongly advised to join and participate in a local support group. It seems that patients and families often find their courage and strength from one another, especially when it becomes easier to share with each other their triumphs and setbacks. Patients who had a gastrostomy tube inserted since last meeting are often greeted with applause as they share their experiences. Suggestions are freely offered by the "old hands" in the group with gastrostomies on how to pin it, how to clean it from the inside, and what kinds of stop-cocks work the best.

Other Consultative Services

A patient stricken with ALS will move through the various stages of grief—initial shock, anger, depression, acceptance—in accordance with his or her individual psychological makeup. Only one thing is certain in all ALS cases; that is, these patients, suddenly faced with the unimaginable, wish to cling to every last possible shred of human dignity. A primary function of the ALS consultant is to provide the patient and family with coping skills, dispensed at psychologically correct moments, that will enable them to come to grips with long-term planning during each phase of total disease progression. This information may be imparted to the agency nurse, the caregiver, or the individual patient as he or she is ready to discuss hopes, fears, life support options, death, and dying.

Direct consultation, i.e., where the consultant makes a home visit to counsel, guide, and instruct the patient, is only one available avenue. Referrals may be made by the consultant to home health care agencies, to local support groups, and round table discussion groups on specialized topics such as high technology ventilator systems, telephone consultation services, and the best sources of equipment that will become necessary as the disease runs its course.

The consultant may act as a liaison between the patient, the family physician, and the insurance companies. Patients may ask the consultant to verify the diagnosis and other findings they have obtained from their own physician. In order to comply with the patient's request, the consultant will obtain and examine the patient's health history and physical assessment via direct contact with the physician. Part of the nursing assessment involves determining the patient's resources for providing skilled home care. In the event the patient is fortunate enough to have full insurance coverage, skilled nursing care can be implemented. A letter of medical necessity provided by the physician must show that the required care has to be rendered by a skilled nurse. Suctioning, which is necessary during dysphagia, and administering gastrostomy feedings cannot be done by nurses' aides in many states. A detailed and informative letter of necessity from a physician can point out life-threatening conditions that will hasten the disease process if they are not medically supervised by a skilled nurse on a daily basis. The physician should advise the insurance company that the care necessary for this patient, along with a family that is willing to supplement some nursing hours, will cost far less than a lengthy hospitalization. In the event that there are no financial resources available, the consultant will advise pulling together the family, friends, and church to take care of their loved one.

The consultant also takes on the roles of professional writer and public speaker toward the goal of educating the public on the unique aspects of this devastating disease. These roles include publishing articles on the newest techniques for combating ALS in newsletters for home health care professionals and speaking on a variety of topics related to ALS at nursing conferences.

Experiences in Japan

Ben Cohen is a 46-year-old American citizen who has been living in Japan since 1974. He is a distinguished potter of Echizen pottery and quite renowned for his work in that country. When stricken with ALS in the summer of 1989, little did he know that his two- to five-year life expectancy could be shortened.

As his body deteriorated physically, Ben waited for bulbar dysfunction to strike. Through his own research, he felt that bulbar dysfunction would progress before the onset of any pulmonary problems. However, sudden respiratory distress and CO_2 narcosis left him with a life-or-death decision. Ben chose life.

Although Ben is married to a Japanese woman, which qualifies him for health care benefits, there are no home health care agencies in Japan. Patients on ventilators there are usually placed in hospitals. Those patients who can no longer make their needs known are fed and kept clothed and dry, but there may be little quality to their lives. For those Japanese who can afford them, private nurses in the home are available but extremely costly, and they must be trained by family and fellow nurses.

The remote fishing village in which Ben lives is limited in medical personnel. The villagers of Kadanji gathered together and made a commitment to bring Ben home and to learn to care for him. A committee was formed of friends, some professionals, and three local doctors to organize the training of local rice farmers, fishermen, and fellow potters.

An ALS consultant was hired by a group of Ben's friends in Los Angeles who had started their own fund raising. This nurse spent three weeks in Kadanji, training anyone who walked through the door. A videotape was produced and translated into Japanese for Ben's caregivers. The video demonstrated the vital services required to sustain Ben's life on a ventilator system. A "how to" video of his breathing treatment, exercise routine, turning and positioning, transferring, and maintenence of his machinery was observed. Ben turned out to be the best student. He was taught to know his body and to listen to it. Ben needed to be the primary teacher of his caregivers, and this task required great patience, trust, and courage. As his caregivers would do return demonstrations, he learned to compliment and encourage the novices as well as tactfully advise the professionals. A daily plan of care was written describing his hour-by-hour routine. ALS patients usually prefer routine and consistency in order to maintain that control in their life. Ben is still alive today and continues to work designing his pottery. Although he can move only his eyes and mouth, he designs his artwork on the computer and employs his wife, Reko, to serve as his hands. His caregivers act as his team when the pottery goes for firing twice a year. Since stricken with ALS in 1989, Ben has displayed his latest artwork in Tokyo galleries three times.

What was done in Japan is also what the ALS consultant does in the United States or, for that matter, anywhere. After consulting with the physician, other team members, the patient, and family, he or she writes a comprehensive detailed plan of care. An hour-by-hour, step-by-step plan is established by reading the care plan, observing the care, and reviewing it on a VCR, which can also be used for demonstrations.

Finding the right personnel to care for an ALS patient is not an easy task. The nurse who needs to see that his or her care is helping the patient get better may become stressed working with ALS patients who are in continual decline. Nurses should be carefully screened for competency and personality. A good knowledge of nursing and how to respond to system breakdown is essential. Nurses and caregivers should be encouraged to work with the patient in determining what nonprescription actions may remedy a given situation before the physician is contacted. Personality also plays a large part in the screening of the nurse who will be the caregiver. Knowing as much about the patient's personality and determining what his or her particular likes and dislikes are enables the consultant to select the best nurse to work well with the patient. There are no stereotypes. Young patients do not necessarily want young nurses. Sometimes they want to be mothered by someone older. Older patients may not want a nurse of their age, but perhaps someone younger.

One thing they all want, however, is the nurse or caregiver who makes them feel secure and hopeful. Hopeful is very often a difficult word for the ALS patient to accept. The caregiver should not destroy the patient's hope—nor is it fair to offer false hope. The best course the caregiver can take is to assist the patient to achieve as much control of life as possible through encouragement and the promotion of decision-making skills. Even if patients can only blink their eyes in a yes-no response, simple things that they decide will give them this control—decisions about what clothes to wear, what to prepare for supper, what bills to pay. A routine should be maintained for as long as possible, be it church, bingo, PTA, baseball, and so on.

The best advice that can be shared with all caregivers for the ALS patient is to facilitate patient dignity. This is one of the few things that ALS should not be allowed to take away. Remember that the patients want to be treated as they were when they were healthy and productive members of society. Their productivity as an ALS patient is only limited by their own desire and determination.

15

Psychosocial-Spiritual Overview

Evelyn R. McDonald, M.S.

The previous chapters have provided a comprehensive exploration of the physical aspects of ALS, palliative treatment for clinical manifestations, and useful environmental adaptations. All of these topics relate primarily to the effects of ALS caused by denervation of the skeletal muscles. However, the experience of ALS goes far beyond the physical body. The patient's psychological, social, and spiritual well-being are challenged every step of the way, and critical issues are faced by the family and even by the health care providers from whom the patient and family seek treatment.

Socrates said, "There is no disease of the body apart from the mind." Simply stated, this means that the activities of the mind (one's thoughts, emotions, and psychosocial and spiritual experiences) and the physical body are not separate, walled off entities but are interconnected, each continually influencing the other. This interactive system creates human beings who are unique in their responses to all of life, including illness.

The patient's psychosocial-spiritual status is of great importance to the health care practitioner. It profoundly affects the patient's experience of having ALS, affects how the palliative treatment offered will be accepted and used, and also influences survival time. Awareness of the psychosocial-spiritual dimension of ALS and assessment of individual patients in this area contribute to a greater awareness of the patient's perceptions of his illness and the effect the illness has on both his daily life and his sense of meaning and purpose.

Other systems in addition to the patient's body/mind come into play in working with the ALS patient. One is the "family system," which is deeply affected by the patient's illness and which in turn affects the patient's experience of living with the disease. Another is the health care system, in which the patient and family are impacted by each person and situation they encounter. The direct providers to the patient form an important part of the health care system; these doctors, nurses, physical and occupational therapists, social workers, and counselors must work as a team in order to ensure treatment of the "whole person."

This chapter examines the relationship between ALS and the psychosocial-spiritual dimension of the patient, the spouse, and the health care practitioner and offers suggestions for appropriate management. Topics include: 1) a discussion of quality of life for the ALS patient; 2) a psychosocial-spiritual profile of a "typical" ALS patient, taking into account length and severity of illness and other crucial factors; 3) an indication of potential problems—and solutions—in the area of the patient's social functioning; 4) a discussion of psychosocial-spiritual assessment tools and interventions; 5) a review of the experiences of spouses of ALS patients and the effects of the disease on the spouse-patient relationship; and 6) suggestions for health care practitioners serving ALS patients.

Observations concerning the importance of psychosocial-spiritual management are based on the author's experience of a decade of meeting and talking with ALS patients, their families, and health care providers, and on the results of the ALS Patient Profile Project, a multidisciplinary team study of 144 ALS patients and 123 spouses or primary caregivers in three cities in the United States.

The Patient

The quality of life cannot be measured simply by evaluating physical function. A person with a well-functioning mind and a degenerating or minimally functioning body can experience a life rich and full of activity.

Mr. W is on a respirator, has a feeding tube, cannot vocalize, and is unable to move his arms and legs, and yet a feeling of fun and vitality surrounds him. He and his wife, along with their nurse, go shopping, participate in community service, travel, visit with a wide circle of friends and family, and sometimes design elaborate practical jokes. Even though he is severely "disabled," he clearly enjoys a high quality of life, one that many people in "perfect health" would envy for its zest and love. He continually finds meaningful ways to help and inspire others and is, in turn, loved by many people.

Perhaps quality of life is more accurately represented by the "spirit" of the patient. In our study, 37 percent of the patients found that something good came from their ALS, and some of the most severely ill patients had lives that they considered fulfilling. Although not every ALS patient achieves such a degree of quality, it is critical that the health care professional believe that such a state is possible and that it can exist throughout the progression of the disease.

How can health care professionals assist in the maintenance of a high quality of life for the individual with ALS?

- By considering the patient in the context of the physical, psychosocial, spiritual, family, and health care systems;
- By being aware of the psychosocial-spiritual dynamics in the ALS patient (see below), which suggest what to look for in the patient as the disease progresses;
- By assessing each patient's psychosocial-spiritual status and providing follow-up where indicated.

Psychosocial-Spiritual Profile

Just who is it that you are encountering when an ALS patient comes to you for treatment? Is there a characteristic personality pattern of the ALS patient that is different from the normal population or other ill populations? Several studies have attempted to answer this question. In a study of ten ALS patients who were compared to patients with inoperable cancer, Brown and Mueller (1) found a lifetime pattern of active mastery along with the belief that they (the ALS patients) are in control of their lives. In contrast, a study of forty ALS patients by Houpt, Gould, and Norris (2) failed to confirm these findings. Additionally, when Peters, Swenson, and Mulder (3) administered the MMPI to forty-four ALS patients, they found that thirty-eight of the patients did not differ from general medical patients.

In our study of 144 ALS patients, we evaluated many different aspects of psychological, social, and spiritual status. This evaluation included tests that measured depression, hopelessness, perceived stress, anger expression, loneliness, health locus of control, life satisfaction, and purpose in life. Surprisingly, patients' scores for each test scale covered a broad range, suggesting great variability in psychosocial-spiritual status. When the average scores for these tests were compared to those of a normal, healthy population, the only differences were that the ALS patients exhibited more depression (60 percent had some level of measurable depression compared to the 16–20 percent typical of a "healthy" population) and had a more external health locus of control. Neither depression nor an external health locus of control is unusual in patients with chronic disease.

The wide variability and overall normality of these results suggest that there is no predictable psychosocial-spiritual profile for the ALS patient. The patient who comes to you for treatment may fall anywhere on the psychosocial-spiritual spectrum from well-being to distress. A person exhibiting well-being will be experiencing high satisfaction with life, a well-defined purpose, a more internal health locus of control, appropriate expression of anger, and minimal levels of depression, hopelessness, loneliness, and stress. A person in distress, on the other hand, will tend to experience high levels of depression, hopelessness, loneliness, and stress, little satisfaction with life, a lack of purpose, a more external health locus of control, and little expression of anger.

Many factors influence where a patient will fall on the psychosocial-spiritual spectrum, including the physical parameters associated with the progression of the disease, social factors, the patient's environment and family relationships, the patient's spirit, and the patient's experience with the health care system.

Response to Physical Challenges

Although the psychosocial-spiritual status of a patient is not solely determined by the physical aspects associated with progression of the disease, the two are related in a number of ways. Awareness of this relationship is necessary for comprehensive care of the patient. Significant physical parameters include mode of onset of ALS, age of the patient, severity of the disease, how long the patient has had the illness, rapidity of decline, and ventilator-dependency (Table 15-1).

Mode of Onset

With regard to mode of onset, we found no significant differences in the psychosocial-spiritual profile between patients whose initial symptoms were bulbar versus patients whose initial symptoms were spinal. The frustration of individuals in both groups was apparent. The particular challenges faced were different,

Table 15-1. Relationship Between Physical Parameters Associated with ALS and Psychosocial-Spiritual Profile[a]

	Psychosocial-Spiritual Profile			P Value[b]
	Distress	Neutral	Well-Being	
Sample	34 (24%)	71 (51%)	34 (24%)	
Age (years)	64 ± 12.3	59 ± 11.7	57 ± 12.0	0.03
Severity of Disease (total ALSSS)[c]	22 ± 7.9	26 ± 7.8	27 ± 8.4	0.03
Length of Illness (months)	48 ± 70.4	48 ± 54.9	72 ± 70.3	0.10
Onset Mode:				0.39
Bulbar	5 (15%)	13 (18%)	3 (9%)	
Spinal	25 (74%)	47 (66%)	27 (79%)	
Ventilator-Dependent	2 (6%)	9 (13%)	5 (15%)	0.47

Psychosocial-spiritual profile based on seven tests measuring depression, hopelessness, perceived stress, anger expression, health locus of control, life satisfaction, and purpose in life.
[a] Sample = 139. Results as n (and %) or mean ± standard deviation.
[b] Based on Kruskal-Wallis one-way ANOVAS and chi-square tests.
[c] ALS Severity Scale (Range = 0–40; the lower the number, the more severe) (4).

however. Patients with bulbar onset often experienced fear and anger over losing the ability to communicate clearly and expressed reluctance to participate in social functions. In patients with spinal onset, the frustration, fear, and anger centered around the apparent or imminent loss of independence. Such a loss could be a major adjustment for the 66 percent of the patients in our study who described themselves as fiercely independent before ALS. Only 18 percent considered themselves fiercely independent at the time of the study.

Age

The older population (those over 65) had higher levels of depression and hopelessness, indicating more psychosocial-spiritual distress. ALS may not be the cause of this depression or hopelessness but may exacerbate a state that existed prior to its onset, especially if the patient had already been facing end-of-life issues. Additionally, many older patients voiced concern about being a burden on their spouse, particularly when the spouse had physical limitations or a chronic illness. Some of these couples were initially reluctant to voice difficulties surrounding physical care. As one woman said, "It meant admitting my own lack of strength and also my fear that we didn't have enough money for help." Being alert to how difficult it may be for the spouse to assist the patient with the activities of daily living will enable the health care professional to work with the spouse on finding creative solutions to ease the burden of care.

Severity of Disease

As one might expect, we discovered a relationship between psychosocial-spiritual profile and severity of illness as measured by the ALS Severity Scale (4). Mildly ill patients had a higher level of well-being than moderately or severely ill patients; in particular, mildly ill patients were less depressed and perceived less stress. Interestingly enough, there was no difference in psychosocial-spiritual profiles between moderately and severely ill patients. Furthermore, psychosocial-spiritual well-being did not decline relentlessly during the eighteen months of participation in the study. While some individuals did show increased distress, an equal number experienced increased well-being, and the majority of patients remained in the same psychosocial-spiritual state throughout the testing period.

Length of Illness

It is particularly interesting to observe the patient's psychosocial-spiritual status in relation to length of illness. The current assumption is that most ALS patients will die within three to five years after diagnosis and will have increasing feelings of depression, hopelessness, and perceived stress plus an ever decreasing purpose in life. Many patients have had experiences similar to Mrs. C, whose neurologist told her, "You have a horrible disease, and if you're planning a vacation, take it now, for soon you won't be able to.'' However, studies report five-year survival rates ranging from 18 to 42 percent, with many individuals surviving far longer than that (5–7). As far back as 1976, Mulder and Howard (8) reported that 20 percent of patients seemed to be resistant to ALS and would live longer than five years. They went on to say, ''It is apparent that other factors, such as the patient's will to live and the support of his family, play significant roles in extending his life.''

Of the 144 ALS patients who entered our study, 31 percent had survived longer than five years. Overall, these long-term survivors exhibited greater psychosocial-spiritual well-being than those who had had ALS a shorter period of time, even though 21 percent were severely affected by ALS. Most of these patients saw a physician only rarely or had not seen one for years. ''Why should I,'' many have asked, ''when the doctor told me I'd be dead years ago and there was nothing more he could do for me?'' The physician who treats only two or three ALS patients in her entire practice and whose first patient followed the ''standard'' rate of decline (becoming progressively more depressed, hopeless, angry, and withdrawn and dying within three to five years) has no experience from which to offer the next ALS patient any hope. Yet there is hope. Some ALS progresses very slowly or ''burns out'' and stabilizes (9,10); it may even reverse, although that rarely happens.

Ms. O, a high-spirited young woman with ALS, which has been stable for nearly ten years, decided (like many of her peers) to live with her boyfriend. Her speech and legs are severely affected by the disease and her arms are very weak, but that did not keep her from setting up housekeeping with this friend, who has cerebral palsy. In addition to the joy of living together, they saw it as a way to share expenses—including a full-time nurse. Ms. O maintains an active life—going to school, swimming, and even parachuting from airplanes just for the fun of it.

Rate of Decline

Rapidity of decline can influence an individual's psychosocial-spiritual well-being. In a patient who is progressing rapidly, changes occur so fast that there is little opportunity to integrate the loss of one function before another loss is confronted. The phase of healthy denial of the disease, which can give an individual time to integrate the diagnosis and call upon her inner resources to deal with it, is not available to individuals who every day experience themselves losing more functional abilities. Especially in these instances, the health care practitioner needs to be sure that the patient, spouse, and family are all getting appropriate and sufficient psychosocial-spiritual care.

What about the individual whose disease is not progressing at an extraordinary rate? A common assumption is that the more severely ill a patient is and the longer he has had the disease, the more psychosocial-spiritual distress he will experience. It was a surprising finding in our study that moderately affected

	LENGTH		
	Short (0-18 months)	Medium (19-60 months)	Long (> 60 months)
Mild	0.73	1.07	1.31
Moderate	– 0.58	– 2.67	1.08
Severe	– 3.90	– 2.22	2.49

SEVERITY

Figure 15-1. Mean psychosocial-spiritual profile scores for 139 ALS patients grouped by length and severity of disease. The more positive the number, the greater the psychosocial-spiritual well-being; the more negative the number, the greater the psychosocial-spiritual distress. Severity measured by the ALS Severity Scale. (4)

patients who had had ALS for from nineteen to sixty months were, as a group, in a state of psychosocial-spiritual distress exceeded only by patients who had a very rapid disease progression (Figure 15-1). This distress was characterized by high levels of depression, hopelessness, and perceived stress and by low purpose in life. Individuals in this group are often considered by the health care practitioner to be ''handling'' the disease, but many are in a psychosocial-spiritual crisis and need intervention by the medical team. Frequently, counseling is offered to the patient at the time of diagnosis. Over time, however, as the patient and family are thought to be adjusting to the disease and its manifestations, less psychosocial-spiritual evaluation and support may be offered. These findings underscore the need to evaluate the psychosocial-spiritual status of patients on a routine basis and not to rely on assumptions or even on previous experience about how ALS patients respond psychologically.

Does increasing psychosocial-spiritual distress in any way accelerate the progression of the disease? At this point there is no clear answer, although there are strong feelings on both sides of the issue. Perhaps having a definitive answer to that question is not as important as understanding that your patient may feel that, given what ALS has already taken away from him, life is not worth living.

Respirator Usage

As the disease progresses, the patient, spouse, family, and health care provider have to face the question of whether or not to use a ventilator as a treatment to prolong life. Many health care providers have strong feelings (both pro and con) about placing patients on respiratory support. They may forcefully encourage it or refrain from discussing it, depending on their personal stance. This stance is often based on their experience with one or two patients or on their projection of what they themselves would do in that situation. Of the ALS patients we evaluated, only 24 percent said they would be willing to use a respirator. Little information has been available about how individuals on ventilators fare psychologically; the prevalent assumption is that life on a ventilator must be psychologically distressing.

Eighteen patients (12 percent) were on respirators when they entered our study. Contrary to expectation, these patients were not, as a group, more psychologically distressed than other ALS patients. They had similar levels of depression, loneliness, hopelessness, and perceived stress, and they considered their lives to have purpose and meaning. They did have a more internal health locus of control than ALS patients who did not need ventilation. While one might expect that only those individuals who had a strong family support system would have elected ventilatory support, we observed that patients who chose to be placed on respirators included those dependent on hired caregivers as well as those with tight-knit families.

Being on a ventilator does *not* condemn a patient to a horrible life, devoid of purpose and isolated from friends and family. In fact, experientially quite the opposite was true for many of our eighteen patients. Working with their families and the health care practitioner, many of these patients found that life was more satisfying than before they went on the respirator and that ventilatory support allowed them to leave the house and participate more fully in life.

Mrs. D, now in her forties, had no use of her extremities and had been on a respirator for several years. When she was first placed on ventilatory support, her physician told the family she would be dead in a few months. Now, several years later, there is no evidence that Mrs. D is any closer to the grave than when the doctor predicted her imminent demise. With the help of home care nurses, she lives a life rich in meaning and purpose. She is a parent, hosts an Al-Anon support group in her home, enjoys reading with a mechanical page turner, and has become an award-winning artist, painting with a brush held between her teeth. She is a lively conversationalist when friends visit. Her goal these days is to live fully, one day at a time. Like Mr. W, Ms. O, and many others, she is not simply surviving with ALS, she is living her life.

Nonphysical Challenges

In addition to the physical challenges of ALS, the disease places many other stresses on the patient and family. Many of these ultimately affect the patient's quality of life and sense of well-being. Individuals with ALS often experience ever-increasing isolation from family, friends, events of the world, and nature.

Many have fewer visitors, just at the time they are less able to get out of the house. This was true for 40 percent of the patients in our study. Living in a culture that values physical perfection, the ALS patient may feel embarrassed or ashamed by the condition of his body and may be reluctant to be seen in public. For many, the main social event is a visit to the clinic or doctor's office. Some patients stop going to church (16 percent in our study), and only a small percentage (19 percent in our study) participate in support groups.

Over time, patients may no longer be able to function in roles that defined their lives and their sense of purpose. The "breadwinner" can no longer work; the one accustomed to cooking can only watch someone else do it. The patient may begin to question her competency as a spouse, parent, friend, or lover, and family relationships may become a source of stress rather than support. Worries about money often increase dramatically. Being a burden on others can be the worst thing about having ALS; this was true for 12 percent of the patients in the study.

Most participants in our study also felt that their lives were devoid of leisure, despite the fact that they watched an average of four hours of television every day. Evidently there was no part of the day that was *experienced* as leisurely—that is, devoted to having fun and to participating in activities that would distract them from their disease.

Quality of Life

The ALS patient faces innumerable challenges in addition to the difficulties of coping physically with the symptoms of the disease. Yet we know that high quality of life is experienced by many persons in all stages of ALS. There are ALS patients who travel with wheelchair and portable respirator, direct video productions, coach football, oil paint, or explore the nature of the universe—despite profound physical limitations.

High quality of life is a function of an individual's perception and is reflected in a sense of psychosocial-spiritual well-being even in the face of severe physical handicaps. Patients in our study were defined as experiencing a high quality of life if their profile showed that they were mildly or not at all depressed, not lonely, had an internal health locus of control, may have perceived stress but confronted it effectively, expressed anger appropriately, maintained a sense of hope, and felt their lives had purpose. These qualities are the cornerstones to experiencing a sense of spiritual well-being and satisfaction with life. It is evident that an essential component of optimal treatment for the ALS patient lies in this psychosocial and spiritual dimension.

The health care professional assessing the psychosocial-spiritual dimension is in a position to discuss the importance of interacting with others to maintain a sense of purpose and belonging. Those patients who have the experience of participating in activities with their family, friends, and co-workers relate that their lives continue to have purpose and meaning.

At the time of her participation in our study, Mrs. G lived in a small trailer (caravan) with her husband and two teenaged children. She was unable to communicate except with her eyes and an alphabet board. She had minimal physical function, and her respirations were labored. Yet, far from being isolated or excluded from life, her children actively sought her advice, and with the assistance of her husband, she planned meals and even parties. Visits from caring friends were also a part of her daily routine. This family went beyond simply coping with the effects of ALS. They lived as a happy and integrated unit, planning for the future while facing the reality that Mrs. G was probably going to die soon.

Assessment and Intervention

The psychosocial-spiritual condition of the ALS patient profoundly influences the experience of the illness, the response to medical care, and the overall quality of life. One of the most compelling conclusions reached in our study is that routine assessment of psychosocial-spiritual status is critical in creating an ongoing plan of treatment for the ALS patient. This assessment provides the basis for a deeper understanding of how to relate to each patient and family and an indication of the need for intervention and referral.

Seven tests were used in the development of our measure of a patient's psychosocial-spiritual profile. However, our statistical analysis showed that using just three of these tests—the Beck Depression Inventory, the Health Locus of Control Scale, and the Purpose-in-Life Test (11–13)—provided almost the same level of accuracy as using all seven. Individually, these three tests measure very different aspects of the patient's psychosocial-spiritual profile: the emotional state, the sense of inner direction or control, and the sense of meaning or connection with the world. Combined, they provide a window into the patient's inner experience of life. As with the more comprehensive measurement of psychosocial-spiritual profile provided by the seven tests, this condensed measure shows that a sense of well-being is related to a higher quality of life and longer survival.

The following guidelines are useful in administering these tests:

1) The spouse should not be present. This often helps the patient feel more comfortable answering the questions as honestly as possible. It is especially important for patients who need assistance in communication.
2) Allow a total of one-half hour for completing the tests.
3) Follow the simple instructions for scoring that are provided with the tests, and use their guidelines for interpretation.

Creative communication techniques may be required for patients who cannot write or speak. Far from being laborious, the process of communicating with people who can neither speak nor write can be both moving and engaging. One strong-willed and independent man who could only move his head had rigged up a Morse code device on the pillow next to his ear. The interviewers were given cards with the complete code and translated as they went along. Another patient typed out her answers with her toe. Other communication devices like the ones described in an earlier chapter can be used. While there is a natural communion that develops as one struggles to understand someone with an alert mind but limited expression, care should be taken not to influence the patient. It is important to recognize that these questionnaires probe deeply and answering them may be quite challenging and sometimes emotional for the patient.

If baseline testing shows a patient to be depressed, treatment for depression should be considered. It is a mistake for the health care professional to label such a patient "normally depressed" and therefore without need of intervention. Depression is frequently a part of the disease process (nearly 60 percent of the patients in our study had some degree of depression), but it is not inevitable. Many severely ill patients are happy or only mildly depressed. Depression can be assessed and, if severe, counseling and/or psychopharmacological support can be offered. Alleviating depression has the potential to greatly improve the patient's experience of quality of life.

Assessing a patient's health locus of control gives the health care practitioner a valuable tool for determining the degree to which the patient would benefit from participating in development of the health care plan. A patient with a high external locus of control may not want to be given multiple options for symptomatic support or treatment, but may want the health care team to be directive, telling the course of action to be taken. On the other hand, if the patient has a highly developed internal locus of control, she wants the health care professional to be a team member who facilitates decision making but recognizes that the patient has the final say.

The assessment of purpose in life can identify those patients who lack a sense of meaning and purpose in their lives. Finding ways to increase purpose in life may seem outside the domain of the health care practitioner (or may even challenge his own sense of purpose in life), but there are steps that can be taken. The family of the patient can be informed of how the patient is feeling and may be able to find ways to involve the patient more in their lives. This may run the gamut from making the extra effort to take the patient on family outings to remembering to seek his input on family decisions, keeping him apprised of happenings in each family member's life, and discovering how his many gifts can still be given. Additionally, the patient, or the whole family, can be referred to an appropriate psychiatrist, psychologist, therapist, or religious counselor. The health care practitioner seeking ways to help patients rediscover meaning and purpose may well discover that she has some narrow ideas about what constitutes a well-lived life. The life of Stephen Hawking, the British physicist whose physical function has been severely limited by ALS for many years, reminds all of us that physical disability in no way limits one's ability to contribute to humanity.

The Spouse

ALS is a disease that affects the entire family and can have profound physical and psychosocial-spiritual consequences for the spouse. In our study, 79 percent of the ALS patients were married. The 123 spouses or other primary caregivers were given the same series of tests as the patients. As a group, their psychosocial-spiritual profile was similar to the norm for adults except that the spouses had higher depression scores (although much lower than for the patients) and experienced a greater degree of loneliness. Some clearly experienced psychosocial-spiritual distress. Approximately 15 percent felt profoundly hopeless and were moderately to severely depressed, while 23 percent experienced a high degree of loneliness, and 47 percent perceived a high degree of stress in their lives.

Many spouses (as well as patients) expressed frustration over how they were informed of the diagnosis. Additionally, they tended to feel isolated and reported receiving minimal information from the physician about what ALS really is and how it progresses. One wife stated that she never understood what having ALS meant; it was not until she went to the library to do her own research that she learned of the devastating effects of this disease, and she felt betrayed by the physician.

As they attempt to cope with an information vacuum, many spouses create their own theories about the cause of ALS. They may blame physical overwork, repression of emotions, chemicals in the garden, or a previous illness. Trying to understand the onset of ALS without clear input from the physician can lead to feelings of guilt. They may feel that they did not intervene soon enough in attempting to change whatever factor they think caused the illness.

The word *abandoned* was used repeatedly by spouses in the study. Many felt abandoned by physicians who said, "There's nothing we can do for your husband (or wife)," and also by friends who were too uncomfortable being around an ill person (who might force them to acknowledge their own mortality).

When the patient's traditional roles in the family alter with the decrease in functional ability, these roles must be taken on by the spouse or other family members. Everyone in the family system will probably experience changes in the roles they play. Careers may need to be suspended. Wives may need to undertake everything from managing household finances to mowing the lawn for the first time in their lives; husbands may find themselves chief cook, dishwasher, and child-rearer.

Approximately 70 percent of the spouses in the study were working prior to their mate's diagnosis of ALS. Nearly one-fourth of them had stopped working by the initial interview in order to care for the patient. The resulting reduction in income, along with medical costs, greatly increased the occurrence of financial difficulties. Prior to ALS, only 3 percent of the spouses were "very worried" about money; after its onset, 18 percent were "very worried." Some spouses (9 percent in the study) started working in order to meet their family's financial obligations, often at a time when they were increasingly needed at home.

Many spouses curtail their volunteer work and church or community activities in order to stay home and care for the patient. The number of spouses doing volunteer work decreased from 47 percent before diagnosis to 31 percent at the time the study began. The percentage not attending church almost doubled (from 26 to 44 percent). These changes and others can lead to a sense of isolation and loneliness, loss of self, and resentment toward the ill spouse. Fortunately, most spouses reported that they had an outlet for their emotions (85 percent) and were able to have some amount of private time (80 percent).

It is apparent that the spouse (or other primary caregiver) is dealing with myriad challenges and that the health care professional needs to be aware of the psychosocial-spiritual status of the spouse as well as the patient. Psychotherapy and/or psychopharmacological support may be needed by the spouse, a need that can go undetected unless a situation becomes extreme. For example, stress that has gone undetected by family, friends, and the health care provider has led in rare cases to physical abuse of a patient by a spouse under too much stress. Detecting such distress can only be done through assessment. A way to start is by administering the same three tests suggested for the patient (for depression, health locus of control, and purpose in life) at initial and all subsequent visits. Appropriate referrals can be made when indicated by these test results.

Additionally, the spouse can be given the opportunity to talk about the effects of ALS on her life. When feelings of isolation, loss of self, and resentment begin to emerge, the health care practitioner can assist the spouse in discovering ways to make time for herself and for her social life. Explaining health care options, such as hospice care, respite care, home health aides, and how other family members or even friends can be trained to care for the patient, can help the spouse to avoid feeling trapped or abandoned.

The health care practitioner also needs to be a facilitator for the spouse and patient in practical matters. She needs to know where they can seek financial assistance, apply for disability, and locate needed assistive devices. When the health care practitioner operates as a facilitator, the spouse and patient have the experience of being cared for rather than abandoned by the medical community.

The Spouse-Patient Relationship

Mr. E and his wife, an older couple who married late in life, had been together only a few years when he began to have trouble swallowing. His speech soon became slurred. After thorough testing, ALS was diagnosed. Initially, Mrs. E seemed to be coping and adjusting, but her anger, resentment, and embarrassment over her husband's condition soon became apparent. She did not want to care for someone who was ill, felt robbed of the life she had expected, and felt a strong desire for her husband to die quickly. Little communication occurred between the two of them, as she could not tolerate listening to him trying to verbalize. Her pain was deep, yet no intervention had been offered by the health care team. The tension between them continued to mount, and Mrs. E's feelings of resentment evolved into profound feelings of guilt. Additionally, she had the intense experience of being inadequate as a spouse. Both Mr. and Mrs. E felt isolated and unsupported by their family and the health care system. Mr. E felt that his life had little value, and Mrs. E felt hopeless. Mr. E died within a few months. Did their hopelessness hasten his death?

This scenario is not uncommon or overdramatized. Our current health care system is not designed to easily and effectively include the spouse-patient relationship that needs to be considered in the overall evaluation and treatment plan. Nurses and physicians are taught that the primary objective of treatment is physical cure. Curing means focusing on the ill individual and attempting to free the body of disease. There is little room in this model for consideration of the family. However, a physically and psychologically healthy family can be a strong ally to both the patient and the health care team. Understanding some of the dynamics of this system, especially those between the spouse and patient, can be of great value to the health care practitioner.

Change in the Nature of the Relationship

The changes in roles necessitated by the decreased functional abilities of the ALS patient can lead to an unrecognized and unacknowledged shift in the relationship between spouse and patient—from that of husband-wife to that of caregiver-patient. For the psychosocial-spiritual well-being of both patient and spouse, the husband-wife relationship needs to be nurtured and maintained. The couple can accomplish this by having other people help with physical care and by continuing previously shared activities, such as seeing movies, playing cards, watching sunsets, having sex, or smelling roses.

Mrs. P, reminiscing about the time period before her husband died of ALS, says poignantly, "Living became the center of our lives, not ALS." That focus on living allowed them to maintain a loving and intimate husband-wife relationship until the end.

Mr. L and his wife were a model of intelligent and mature coping with the reality of impending disability and death. They never talked about what *he* was going through, but rather about what *they* were experiencing. They talked openly about his death and the challenges of each stage along the way. They made sure that they had a variety of experiences together and created the memories that she would be able to cherish once he was gone. They discussed what her life might be like after his death so he was able to feel part of it. Rather than being morbid, this intimate honesty allowed them to live together fully in the time they had.

Every couple, of course, has its own style of enjoying the relationship. In both these cases, the couples were successful to the degree that they saw the disease as a shared experience and were able to communicate sufficiently so that resentment, guilt, or other negative emotions did not build up over time.

Experience of the Disease

The stressful aspects of life with ALS may be quite different for the patient and the spouse. When asked what their major stressor was, 83 percent of the spouses listed health issues, while only 55 percent of the patients did. Some patients (12 percent) were most concerned about financial matters, but only a few spouses (2 percent) listed this as the major stressor. One can see how communication difficulties may arise when the spouse wants to talk about the patient's health at a time when his attention is focused on financial concerns, or when the spouse is preoccupied with coping with the disease while the patient wants to focus on living, not on the illness. In fact, relationships themselves were a major stressor for some patients (18 percent) and spouses (12 percent).

As a group, the spouses in the study were more lonely than the patients. Having given up previous activities such as pursuing a career, lunching with friends, or competing on a bowling team, the spouses often felt housebound. At the same time, they spoke of a reluctance to leave the house because the patient could not. This sense of loneliness and isolation sometimes escalated to resentment and guilt. Assisting the spouse to see the importance of maintaining activities with friends (and helping the patient understand and support the spouse in such pursuits) is one way the health care practitioner can help the spouse lessen the experience of loneliness.

When spouses have a more internal health locus of control than patients, they may want to be more involved than the patient in the health care plan. It sometimes happens that a spouse talks to the patient about the collection of material regarding ALS, and cannot understand why the ill partner does not want to know more about the disease. Or the spouse may want an in-depth explanation from the physician of all the phases and complications that his partner will probably go through, along with a discussion of the various forms of supportive treatment that are available, whereas the patient does not want to participate in the process. The opposite may also be true. The spouse may simply want to be told what to do to help the mate without taking part in decision making.

One wife stated, ''I read everything I could about the disease and all aspects of healing—medical, spiritual, and holistic. I couldn't understand why he (the patient) didn't want to do this reading with me, and I got frustrated by that. It took a while, but I realized I needed to accept him exactly as he was—and that included the way he wanted to approach the disease. This was a turning point for me and actually drew us closer.''

Timing of Psychosocial-Spiritual Distress

One of the findings in our study was that the patient and spouse often experienced psychosocial-spiritual distress at very different stages of the illness. The health care provider may assume that the patient and spouse manifest the stress of ALS in the same manner at the same time, i.e., if the patient seems depressed and lonely, then the spouse is likely to have similar feelings. In a very general sense, this may be true. For example, in our study spouses of the patients experiencing the most psychosocial-spiritual distress tended to feel more depressed, hopeless, lonely, and stressed than spouses of the patients with the greatest sense of well-being.

However, there were noteworthy differences. For example, patients who had had ALS longer than five years and patients whose disease remained mild regardless of length of illness were often mildly depressed while their spouses had no measurable depression, leading to friction between the patient and spouse.

Mr. S had had ALS for seven years. He needed assistance walking but could manage feeding and dressing himself. Though minimally affected by ALS, he remained moderately depressed and exhibited a strong need to remain in control, and his control mechanism was time. If he needed to be ready for an appointment by 11:00 A.M., he was rarely dressed and ready to go before noon. His wife, who was not depressed and in fact was feeling hopeful due to the slow progression of her husband's disease, had little tolerance for his lack of participation, including his resistance to going out or having company. There was open hostility between them. "I can't understand why he'd be distressed," said Mrs. S. "There's a lot he could be doing." Mr. S, on the other hand, felt that his disability stripped him of the capacity to enjoy life or participate with others. Neither experienced a satisfactory quality of life.

The S's experience of life might have been enhanced by an evaluation of their psychosocial-spiritual status and by intervention initiated by the health care practitioner. They might have been taught ways of communicating that would have allowed each to understand the other's emotional-spiritual state and be more accepting of the other's actions.

Another difficult period for the spouse/patient relationship can occur when the patient has been ill a medium length of time (nineteen to sixty months) and is moderately affected by ALS. In the study these patients were, as a group, in a psychosocial-spiritual crisis. Their spouses, however, were not. While the patients were experiencing their lives as devoid of purpose and meaning, were moderately depressed, and had high levels of hopelessness, their spouses were not hopeless or even mildly depressed and were experiencing purpose and meaning in their lives. Additionally, while the patients depended on the medical practitioners to manage their health care, their spouses wanted to be more involved in the patient's care.

These differences in experience can lead to mistaken assumptions on the part of the health care provider. Very often the patient and spouse are seen together by the physician, and it is not uncommon for the spouse to "talk" for the patient, particularly if speech is impaired. Often the patient will not openly acknowledge feelings and experiences with the spouse present. When this dynamic occurs with patients already in psychosocial-spiritual crisis, it can be a serious matter and can be a crucial juncture in the treatment of the patient. If the crisis goes undetected, the patient may become increasingly distressed, fall into despair, and withdraw from family, friends, and life.

There is one time period in the study during which the spouses exhibited more psychosocial-spiritual distress than the patients, i.e., when the severely ill patient had survived longer than five years. Surprisingly, these patients, as a group, exhibited a state of well-being characterized by lack of hopelessness and depression, low perceived stress, and high life satisfaction. Meanwhile, their spouses, although not in psychosocial-spiritual crisis, showed a tendency toward more hopelessness, depression, and perceived stress and a more external health locus of control. Perhaps the spouse recognizes the long-term nature of the care that must be given to the severely ill patient and has depleted inner resources from the valiant attempt to care for the patient over the preceding years.

Effective psychosocial-spiritual intervention has the potential to dramatically alter the patient's perceived quality of life. Although disease progression may not be altered, when depression is lightened and a sense of hope about coping with his destiny is instilled, the patient may once again participate more fully in life, alleviating the anguish of the couple's isolation. As one person stated, "He (the patient) becomes frustrated if he isn't able to do the things he wants for his family. If he can do them through us (family and friends), he may still have frustrations, but he's not into despair."

For some couples, mutual understanding develops as they cope with the diagnosis and talk about their feelings and fears. However, many couples need assistance with communication skills. During chronic illness, unhealthy dynamics already present between family members may become intensified, which is what happened with Mr. and Mrs. E, discussed at the beginning of this section. Mrs. E reported that communication about feelings was difficult prior to ALS and that after the diagnosis it seemed impossible to talk about their fears and concerns. If a couple having very different emotional experiences has not previously developed skills in listening to and understanding each other, friction and feelings of isolation may develop. Simply learning to listen can increase understanding, tolerance, and love of another person. The help of a qualified counselor can be invaluable in such a situation.

There is a period when the patient and spouse are likely to be having a *similar* experience—when a patient has had ALS less than eighteen months and is severely ill. For spouses in the study, the highest levels of hopelessness, depression, and perceived stress and the least sense of purpose in life occurred in spouses of these patients. This was also the time of greatest distress for patients. Here both patient and spouse need all the physical, psychological, social, and spiritual support that the health care team, family, and friends can provide. Spouses and patients in this situation reported that knowing their physician was available to be called, even to make home visits, was very important in helping them feel supported and cared for by the health care system. This can be an extremely difficult time for the health care provider, who is trained to cure illness and is now faced with a seemingly hopeless situation—one in which he not only may experience failure but also may be forced to examine his own mortality. Hope, however, still exists—the hope that one can deal with one's destiny. Assisting the patient and spouse in realizing their inner strength and sustaining or developing a nurturing support system is essential in maintaining the psychosocial-spiritual well-being of the patient and the spouse and in supporting the patient-spouse relationship. This can be one of the most rewarding times for a practitioner who realizes that caring—not curing—is what he is able to provide.

Differing Perceptions of the Patient's Experience

A complicating factor in the whole realm of mutual understanding and communication is that the spouse often perceives the patient's experience quite differently. Spouses in the study tended to rate their ill partners' level of life satisfaction lower than the ill partner rated it. Spouses' ratings of the patients' self-acceptance and acceptance of help were very often much lower than the patient's own evaluation. Spouses also thought that patients were more worried about money than patients themselves reported. Furthermore, the spouses felt that the patients were not as honest in communicating how they felt as the patients reported they were.

Many dynamics can play a role in these differences. For example, the patient may be in denial, not ready to acknowledge or accept the current reality of her life. The different emotional states of the patient and spouse, reported previously, may cause them to perceive their partners through the filter of their own emotional state. The key point here is for the health care practitioner not to accept as fact either the patient's or spouse's view about the other.

Each Patient and Spouse Is Unique

While the length of time the patient has had ALS and the severity of the disease give some clues as to how the patient and spouse may be dealing with the disease at a psychosocial-spiritual level, the uniqueness of their makeup as human beings and the emotional health of each at the time the illness began are essential factors in determining their individual responses to the effects of ALS in their lives and on their relationship. This response can change over time as their psychosocial-spiritual status changes in response to all aspects of life.

It is important that the health care provider not necessarily look to the spouse to provide the psychosocial-spiritual support that is needed by a patient, because the spouse may also be in need of support. The only way to know how the patient and spouse are really doing is to assess the psychosocial-spiritual status of both. The health care practitioner then has the option of proposing counseling and/or psychopharmacology as a normal and natural part of the treatment plan for both the ALS patient and the spouse.

The patient, the spouse, and the spouse-patient relationship comprise three independent yet interconnected systems. Each system faces challenges in responding to the diagnosis and effects of ALS. The healthier the couple's relationship prior to illness, the more likely it is that they will be able to communicate openly and enlist the support of friends and other family members. As one husband and wife put it, "Certainly we were close before, but we've grown much closer." While many of their friends drifted away, others became an integral part of the family life, lending their skills to design and implement assistive devices, being there to listen, and relieving the spouse from the demands of physical care so that she could have some time for herself.

The Health Care Practitioner

ALS affects not only the patient and family but also the medical practitioner, who needs to be aware of the stresses experienced while working with ALS patients and families. A pervasive sense of failure can linger in the mind of the physician. Establishing a relationship with someone who is slowly dying can be difficult and emotionally taxing. Too often the health care practitioner attempts to deny his feelings and avoids developing a partnership with the patient, spouse, and family.

However, the patient is impacted by the emotional well-being of the health care practitioner. In areas where psychosocial-spiritual distress is common among clinic staff serving the ALS community, ALS patients as a whole appear to do less well. The health care practitioner needs to be able to recognize when he needs emotional support and then get it.

Physicians and nurses have been trained to *cure* disease, not to aid in *healing*. The difference between disease and illness was stated clearly by Eric Cassell of Cornell Medical College: "Disease is a clinical entity. . . . Illness, on the other hand, is a patient's experience of the disease's symptoms and treatments." Curing is referred to as "restoring the patient's physical body back to its pre-disease condition." When cure is not possible, many health care practitioners feel there is little they can offer the patient and therefore withdraw from the relationship. According to Cesa-Bianchi and Ravaccia (14), many physicians "cope exclusively with technical problems, ignoring the emotional aspects of an incurable illness."

Yet Beisecker, Cobb, and Ziegler (15), in research on patients' perspectives and the role of physicians, noted that patients derive hope and encouragement from the simple act of talking with a physician regarding any problem. Patients and spouses in our study also talked about the need to know that their physician cared about them as individuals and would take time *first* to listen to them and *then* to answer their questions. The development of a relationship with the patient and spouse enables the health care practitioner to include them in "healing the illness experience." This process involves guiding the patient and spouse as they learn to live with ALS and develop a life that is worth living, even when ALS has left the patient severely physically debilitated.

In this light, medical success needs to be redefined. Facing the possibility of a patient's death on a daily basis is common for the health care practitioner who is part of an ALS team, and it is easy to feel hopeless and unsuccessful if death is seen as a failure. But success comes not just in curing the disease or keeping the patient alive, but also in assisting the patient and family in having an illness-experience that goes beyond coping to creating lives of quality and dignity.

Individuals with ALS and their families can live exceedingly rich lives. We discovered many such people in our study, not only individuals who had an extraordinary gift for successfully coping with a "terminal" illness, but also persons who seemed simply average.

At the time of his diagnosis with ALS, Mr. J was an apartment manager. He was single and in his forties. Ten years later, he has lost all ability to talk or walk, has difficulty swallowing, and has only limited use of his arms. On the surface, he has little reason to be happy and much reason to be lonely, depressed, and hopeless. But when you walk into his room in the nursing home, you find it filled not only with an array of bright cloth and ceramic frogs brought by loving friends but also with an air of joy and peace. His face lights up with a huge smile at the sight of a guest, and he is eager to share his thoughts or a joke, bending earnestly and patiently over his writing board. His inner spiritual life has become increasingly important to him since his diagnosis, and he spends a good deal of his time reading the Bible. He is clearly a man at peace with his life, and he transmits his happiness to those around him.

In many cases, quality of life has little to do with physical disability. Many patients and families maintain high quality lives at all stages of physical disability and all lengths of illness. The key lies in their psychosocial-spiritual well-being. Today, the health care practitioner can do nothing to alter the progressive disability encountered in this disease except to provide palliative treatment; but he can assist the patient and family in raising their level of psychosocial-spiritual well-being. Sometimes the health care practitioner simply needs to cooperate with a patient who is determined to care for himself.

Mr. H could only be called a curmudgeon—with a bit of scoundrel mixed in. As a veteran, he knew he was entitled to health care, and he made sure he got it. Periodically he checked into the V.A. hospital for respite care. Since the hospital was several hundred miles away from his rural home, he wangled a van ride from the system. His apartment in the basement of his home had concrete floors for easy use of an electric wheelchair. Although his arms were nearly useless, he had devised a series of slings and pivots on the arms of his wheelchair so he could feed himself and, more importantly, get a fresh chew of tobacco. He had acquired a parachute harness through his military connections and was figuring out a system to rig himself up and actually walk around—after a fashion.

Adaptations to ALS are as varied as human psychology. If a patient and his family system were healthy—psychologically, socially, and spiritually—prior to onset of the disease, they have a good chance of finding unique, creative, and meaningful ways to deal with this challenge. If they were not, or if their psychosocial-spiritual well-being has deteriorated, the health care practitioner should look for ways to reawaken their will to be alive and enjoy life.

The health care practitioner is indeed in a position to provide the hope that ALS patients and their spouses so desperately need. This hope lies not necessarily in believing that "they'll find a cure," but in knowing what research is happening, participating in clinical trials when possible, but most of all receiving encouragement that they can still lead meaningful and high quality lives.

The health care practitioner is not being asked to fulfill all the needs of the patient, spouse, or family but to be in relationship with them, to be aware of what they are going through, and to facilitate their movement through the complex health care system. The patient should be invited to be an active part of the "wellness team." Dr. Forbes Norris reminded the health care practitioner, "Never forget that the patient is in charge throughout the illness." The informed patient will be able to grapple more effectively with the difficult questions around life support and other treatment options.

As discussed throughout this chapter, there are numerous interventions available for the health care practitioner to use when integrating the psychosocial-spiritual status of the patient and spouse into the treatment plan. Assessing depression and offering treatment when indicated is particularly important. Providing opportunities for the spouse to talk about the personal effects of ALS can yield benefits for the whole family. Attention to the psychological, social, and spiritual well-being of the patient and family, with quality of life as the goal, can help the health care practitioner find success in treating patients and families with ALS.

Summary

Although ALS is a devastating disease, it is possible for the patient, family, and health care practitioner—working together and armed with knowledge, hope, and the willingness to venture into the psychosocial-spiritual realm—to experience healing even though cure is not possible. When the emphasis is on maintaining quality of life and healing the illness experience, everyone in the family system plays a vital role.

The health care practitioner plays a particularly important role in determining how patients and families respond to the experience of ALS in their lives and in assisting the patient and spouse to reach the highest level of psychosocial-spiritual well-being achievable. There are several important points for the medical practitioner to keep in mind in moving from a curing to a healing approach.

First, a life-threatening illness can have positive aspects (37 percent of the patients in our study said that something in their life, such as relationships with family, had improved during the process of learning to cope with ALS and their own mortality).

Second, a significant number of ALS patients do live a long time and a significant portion do not decline rapidly. Some patients will have five, fifteen, or even more years of life ahead of them, and perhaps even outlive the practitioner.

Third, there is no characteristic personality profile of the ALS patient, and psychosocial-spiritual status is not solely related to severity of disease or length of illness. In fact, the most severely ill patient in our study had one of the healthiest psychosocial-spiritual profiles, and the group of patients with the longest survival time had the healthiest psychosocial-spiritual profile of all (16). ALS patients of any disease severity or length of illness can (and many do) lead rich and rewarding lives.

Fourth, the patient and spouse rarely have the same psychosocial-spiritual response to the effects of ALS. Their levels of depression, hopelessness, and perceived stress, along with their sense of purpose in life, may differ greatly. There are stages at which intense psychosocial-spiritual support is needed. A simple routine assessment of the patient's and spouse's psychosocial-spiritual status using the three tests suggested earlier in this chapter—the Beck Depression Inventory, the Health Locus of Control Scale, and the Purpose-in-Life Test—can provide invaluable insights into the psychosocial-spiritual needs.

Health care professionals who experience or learn about patients whose lives remain whole despite living with the disabilities induced by ALS are more likely to develop a willingness to enter into a dynamic relationship with ALS patients and their families. The practitioner holds the key to an integrative system of care, including one of the most important elements: psychosocial and spiritual support.

References

1. Brown WA, Mueller PS. Psychological function in individuals with amyotrophic lateral sclerosis (ALS). *Psychosom Med* 1970, 32:141–52.
2. Houpt JL, Gould BS, Norris FH. Psychological characteristics of patients with amyotrophic lateral sclerosis (ALS). *Psychosom Med* 1977, 39:299–303.
3. Peters PK, Swenson WM, Mulder DW. Is there a characteristic personality profile in amyotrophic lateral sclerosis? *Arch Neurol* 1978, 35:321–22.

4. Hillel AD, Miller RM, Yorkston K, McDonald E, Norris FH, Konikow N. Amyotrophic lateral sclerosis severity scale. *Neuroepidemiology* 1989, 8:142–50.

5. Rosen AD. Amyotrophic lateral sclerosis: clinical features and prognosis. *Arch Neurol* 1978, 35:638–42.

6. Mortara P, Chio A, Rosso MG, Leone M, Schiffer D. Motor neuron disease in the province of Turin, Italy, 1966–1980: survival analysis in an unselected population. *J Neurol Sci* 1984, 66:165–73.

7. Caroscio JT, Mulvihill MN, Sterling R, Abrams B. Amyotrophic lateral sclerosis: its natural history. *Neurol Clin* 1987, 5:1–8.

8. Mulder DW, Howard FM. Patient resistance and prognosis in amyotrophic lateral sclerosis. *Mayo Clin Proc* 1976, 51:537–41.

9. Norris FH. Ten commandments of MND. *International Information Exchange Bulletin* January 1992, 11–13.

10. Tandan R, Bradley WG. Amyotrophic lateral sclerosis: part 1. clinical features, pathology, and ethical issues in management. *Ann Neurol* 1985, 18:271–80.

11. Beck AT, Rush AJ, Shaw BF, Emery G. *Cognitive Therapy of Depression.* New York: Guilford Press, 1979.

12. Wallston BS, Wallston KA, Kaplan GD, Maides SA. Development and validation of the Health Locus of Control (HLC) scale. *J Consult Clin Psychol* 1976, 44:580–85.

13. Reker GT, Cousins JB. Factor structure, construct validity and reliability of the Seeking of Noetic Goals (SONG) and Purpose in Life (PIL) tests. *J Clin Psychol* 1979, 35:85–91.

14. Cesa-Bianchi M, Ravaccia F. Psychological preparation of the physician for ALS patients. *Adv Exp Med Biol* 1987, 209:311–312.

15. Beisecker AE, Cobb AK, Ziegler DK. Patients' perspectives of the role of care providers in amyotrophic lateral sclerosis. *Arch Neurol* 1988, 45:553–56.

16. McDonald ER, Wiedenfeld SA, Hillel A, Carpenter CL, Walter RA. Survival in amyotrophic lateral sclerosis: the role of psychological factors. *Arch Neurol* (in press).

16

The Effect of Cultural Expectations on Progression Responses in ALS

Ann Kuckelman Cobb, Ph.D., R.N.

Introduction

The purpose of this chapter is to examine variation in coping as ALS progresses and to relate these responses to the cultural context in which they occur. Five anthropological concepts and five coping concepts organize the discussion. Data are drawn from ten years of clinical and volunteer experience with ALS patients and caregivers and four previous research projects (1,2,3,4,).

ALS and Other Chronic Diseases

When clinicians and researchers write about coping with chronic illness, the diseases most often referred to are conditions such as diabetes, hypertension, arthritis, and cancer. Although each of these is a progressive disease and requires some ongoing adaptation, the progress is often much slower than may be the case with ALS. There is usually time to make an adjustment, one that may be an effective means of coping over a long period of time, before another adaptation is required. This is the feature that most sets ALS apart from other chronic illnesses. The progressive loss of physical function, combined with increasing limitations in performing social roles, are characteristics of ALS that present a continuous demand for adaptation on the part of both family members and persons with ALS. Although there is individual variation in the progress of the disease, patients and families still live with the knowledge that the overall course is usually a relentlessly downward trajectory. They must, therefore, not only cope with whatever the current limitations are, but also deal with limitations to come.

Coping with ALS has been discussed, as have many other illnesses, in terms of stages (5,6); however, the metaphor of the spiral, or the recurring cycle, is more appropriate. While attempting to contain the current disability and its effects, the person with ALS and family members as well are in constant anticipation of the next loss. When that actually occurs, a cycle is set in motion, of grieving the loss, attempting new coping responses, and reaching another temporary equilibrium.

Scott et al. (7) present a conceptual framework based on the spiral. They argue that in chronic illness patients experience a loss followed by a period of adjustment, then one of equilibrium, followed by another loss that calls for another adjustment. This is clearly the pattern in ALS, except that in some cases the losses follow so quickly, one upon the other, that no real equilibrium is reached, and the trajectory is much more precipitously downhill. In these instances, coping may simply be a "keeping together" on a day-to-day basis, with little if any respite from the stresses involved.

Overlaid on this pattern of cyclic loss and adaptation are three important factors that can contribute to or impede the adaptive process. The first is individual, the second social, and the third cultural. Much is written about psychosocial adjustment to chronic and/or terminal illness (5, 8, 9,10,11,12,13). This literature takes into account the first two factors and is briefly mentioned here. The third, or cultural factor, is the focus of this chapter and is discussed at length after some cursory remarks about individual and social factors influencing coping with ALS.

The Individual and the Coping Response

There have been several studies of psychological parameters of ALS (5,14,15), which have been aimed mainly at identifying distinctive personality characteristics of ALS patients. For the most part, there has been little success in finding differences between individuals with ALS and persons with other illnesses. Clinical observation and data collected for an earlier study (2) suggest that people are ill as they are well. That is, they tend to deal with ALS generally in the same way they have dealt with other life crises. If they are indecisive, they are likely to be indecisive regarding what to do about specific problems that arise in ALS. If they approach things matter of factly and tend to be problem-solvers regarding other issues, they will probably have the same basic attitude toward management of ALS. If they tend to be nonconfrontive, to deny that problems exist, they may overutilize denial as a coping mechanism. This does not mean that they cannot be helped to adopt a new way of coping. What it does mean is that clinicians who are helping families to plan interventions need to know how persons with

ALS usually cope with problems, and both to build on the strengths of these existing patterns and introduce change when a given approach is no longer effective.

Social Factors That Influence Management of ALS

Cobb and Hamera (2) have discussed the social context in which coping with ALS must occur. Social influences include such factors as laws governing decision making in catastrophic illness, levels of technology available in a given society, availability of institutional support services and who pays for them, and federal and state policies regarding management of disability issues in relation to employment. These are extremely complex issues and deserve attention both in research and clinical management, since they impinge sometimes very directly on how patients and families are able to cope with ALS.

Cultural Factors That Influence the Management of ALS

Sickness and suffering are universal human concerns, although there are differences in how each culture defines and manages a particular illness. Disciplines such as medical anthropology, medical sociology, and transcultural nursing are devoted to conceptualizing and reporting on these variations cross-culturally. However, an equally important concern of these disciplines is the recognition of the cultural origin of one's own expectations regarding illness and its management. Accordingly, this discussion is organized around the anthropological concepts of 1) cultural expectation, 2) reciprocity, 3) belief systems, 4) social networks, 5) "drums of affliction," and 6) stigma. Each of these is examined in reference to progression responses in ALS in relation to the five major coping mechanisms outlined by Cohen and Lazarus (16): 1) information seeking, 2) direct action, 3) inhibition of action, 4) intrapsychic processes, and 5) turning to others for support. The goal is to demonstrate ways in which ALS violates generalized American cultural values, creating problems for health professionals as well as for ALS persons and their family caregivers.

Cultural Expectations

Every culture has a set of written and unwritten rules for behavior, which are termed *norms* or *cultural expectations*. Because they are such widely shared assumptions and so much a part of what is seen as "normal" behavior, people often become aware of them only when they are violated. Agar (17) terms such occurrences *breakdowns in code*. For example, the American values of independence, mobility, individual control, and competence are all compromised for the person with ALS (2). Americans expect people to be responsible for their own actions, to ask for assistance only when absolutely necessary, and to maintain as much control over their own lives as possible. The underlying cultural code is dramatically and painfully laid bare when persons with ALS are no longer able to meet these expectations.

There are also norms for being sick. That is, it is acceptable to be ill as long as one seeks proper care, follows directions, and returns to previous social responsibilities within a reasonable length of time (18). But as a culture, we have a low tolerance for prolonged relinquishment of social roles and functions, and persons with chronic illnesses are in violation of the expectation that an individual be "productive." There is pressure to return to one's responsibilities as quickly as possible, and much of our rehabilitation efforts are aimed at restoration of function (10).

Many ALS patients do manage to continue to be productive. The British physicist Stephen Hawking and the late Senator Jacob Javits are outstanding examples. However, it should not be overlooked that one of the reasons we admire such people is that it is a shared cultural expectation—one that we learn from birth. Ours is a culture with an emphasis on "doing" rather than "being" (19). It takes tremendous effort on the part of families to help persons with ALS continue to "do," and this may be an important part of coping, especially in the early stages of the disease, and depending on what the person's occupational role has been. A mail carrier or an auto mechanic may have the work role subverted early in the course of the disease, as leg and hand function diminishes, while someone whose work primarily involves thinking and organizing may continue for some time to feel productive and to be seen as such by others.

Given these cultural expectations, denial of loss of function may be expected as a coping response that occurs early in the progress of ALS. Eventually, however, inhibition of action may be a more realistic one. ALS patients " . . . may progressively have to give up actions not only when they cannot do them, but when the action becomes more and more dangerous to their well-being" (20).

This giving up of an activity can be related to the concept of the spiral of loss, grief, and adaptation noted earlier. As a family member in one of our studies said, "It was really a shock the day he could no longer release the catch on his recliner chair to get himself out of the chair. Now he has to wait for someone to come help him whereas before he could get up and walk every twenty or thirty minutes, and keep comfortable." There is, then, a practical component to the doing ethic that is so much a part of American culture. The person is motivated to take direct action, and as long as he/she is able to do so, is more in control of maintaining comfort.

Intermediate in the course of the disease, direct action may take the form of simply completing physical care needs. One of our patients expressed this in the following way:

> "It's not like I have any free time. By the time I get up and brush my teeth and have breakfast, sit in my chair, get up and get a drink, three hours have passed! I mean,

it takes me THREE HOURS to do this! And it's not that my days go very slowly. I'm just completely occupied with just trying to take care of myself.''

This particular patient liked to read, but his hands were getting too weak to hold a book, his eyes were burning, and he was spending all his energy just to complete activities of daily living. We suggested Talking Books, which he initially resisted. But when he found they were produced more like radio drama than like someone simply reading aloud, he subscribed and found great pleasure in them. Recent enthusiasm for books on tape among busy commuters in the general population may also reduce the stigma attached to their use by people experiencing health challenges. There is some evidence (2) that assistive devices are most readily accepted by some ALS patients when they are not specific to the context of illness, e.g., electric toothbrushes, conference phones.

As the disease progresses, patients may need to be given permission to simply ''be.'' They may need assurance that their value as human beings is not tied to what they are able to do. This may be difficult since Americans share the value of the work ethic, but recognizing it as a significant influence can assist in reevaluating how it is expressed and managed.

At the end, persons with ALS may also need to be given permission to give up. Again, American culture values the ''fighter,'' the one who does not give in to adversity, and patients sometimes feel they are letting everyone down when they finally feel the need to succumb. They need assurance that it is acceptable to let go.

Reciprocity

The next concept to be discussed is reciprocity, the give and take that is a part of social life. Many years ago Marcel Mauss (21) did a classic study of gift exchange in a variety of cultures and concluded that universally, when a gift is given, there is an implied obligation to give something in return. In a longitudinal case study of two ALS patients, Cobb and Hamera (2) found that both subjects expressed some form of the cultural axiom, ''It's better to give than to receive,'' indicating their difficulty with imbalance in exchange.

There are changes over time with how persons with ALS feel about reciprocating. Many ALS patients describe an in-rushing of care and concern on the part of friends when they are first diagnosed. This may be followed by a dramatic withdrawal, especially as the person's ability to communicate becomes diminished. Eventually only the most loyal of friends may continue to visit. In these circumstances, it may be fairly easy to accept the early attention and gift-giving, usually in the form of foods and favors, especially if the person with ALS has been involved in a community and has ''given'' in the past. But as the disease progresses, and the ALS person is forced to become more and more dependent on caregivers, it is sometimes difficult to accept help and gifts, and to feel he/she has anything to give in return.

Some patients manage this rather well over a long period of time, using such coping mechanisms as direct action, turning to others, and intrapsychic processes. Early in the disease, when physical functions are not too inhibited, ALS patients may take on household tasks previously allocated to a spouse or children. As functional abilities deteriorate, many of our patients have designed assistive devices to help caregivers in managing their care. Some have written books (22). They continue to take direct action by using their cognitive abilities, combining this with another coping mechanism, turning to others. While they may no longer be able actually to hold a pencil and write, they can accept the help of someone taking dictation, because of the perceived potential benefit to a large number of people through the publication of books or articles about ALS.

It is during the final stages of the disease that it is most difficult for ALS persons to feel that they reciprocate, i.e., that they have anything to give. The coping mechanism of intrapsychic processes may be the only one possible at this point. That is, they may need to refocus their attention or reappraise the situation so that they may see themselves in some way as giving. Again, some patients are able to do this by continuing to use their cognitive abilities, such as by dictating letters of encouragement to others. But for some, even this will be difficult.

Belief Systems

Beliefs and values are two of the major components of culture. Religion is sometimes listed as a coping mechanism by those who write about chronic illness. But the concept of *belief system* is much more comprehensive and, if focused on health beliefs, refers to what people think is the cause of their illness, how it should be treated, and the terms by which they evaluate the treatments received. As a culture, we share a general belief in science and the scientific treatment of disease. There is an expectation of cure (23). But when chronic illnesses arise, for which there is no curative treatment within the scientific system, people may turn to other systems. Gould (5) has argued that after the initial stage of shock at being given the diagnosis of ALS, patients may enter a stage in which they search for and experiment with many forms of alternative treatment. Our patients have used chiropractic, macrobiotic diets, various forms of IV injections, snake venom, and perhaps many others that they have not told us about. In our clinic, we have assumed a nonjudgmental stance about such treatments in order to keep the lines of communication open between patients and professionals, and so that we may know whether there is any perceived benefit from these treatments.

Kleinman (24) has suggested that there are differences in explanatory models that lay people and professionals hold regarding disease/illness. He advises (25) that clinicians should not assume that patients share their beliefs about cause and treatment, but instead should directly ask, "What do you think has caused your illness?," "How do you think it should be treated?," "How long do you think it will last?" Although these questions are meant to bring out differences, especially between the professionals and the patients, they might also be useful for ALS patients in identifying potential areas of conflict and in identifying coping mechanisms. Similarly, Tripp-Reimer et al. (26) and Neuman (27) have developed nursing assessment tools that allow for the identification of areas of patient-professional conflict that may be useful in communicating with ALS persons.

One of the intrapsychic processes used for coping with ALS, then, may be a well-developed and tightly interconnected set of beliefs about cause and cure. In some instances, this may be totally secular, such as the belief that there is a biological deficit—some missing element—for which taking megadoses of certain vitamins would seem to be a reasonable treatment. In other cases, ALS patients may believe that the illness is a punishment from God, or that God "punishes those whom he loves," and consequently may feel that, regardless of what professionals do, the possibility of healing is in the hands of God.

Professionals in a clinic setting may see this belief as a form of denial, and perhaps it can be called that. But there is a growing consensus in the literature that denial can be an effective coping device, especially in the short term (5). For example, one of our patients wrote a beautiful letter just before her death. In it she said that she still was hoping for a healing, but if that did not happen and she got to heaven and found that there was a healing committee, she was going to ask right away to serve on it. Her belief in God and in the possibility of a miraculous healing sustained her to the end. On the other hand, one of the patients we interviewed for our study (2) placed her faith in medical science, hoping until the very last for a cure that would be beneficial to her, even when to the objective observer the atrophy had advanced beyond any possibility of reversal.

The concept of belief systems, then, encompasses more than just religious belief. It can include the interlocking set of explanations for cause, treatment, and cure that ALS patients utilize throughout the course of their illness. Sometimes they are different from beliefs that professionals have, but it is important to remember that they are logical and consistent to the patient and can function as a major coping mechanism from diagnosis to death. They are connected to all five of Cohen and Lazarus's (16) coping strategies. That is, it is on the basis of what people believe about their illness that they seek information, take direct action, inhibit other actions, utilize various intrapsychic processes, and turn to others for assistance.

Social Networks

The concept of social networks (28,29,30) and coping by turning to others for assistance are closely related. If we define social networks as the web of relationships an ill individual has, then social support is the outcome health professionals hope to help patients obtain by turning to people in their network for assistance. In preindustrial societies, every individual had a totally dense network. That is, he or she had kinship, friendship, or work relationships with many other individuals in the society. In our culture, however, people may have networks that are very small in structure—containing very few people—or they may not be very dense. That is, the person may know many people, but the ties may be only a single strand, e.g., a work relationship, rather than many-stranded, in which the person may live in the same neighborhood with the ill individual, work at the same company, attend the same church, and even be related. Such a dense or many-stranded network is more likely in a small rural community than in our mobile urban areas. And it is the density of a network that largely determines the kinds of assistance network members are willing to contribute, how often they can be expected to be called on for help, and over what period of time.

Assessment of the quality of the social network is important early on in the course of ALS, because it can help to predict how well family members will be able to continue over time to cope with the increasing demands for care made on them as the disease progresses. The social network is one potential source of physical and psychological respite for family caregivers.

An example of a dense network from our clinic was Mary, who moved with her husband to Kansas City so that they could live in a residential community made up of church members. Her husband became employed as a caretaker for the church, and they attended services every Sunday, with Mary continuing for a long period of time to edit the church newspaper. They were in close physical proximity to family, church members, and work associates, and were able to make contributions in which they could maintain some reciprocal balance, at least for a time.

In contrast, our local ALS chapter has worked with ALS persons who not only lived alone, but had few close contacts of any kind. In one instance, George, an impeccable, articulate, black man who had always lived alone, managed for as long as he could, mostly with the help of ALS society volunteers and auxiliary home care workers, then was welcomed back to Texas by his extended family, who cared for him until he died several months later. In other cases, persons have had to go to long-term care facilities when they were no longer able to care for themselves alone. And there are those instances in which the primary social network, i.e., spouse and children, dissolves in the face of the stresses that ALS produces.

Drums of Affliction

"Drums of affliction" is a term coined by Turner (31) to describe certain African ritual groups and the activities they perform to assist community members suffering from particular difficulties. Although African ritual activity may seem far removed from the concerns of persons with ALS in the United States, Janzen (32) has argued that there are similarities between the groups Turner describes and contemporary Western support or self-help groups. Characteristic of both is that people become members by virtue of being a victim of some kind of difficulty, which often comes on rather suddenly and is not, in essence, solvable. Members, therefore, have a shared life experience, and much of the content of belief, ritual, or discussion in such a group revolves around how to deal with this life problem.

Janzen (32) goes on to say that what is therapeutic about these kinds of groups in any culture is that the affliction becomes reframed in such a way that those afflicted become, in some sense, healers. That is, by group sharing and problem solving, participants become empowered. They learn how to deal with day-to-day problems; they can see themselves, at least within the group, as "special" rather than "different"; they are given an opportunity to reciprocate with new members, to offer them the wisdom of their experience in dealing with the affliction.

ALS support groups serve all these functions, just as the drums of affliction do for the Ndembu. There has been an ALS support group in the Kansas City area for almost fifteen years. It began with much concern that ALS patients would be depressed at seeing others in more advanced stages of the disease, and indeed this has happened for some people. Their response has been either not to return to the group or to wait and try it again later. For the vast majority, however, the group calls into play most of the five coping mechanisms discussed here.

For example, in the early stages of ALS, the support group acts as a resource for those who are seeking information. Careful as physicians and nurses in the clinic situation may be to provide information at the pace that patients and family members are able to handle it, this is extremely difficult in the short time allotted to a clinic visit. Individuals also need time to absorb the impact of being given the diagnosis and may not be ready to ask questions until some weeks after the clinic visit (3). It can be very helpful to ALS patients and families to know there is a support group with a library of information, as well as volunteers with whom one can talk.

As the disease progresses, both patients and family members learn kinds of helpful direct action to take, and in the group they may also learn what kinds of actions need to be inhibited to conserve energy and to preserve their relationships with each other. People often go to the group for just this kind of practical advice, but they find that the intrapsychic processes involved in coping with ALS also form a significant part of the exchange. For example, in one of the early support group meetings, efforts were made to assist members in dealing with the death of an individual who was particularly important to the members. The suggestion was made to break into small groups and "get our emotions onto the table" by looking first at the three emotions of grief, fear, and frustration; then, "on a more positive note," to look at acceptance, hope, and support. This kind of sharing of feelings is an important aspect of coping, which of course become more and more difficult as the person loses the ability to communicate.

Facilitators in ALS support groups (as well as caregivers in hospitals, clinics, and homes) must be careful to allow the time needed for patients to spell out or to use other means of communicating what they have to share if they have lost the ability to speak. This loss is one of the most traumatic aspects of having ALS, and the only place the ALS person is given adequate time to fully express a thought may be in the support group. One of our patients said, "My family tries, but by the time I've gotten across what I want to say, the conversation has moved on to something else." This may be less true when the ALS person is talking one-on-one with someone, but in a group they often feel like "the silent ones." Not to allow time for them to speak in their own way is to deny their basic humanity. The orientation to time in American culture reflects a culture in a hurry. "Time is money," and it is necessary to become aware of how ingrained these attitudes are, and the ways in which they manifest themselves, if persons with ALS are to really be given help in coping with ALS as the disease progresses.

Thinking of ALS support groups in relation to African "drums of affliction" helps to demonstrate that in other cultures as well as in our own there is a recognition of the need to transform a difficult and painful life situation into one more manageable. This can be done through gathering together in support groups, which can serve as a major coping mechanism both for patients and for family members throughout the course of the disease and beyond. Many surviving spouses have continued to remain associated with the ALS group for extended periods after the death of a family member. They do an invaluable service in sharing their accumulated wisdom of this traumatic life experience.

Stigma

Every culture has culturally determined standards for physical beauty as well as for norms of behavior. Because ALS causes atrophy of certain muscles, the physical appearance of persons with this disease changes. Speech also changes because the muscles of the tongue are affected. ALS persons often feel stigmatized (33), partly as a result of these physical changes. Some fear going out in public because gait may be unsteady in the early stages of the disease and there is a danger of injury from falling. Besides the concern of physical injury, there is the social stigma involved with the belief that others may think they are inebriated.

The emotional lability associated with bulbar ALS violates cultural norms that dictate when it is appropriate to laugh or to cry. If persons cannot control this emotional expression, they may withdraw from social interaction because of the stigma they feel this causes. As the emotional lability decreases with the progression of the disease, difficulties with chewing and swallowing may also cause persons to avoid eating in public places, causing further isolation. Some families have coped with this by inviting people in, selecting from among their friends those who are sensitive to the effects of changes in body function and self-image. But coping with one's self-image is an ongoing challenge for the person with ALS throughout the course of the illness.

Conclusion

It is difficult to have a terminal, progressive degenerative disease like ALS, with no known cause or cure, which sometimes progresses so rapidly that there is little time to recover from and adapt to one loss before another must be confronted. It is difficult to be chronically ill in a culture that stresses individual achievement, responsibility, and productivity, when the disease robs persons of the ability to function in these ways and causes physical changes that add to a feeling of stigma. But if health professionals, family members, and friends recognize that these are value patterns that are learned almost unconsciously throughout our lives, and that recognition of them is an important step in evaluating how they affect the way we deal with persons who have ALS, we can become better care providers. The kinds of coping required of both family members and patients over the course of ALS are numerous and varied, and it requires all our sensitivity as clinicians to appropriately assist families in dealing with this devastating illness.

References

1. Hamera E, Cobb AK. Nurse anthropologist as humanist in residence. *Kansas Nurse* 1982, 57:19–20.
2. Cobb AK, Hamera E. Illness experience in a chronic disease—ALS. *Soc Sci Med* 1986, 23:641–650.
3. Beisecker AE, Cobb AK, Zeigler DK. Patients' perspectives of the role of care providers in amyotrophic lateral sclerosis. *Arch Neurol* 1988, 45:553–556.
4. Reckling J, Fernengel K, Berg J, McCann V, Cobb AK. The ALS caregiver's experience: an impelled journey. Poster presentation, *Ann Midwest Nurs Res Soc*, Cleveland, OH, 1990.
5. Gould B. Psychiatric aspects, In: Mulder, DW, ed. *The Diagnosis and Treatment of Amyotrophic Lateral Sclerosis.* Boston: Houghton Mifflin, 1980.
6. Heinemann AW. *Adjustment Following Disability: A Retrospective Investigation.* PhD Diss. Univ Kansas.
7. Scott DW, Oberst MT, Dropkin MJ. A stress-coping model. *Adv Nurs Sci* 1980, 3: 9–23.
8. Comaroff J, Maguire P. Ambiguity and the search for meaning: Childhood leukemia in the modern clinical context. *Soc Sci Med* 1981, 15B:115–123.
9. Fox R. The sting of death in American Society. *Soc Sci Rev* 1981, March, 42–59.
10. Greenwood JG. Disability dilemmas and rehabilitation tension: A twentieth century inheritance. *Soc Sci Med* 1985, 20:1241–1252.
11. Jessop DJ, Stein REK. Uncertainty and its relationship to the psychological and social correlates of chronic illness in children. *Soc Sci Med* 1985, 20:993–999.
12. Kaufert PL, Kaufert JM. Methodological and conceptual issues in measuring the long term impact of disability: The experience of poliomyelitis patients in Manitoba. *Soc Sci Med* 1984, 19:609–618.

13. Sivak ED, Gipson WT, Hanson MR. Long-term management of respiratory failure in amyotrophic lateral sclerosis. *Ann Neurol* 1981, 12:18–23.
14. Houpt J, Gould B, Norris FN. Psychological characteristics of patients with amyotrophic lateral sclerosis (ALS). *Psychosom Med* 1977, 39:299–303.
15. Peters PK, Swenson WM, Miller DW. Is there a characteristic personality profile in amyotrophic lateral sclerosis?'' *Arch Neurol* 1978, 35:321–22.
16. Cohen F, Lazarus RS. Coping with the stresses of illness. In: Stone GC, Cohen F, Adler NE, eds. *Health Psychology: A Handbook.* San Francisco: Jossey-Bass, 1979.
17. Agar, MH. *Speaking of Ethnography.* Beverly Hills, CA: Sage Publications, 1986.
18. Parsons T. Definitions of health and illness in the light of American values and social structure. In: Jaco EG, ed. *Patients, Physicians and Illness,* 2nd ed. New York: Free Press, 1972.
19. Kluckhohn F, Strodtbeck F. *Variations in Value Orientations.* Evanston, IL: Row, Peterson, 1961.
20. Burkhardt CS. Coping strategies of the chronically ill. *Nurs Clinic North Am* 1987, 22:543–549.
21. Mauss M. *The Gift.* New York: Norton, 1967.
22. Hamilton L. *Why Didn't Somebody Tell Me About These Things?* Shawnee Mission, KS: Inter-Collegiate Press, 1984.
23. Young A. The relevance of traditional medical cultures to modern primary health care. *Soc Sci Med* 1983, 17:1205–1211.
24. Kleinman A. Concepts and a model for the comparison of medical systems as cultural systems. *Soc Sci Med* 1978, 12:85–93.
25. Kleinman A, Eisenberg L, Good B, Culture, Illness and care: clinical lessons from anthropologic and cross-cultural research. *Ann Int Med* 1978, 88:251–258.
26. Tripp-Reimer T, Brink PJ, Saunders JM, Cultural assessment: content and process. *Nurs Outlook* 1984, 32:78–82.
27. Neuman B, The Betty Neuman health care systems model: A total person approach to patient problems. In: Riehl JP, Roy C, eds. *Conceptual Models for Nursing Practice,* 2nd ed. New York: Appleton-Century-Crofts, 1980.
28. Mitchell JC, ed. *Social Networks in Urban Situations: Analyses of Personal Relationships in Central African Towns.* Manchester: Manchester University Press, 1969.
29. Bott E. *Family and Social Network: Roles, Norms, and External Relationships in Ordinary Urban Families,* 2nd ed. New York: Free Press, 1971.
30. Tolsdorf CC. Social networks, support, and coping: an exploratory study. *Fam Process* 1978, 15:407–417.
31. Turner V. *The Drums of Affliction.* Oxford: Clarendon, 1968.
32. Janzen JM, Drums . . . anonymous: Towards an understanding of structures of therapeutic maintenance (Unpub). Rochester Plan University Lecture.
33. Goffman E. *Stigma: Notes on the Management of Spoiled Identity.* Englewood Cliffs, N.J.: Prentice-Hall,1963.

17

The ALS Caregiver's Experience: An Impelled Journey

Ann Kuckelman Cobb, R.N., Ph.D., JoAnn B. Reckling, R.N., M.N., M.A., and Karen J. Fernengel, R.N., M.N.

Introduction

Doctoral students in nursing at the University of Kansas take a course in qualitative research methods as part of their curriculum. During this experience, they conduct interviews, make observations, record field notes, and do participant-observation in a naturalistic setting around a particular research question. They are frequently allowed to select a question related to their own interests, but may also be asked to participate in research of concern to the course instructor. In the Fall of 1989, the first author (Cobb) asked the class to focus on the experience of caregivers of persons with ALS. Although the primary goal of the class was to teach methods of data collection and analysis in qualitative research, some substantive issues related to progression responses, coping, and caregiving in ALS were identified.

Methods

Three methods of data collection were used: a focus group interview, long individual interviews of ALS caregivers, and participant-observation in the homes of ALS patients and caregivers. As a demonstration on how to conduct focus group interviews, seven caregivers were asked to come to the School of Nursing to be interviewed as a group by the course instructor, with the students observing the process. The interview was audiotaped and transcribed, with the written permission of the respondents, and each student received a copy of the transcript for analysis. Each student then arranged to meet with one ALS caregiver for a long individual interview, to follow up on issues identified in the focus group, and to uncover other dimensions of caregiving. Students also did eight hours, divided into two sessions, of participant-observation in the home of the person interviewed and with the ALS patient. The goal was to obtain a vivid and realistic picture of what it is like for patients, family members, and other caregivers to manage ALS at home.

Analysis of the data was a two-stage process. Students individually analyzed the focus group data and the data each had obtained from the long interview. The data were then combined into a single set and analyzed by the group under the guidance of the instructor. Transcripts of interviews and field notes were examined for patterns that expressed the essence of the caregiver's experience of caring for a family member with ALS.

Results of qualitative research are presented in nonnumerical, narrative form. The goal is to describe a phenomenon from the perspective of the participants; to present accurately, vividly, and succinctly what they see as important in the situation being examined.

Results

Five categories that characterize the experience of family caregivers for persons with ALS were identified (Table 17-1).

Table 17-1. Summary of Categories and Definitions

Category	Definition
"Taking It"	—Experiencing an awareness of unanticipated, uncontrollable, and/or unknown events from which an ALS caregiver has no escape.
"Staying Afloat"	—Surviving: tolerating the situation and attempting to maintain normalcy, but efforts to maintain balance occur in the face of continuous conflicting tensions, and with a sense of impending crisis.
"Losing Ground"	—Experiencing loss, as for example in relationships, self-control, privacy, tolerance, and one's own health.
"Regrouping"	—Regaining a degree of control either by acquisition of physical and/or informational assistance from outside, and/or spiritual and/or emotional assistance from within or without.
"Holding Together"	—Doing what you can with what there is. Making the most of the situation at hand, understanding it and accepting it and adjusting to it.

We labeled the first category *Taking It*, a phrase often used by our respondents. *Taking It* was defined as experiencing an awareness of unanticipated, uncontrollable, and/or unknown events from which an ALS caregiver has no escape. *Taking It* had two subcategories: 1) taking it *in* and 2) taking it *on*. The first was defined as an awareness of feelings, thoughts, and sensory perceptions associated with experiencing the unanticipated, uncontrollable event. The second refers to committing to the situation, making the continuing choice to stay, to help, knowing that one does not really know what it will be like. This category of *Taking It* is an overarching one, which does not subsume the four discussed below.

The other four categories represent a cyclic process and most clearly relate to the issue of progression responses in ALS.

Holding Together describes the optimum link in the process, when caregivers are managing relatively well. *Staying Afloat* implies managing, attempting to maintain normalcy, but with a feeling of impending crisis. *Losing Ground* describes the caregiver's ongoing experience of loss. When *Regrouping* occurs, there is some regaining of a sense of control, using devices such as physical or informational assistance from outside and spiritual/emotional assistance from within or without. If *Regrouping* is successful, even on a temporary basis, *Holding Together* again occurs. *Taking It* may be reentered repeatedly from any of the other categories as new changes are encountered. At the microlevel, the cycle may repeat several times within a single day. At a macrolevel, this process characterizes the overall pattern of the experience of ALS caregivers and patients in managing ALS (Figure 17-1).

MODEL OF THE ALS CAREGIVERS' EXPERIENCE

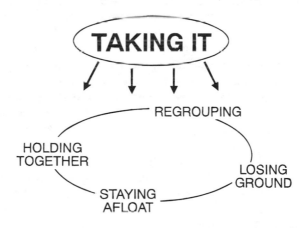

Figure 17-1.

In what follows, the components of the model are related to progression responses of the family and ALS patient as the disease progresses, and to coping responses commonly cited in the literature. In Chapter 16, Cobb discusses five methods of coping as outlined by Cohen and Lazarus (1), including 1) information seeking, 2) direct action, 3) inhibition of action, 4) intrapsychic processes, and 5) turning to others for support, and relates these to cultural influences on ways patients and families cope with ALS as the disease progresses. In this chapter, we focus on the five categories in the model (Figure 17-1) we derived from our research, and again relate them to Cohen and Lazarus's (1) coping methods. We also discuss them in relation to two other concepts: hope and courage.

First, let us say something about hope. Several years ago, Cobb conducted a videotaped interview with Keith Worthington, an ALS patient and founder of what has become the Kansas City Chapter of the ALS Association. Keith was then on a respirator. One of the things that came out very clearly in that interview was his statement, "It is very important to have a physician who does not subscribe to the 'no hope' school of thought." There has been an ongoing argument in the literature about the relationship between hope and denial—when is hope a form of denial, and does denial thwart efforts to provide appropriate health services. Consensus, if there is any, seems to be that denial, at least at certain stages in an illness, can be a positive coping mechanism, i.e., it can help to preserve hope and prevent despair (2,3). Others (4) have suggested that the concept of denial is vague and sometimes inappropriately used in clinical settings. Wright and Shontz (5) conducted research identifying the dimensions of hope in children with disabilities. More recently, Kim used Wright and Shontz's framework in discussing hope as a mode of coping in ALS (6). We will be drawing from both of these works in relating them to our model of the ALS caregiver's experience.

The other concept we wish to bring in is the concept of courage. Shelp (7) discusses courage as a moral virtue in the patient-physician relationship. We take liberties with what he said by generalizing his statements to include more than just physicians, but it seems clear that courage is a virtue required of all parties in the ALS encounter—patients, family members, and professionals of all types. Shelp defines courage as ". . . the disposition to voluntarily act, perhaps fearfully, in a dangerous circumstance, where the relevant risks are reasonably appraised, in an effort to obtain or preserve some perceived good for oneself or others, recognizing that the desired perceived good may not be realized" (p. 354). However, courage is not necessarily action; it can also apply to *enduring*. The essence of courage is the mastery of fear for the preservation of good. In his definition of courage, risk implies vulnerability, and the ultimate vulnerability is death. Sickness causes one to come face-to-face with death and to find meaning in a situation in which meaning is threatened. Caregivers can help to impart that meaning. Shelp (7) states that physicians tend not to disclose their doubts to patients and colleagues, so as to sustain an image of strength, superiority, or power. He suggests that a better image is that of a "sustaining presence," which allows for strength *and* weakness; this implies that one wants to help, is loyal to the other party, and is honest about one's limitations. The sustaining presence of caregivers can state that the patient is affirmed by others and therefore worthy of self-affirmation. We "learn of courage as [we] abide by patients when there is little or no more [we] can do" (7). If courage is a moral virtue relevant to the patient encounter, encouragement can be thought of as a way of enhancing coping in ALS.

The Model

Taking It

We defined *Taking It* as experiencing an awareness of unanticipated, uncontrollable, and/or unknown events from which an ALS caregiver has no escape. Examples of such events are the diagnosis delivered to the ALS patient, the fear it engenders, situations in which everything happens at once, loss of yet another function by the patient, loss of sleep for the caregiver, and so on. Needless to say, the patient undergoes a similar experience. The subcategory *Taking It In* is the awareness of feelings, thoughts, and sensory perceptions associated with the above. Our study participants said, "Life has changed drastically," "Neither of us realized what we were getting into," "Very traumatic, unbelievable,"

Taking It and *Taking It In* are clearly apparent in the early stages of ALS, when the patient and family have just been given the diagnosis and are faced with the task of processing just what it may mean to them, their relationships, their work, and social roles. One caregiver said, ". . . when they told me 'amyotrophic lateral sclerosis,' I thought, Doc, what are you talking about?" At this point, intrapsychic processes of denial of the full ramifications of the disease may be necessary to maintain hope. When patients or family members say, "Neither of us realized what we were getting into," this screening of reality acts as a protective device for the moment. Wright and Shontz (5) term this a dimension of hoping in which one achieves a hopeful attitude by intentionally keeping the future undifferentiated in the face of formidable reality. It is the "one day at a time" attitude, and Kim (6) suggests that an appropriate professional intervention is to support and validate such statements.

Taking It On, the next subcategory, means committing to the situation, making the continuing choice to stay, to help, knowing that one does not really know what it will be like. One of the caregivers interviewed for the study was a 72-year-old woman whose 41-year-old son had ALS. The son was separated and eventually divorced, so this woman and her retired husband took on the responsibility of caregiving as the disease progressed. They had been looking forward to retirement, but willingly came to assist their son when the need became apparent. What they had not bargained for was caring for the grandchildren as well. The woman told us, "They have three children and when [husband] and I decided to come, we didn't realize that three children would be part of our responsibility too, at times, because they only live a mile from our house, and, of course, they are the light of [son's] life, each day that he can see them." This couple made the continuing commitment to stay, despite this unanticipated additional burden. The respondent stated, "You do have to adjust your thinking and your doing in many ways. [Husband] and I are both seventy-two, so it's been an adjustment for both of us, but we're so happy we can do it and wish we could do more."

This example is very much like what Shelp (7) is describing when he speaks of courage. Freedom of choice is one dimension of courage, and although it seems as if patients and families have no choice, we in fact know of family members who choose not to stay. Those who do, who *take on* the responsibilities and the risks to their own health, are exercising moral courage. Patients have less choice, but they exercise courage in living each day and in facing their own death and finding meaning in it. Professionals, too, must have the courage to *take it on*—to be that "sustaining presence," to affirm the selfhood of the ALS person even as abilities decline, even when the professional is challenged by knowing there are not specific curative treatments to offer. Both professionals and family caregivers, like the patients, must be willing to endure, to admit our limitations, making the continuing choice to stay.

Once one has *taken it on*, coping mechanisms such as information seeking and direct action are called into play. Professional caregivers must be sensitive to patient and family readiness to learn more about ALS (8), and the readiness to seek help through the coping mechanism of turning to others for support, such as through attendance at support groups. It should be recognized that going to the first support group meeting may be a significant act of courage for the patient. That is, the patient knows that he/she will be seeing other persons in more advanced stages of the disease, and the risk is one of being robbed of hope. Persons with ALS sometimes come to support groups at least initially as a way of giving something to the family caregivers, whom they recognize as needing a night out, time with people who also are enduring the stresses of caregiving. The risk to their own self-image as they see the effect of the disease on others is high, but so, too, is the possibility of increasing hope when they realize that their own assets and abilities compare favorably with those of others. One role the professional caregiver can play with regard to assets and abilities is to assist the person with ALS to review and value remaining physical, interpersonal, and role-function potentialities (6).

Staying Afloat

This category is defined as surviving: tolerating the situation and attempting to maintain normalcy, but efforts to maintain balance occur in the face of continuous conflicting tensions, and with a sense of impending crisis. One of our respondents said, "You keep hoping he isn't going to get worse, but on the other side of your mind, you know that he is," This "hoping" statement is another example of what Wright and Shontz (5) refer to as "the unpromising future," a version of living in the present as a way to maintain hope. The feeling of just surviving may be most acute in the early phases of the progress of the disease, when patient and family are trying to become accustomed to growing physical and social limitations and to the knowledge of the severity of the illness. It would also characterize more advanced stages of the disease, when there are tremendous demands on physical, emotional, and financial resources, and a growing awareness of reaching the limits of these resources. One respondent, a woman in her thirties, whose 34-year-old husband experienced rapid deterioriation from ALS and was in advanced stages, said, "My problem is . . . with two small children and trying to take care of the house and, the yard and the car and the bills and the doctor visits and the kids being sick, and, you know, running one to soccer, and . . . I *can't* do it all. I *have* been, but I'm ready to go crazy. . . ." She was attempting to maintain normalcy, but was barely staying afloat, aware that finances and her own personal resources were stretched to the limit.

Losing Ground

This category of the model describes the experience of loss as, for example, in relationships, self-control, privacy, tolerance, and one's own health. Both persons with ALS and their caregivers experience all of these losses. As communication and other physical abilities decrease with the progress of the disease, relationships alter. There may be a reversal of roles between spouses and a loss of self-control and tolerance in the face of almost impossible demands. Ironically, two of the coping methods that may be useful in these circumstances, i.e., direct action and turning to others for support, have the undesirable effect of invading the privacy of both patient and caregiver when the ALS person is cared for at home. Caregivers we interviewed sought and received help from a variety of care providers such as nurses, home health aides, volunteers, and friends, yet for all the assistance received, they suffered from the loss of privacy they felt with these helpers coming into their home. One caregiver said,

> "I feel like I have a revolving door. I have no privacy. Every time I turn around somebody is coming in. I just had to finally accept that. I haven't liked it, but I've had to accept it. My home is just not my home anymore. We leave the garage door up all day. And they [care providers] know to just walk through the garage door and come in through the family room door and there we are. People are coming and going all the time, somebody is always coming or going. And . . . you cannot take care of him alone . . . you give up your privacy . . . you give up the control of your own life."

Perhaps it can be viewed as an act of courage on the part of family caregivers to allow this invasion of what is in some sense a sacred space, for the good of the other, i.e., the person with ALS. Similarly, professionals who take themselves into the home setting where they are without the normal sense of control afforded by a clinical context are also exercising moral courage. They are that "sustaining presence," willing to risk a certain amount of vulnerability, willing to affirm the selfhood of the ALS person, by continuing care when cure is not possible.

In relation to the category of *losing ground*, what sets ALS apart from other chronic and/or terminal illnesses is the rapidity with which losses can occur and the relentlessly downward trajectory of the progress of the disease. Scott et al. (9) have presented a model of coping based on the metaphor of the recurring spiral, in which there is a loss, followed by grieving of the loss, then attempting new coping responses, and reaching another temporary equilibrium. Wright and Shontz (5) identify *mourning* as an aspect of hoping, but with ALS in some cases the losses follow so quickly one upon the other that there is no time for mourning, and no real equilibrium may be reached. One respondent said, "It has progressed so fast in [husband] that we've never had a little group of time to adjust to it before he loses something else. He's losing everything all at once." When the progress of the disease is not so precipitous, there may be time to give vent to the realistic and deeply felt sorrow when *losing ground*, providing an opportunity for *regrouping* to occur.

Regrouping

This category involves regaining a degree of control either by acquisition of physical and/or informational assistance from outside, and/or spiritual and/or emotional assistance from within or without. Examples are obtaining assistive devices, getting information and supervision in using equipment, benefitting from reassurance, sharing in support groups. Regrouping is the category most clearly related to coping. It is action-oriented and may include information seeking, direct action, intrapsychic processes, and turning to others for support. Inhibition of action may also take place when regrouping involves preventing the person with ALS from carrying out activities that he or she can no longer safely perform without potential harm to self or others. Regrouping is the attempt to reach a state of equilibrium in the spiral of loss, even if only for a short period of time. One respondent reported obtaining outside assistance through hospice services.

> "We also have a hospice nurse who has been a godsend. I rejected this in the beginning very much. . . . But . . . I just can't say enough for her. She comes twice a week and takes J's blood pressure and last winter he was on the verge of a cold and she got some antibiotics for him right away. She's just a delightful person, and she puts my mind at ease. If he's not breathing just like we think he should be, she checks his lungs and reassures us."

Holding Together

This category in the model is defined as doing what one can with what there is; making the most of the situation at hand, understanding it, accepting it, and adjusting to it. In our model, it is the closest concept to a state of equilibrium. It is a more positive state of coping than *staying afloat*. The feeling component of *holding together* includes perception that one is in fact making the most of the situation. The doing component includes such things as willing self-sacrifice, loving, giving, grieving together, and being able to support other caregivers. Holding together has both a descriptive and metaphorical meaning. Metaphorically, the emphasis is on "together," that is, the ALS patient and family are at a place where they are not being pulled apart by the demands of their situation. They in a sense encircle one another, forming a kind of mandala of support such that there is a sense of enduring together, with a margin of strength left over to give to others in similar circumstances. This state is most likely to occur when the progress of the disease is slower, when there is some time to adjust to changes, and is also affected by the type of resources available to the family. In our interviews with ALS caregivers, those who were caring for a spouse, had grown children, were retired, and were financially comfortable were most likely to feel that they were "holding together." In contrast, the young mother of two small children, whose 34-year-old husband was in advanced stages of the progression of the disease and was being cared for by her at home, and who was running out of funds, was barely *staying afloat*. She was using coping methods such as turning to others for support, but had the sense that such support was not unlimited. She also attempted to inhibit her husband from lying in one position in the knowledge that his skin was beginning to break down, but was frustrated in this by his refusal to cooperate. She understood that his action was one small way of continuing to assert himself, but foresaw further crises for them both if he persisted. Eventually, shortly before he died, she took direct action by placing him in a nursing home when she could no longer both provide direct care to him and manage the needs of their two small children.

When families are *holding together*, there is room for active hoping. There is some time and energy to review with the ALS patient the remaining assets and abilities, and health care providers can be a part of this review process. It is an active intervention that can be taken, particularly if family caregivers do not do it. Another aspect of hoping in which the health care provider can be actively involved is in encouraging the person with ALS to see the illness as an opportunity for personal growth (6). It is not so much a matter of telling the person that such growth is possible, but rather, supporting and reinforcing insights that the patient has. Kim (6) gives an example: the patient might say, "Through my loss of muscle coordination, I learned to take time in doing tasks and the experience of ALS taught me to discover other sides of myself." To support such a statement is to reinforce hope.

With regard to courage, Shelp (7) states that Eric Cassel sees as one of the duties of a physician the relief from suffering through imparting meaning to a situation where meaning is threatened. Shelp goes on to say that how that is done is an open question, but that doing it well may require greater energy and creativity than performing well in physical diagnosis and treatment. To quote him,

> "In the experience of sickness and suffering the weak and strong are bound together in a therapeutic alliance. Rather than being abandoned, the sufferer is a central concern. The one who suffers may be supported in his or her sickness as a means of affirming his or her place in the community. Alternatively, his or her decision to endure no more may be respected and he or she may be assisted in dying as a means of affirming those cherished powers that gave life meaning but that now are gone" (7).

Application of the Model

The model presented in this chapter is intended to describe, primarily in the words of the caregivers interviewed, their experience of caring for a person with ALS as the disease progresses. We are suggesting that the model describes a cyclic process that families go through over the course of the disease, from *taking in* the diagnosis and its ramifications, through *taking it on*, committing to stay without really knowing for certain what that entails, through the hard times of barely *staying afloat* and then *regrouping* through a variety of coping methods until there is a little space of adjustment that we have called *holding together*. We are also suggesting, however, that the model represents a microprocess for the caregiver, in which this cycle may repeat itself several times in a single day—from getting up in the morning committed to doing whatever needs to be done that day to perhaps facing a barrage of unanticipated demands and crises, finding at least some temporary solutions or help, and maybe finding a little breathing space in the day where one has time for oneself. On a given day, the cycle may feel more like a continuous spin. Through it all, both patient and family caregiver may call on the several coping methods discussed. But just as *taking it* is an overarching category in our model, so the elements of hope and courage are continuous themes in coping with ALS. And they are not for ALS families alone. Health professionals can intervene positively by supporting and reinforcing realistic hopes and by listening empathetically even when hopes are not realistic from our own point of view. We can *hope with* those for whom we care. As for courage, we agree with Shelp (7) that:

"Courage is required of those who choose a profession that embodies care and concern. And 'encouragement' is properly one of [health professionals'] duties." Being a "sustaining presence" ourselves helps family members to do the same.

> Sharing in another's life does not consist of burdening the other with requirements. Rather, it consists of eliciting the recognition of personal values and capacities that may go unrealized otherwise. Eliciting courage is not the same as imposing values and norms. For [health professionals] it is assisting patients in not letting fear overtake them

so that the opportunities present in sickness and dying are not lost to them and others. As 'sustaining presence,' the [health professional] shares responsibility for the process and the results. No one bears it alone. Learning to live includes learning even in dying. Without courage the evils in the contexts of sickness and dying go unchallenged.'' (7).

Let us be courageous and hopeful *together*.

Acknowledgments

The authors wish to acknowledge the contributions of Valerie McCann and Jane Berg, who assisted in collection and initial analysis of data.

References

1. Cohen F, Lazarus RS. Coping with the stresses of illness. In: Stone G, Cohen F, Adler N, eds. *Health Psychology—A Handbook*. San Francisco: Jossey-Bass, 1979.
2. Wright BA. The question stands: Should a person be realistic? *Rehab Counsel Bull* 1968, XI:291–296.
3. Herth K. Development and refinement of an instrument to measure hope. *Schol Inq for Nurs Pract* 1991, 5:39–51.
4. Shelp EE, Perl M. Denial in clinical medicine: A reexamination of the concept and its significance. *Arch Int Med* 1985, 145:697–699.
5. Wright BA, Shontz F. Process and tasks in hoping. *Rehab Lit* 1968, 29:322–331.
6. Kim TS. Hope as a mode of coping in amyotrophic lateral sclerosis. *J Neurol Nurs* 1989, 21:342–347.
7. Shelp EE. Courage:A neglected virtue in the patient-physician relationship. *Soc Sci Med* 1984. 18:351–360.
8. Beisecker AE, Cobb AK, Ziegler DK. Patients' perspectives of the role of care providers in amyotrophic lateral sclerosis. *Arch Neurol* 1988, 45:553–556.
9. Scott DW, Oberst MT, Dropkin MJ. A stress-coping model. *Adv Nurs Sci* 1980, 9–23.

18

Amyotrophic Lateral Sclerosis: Legal and Ethical Issues

Mark R. Glasberg, M.D.

Over the past two decades, there has been an increasing concern about the needs of terminally ill patients. A revolutionary change in many of society's viewpoints has occurred during the last five years. Current articles in the media have informed the general public that most people die after an extended period of gradually deteriorating health. There is almost always additional therapy available to prolong a patient's life, and most hospital deaths follow decision making at the end of life, at which time someone must decide how long life will be prolonged, to what quality, and even when death will occur. Generally, at this time, the patient's family and physician explore whether it is appropriate to terminate or withhold treatment in order to hasten death.

Currently, terms that were virtually anathema a few years ago, such as *physician-assisted suicide* and even *euthanasia*, are now becoming acceptable. Within the past two years alone, we have seen a landmark Supreme Court decision in the Nancy Cruzan case, the suicide machine of Dr. Jack Kevorkian, physicians such as Dr. Timothy Quill going public regarding assisting patients with suicide, and a euthanasia referendum in the state of Washington almost approved (44 percent voted for the referendum).

All health care professionals taking care of ALS patients are obligated to be aware of legal and ethical issues in order to provide optimal care to their patients. Since neither treatment that can improve the disease nor a cure is available, it becomes even more imperative that patients and families are properly informed about their ethical and legal rights. They need to be adequately informed about feeding tubes and ventilators, go through the valid consent process, be adequately counseled regarding a living will and Durable Power of Attorney for Health Care, and be adequately advised regarding terminal care. Autonomy, the right to control one's own health care decisions, is a key principle for an ALS patient. Needless to say, if the health care professional cannot adequately inform ALS patients of their ethical and legal rights, then the achievement of autonomy will become markedly more difficult.

Informing Patients of the Diagnosis

Confronted with a newly diagnosed ALS patient, some physicians feel it is best to delay telling the patient the diagnosis as long as possible. In support of their position, they argue that it would be psychologically damaging to the patient to have the burden of the diagnosis of such a bad disease, and the patient may misinterpret what the physician has told him. Also, since the physician can never be 100 percent certain of the diagnosis, perhaps he should not tell the patient (1).

Such diagnostic deception is not helpful and may cause harm to the patient in several ways. Patients may worry that they have an even worse disease than they actually have. They are also deprived of the ability to plan their lives based on the known prognosis of the disease. Additionally, they tend not to believe that physician and may "doctor shop," undergoing expensive, repetitive testing, until at last they are given a diagnosis. Finally, patients will eventually discover the deception and may subsequently disbelieve any of that doctor's future statements., or even those of another physician.

Patients should be told about the diagnosis in a sensitive, understanding, and compassionate manner. They should be educated about the disease and told about current research and experimental drug studies. They should also be put in touch with the Amyotrophic Lateral Sclerosis Association (ALSA) and the local chapter and should be given written information.

Consent

The concept of valid consent and refusal provides that competent adults can accept or refuse all treatments. Therefore, the patient's decision regarding life support is facilitated through the process of valid consent (2). The physician should carefully review the patient's treatment options with him without undue bias, and consent should be obtained without coercion. This does not mean that the practitioner cannot strongly recommend a particular treatment plan; indeed that should be done when indicated, as long as risk and benefit ratios are not exaggerated to convince the patient to agree. The patient should never be threatened that a health care professional will refuse continued medical care unless a specific treatment plan is followed.

Professional Ethics

Neurologists, as well as all physicians, are bound by a set of ethical duties to their patients and their patients' families (3). In addition to obtaining valid consent from patients, a physician is obligated to follow the rational decisions of competent patients. They also have the duty to maintain patient confidentiality. Compassionate caring is another important ethical duty. In particular, in ALS, the physician/patient relationship becomes therapeutic when the physician cares for the patient and treats him with kindness, respect, and empathy (4).

There are specific duties that physicians owe to dying patients, such as doing whatever they can to be sure that the patient does not suffer from pain or any undue distress, and that his wishes are obeyed. However, physicians do not have the ethical duty to provide unproven treatments that will be of no benefit to the patient, particularly if they may be harmful (5, 6). Also, terminally ill patients may ask their physician to mercifully put them to death to end their suffering. Some physicians may feel motivated to comply because they cannot cure the patient and they feel the imperative need to relieve suffering. These patients have the clear right to refuse all life-prolonging medical therapy, including food and water.

Physicians may believe they have a moral duty to continue hydration and nutrition in dying patients to attempt to maximize their comfort. However, terminal patients lose hunger and thirst drives as part of their natural dying process. If physicians attempt to medically hydrate their dying patients, then patients may develop pulmonary edema from overhydration and die in more discomfort than was present without hydration. Hydration should be provided only to thirsty terminal patients (7).

However, physicians have no ethical duty to assist in suicide, even when a competent patient makes such a request. It is indeed wrong to do so (8). Active euthanasia programs, such as those in place in the Netherlands, are not yet approved in the United States (9). However, physicians are certainly obligated to provide complete analgesia for terminal patients. Even if it might hasten death, this is not viewed as euthanasia.

Refusal or Withdrawal of Treatment

Decision making regarding level of care for ALS patients is based on three ethical principles and moral rules (10, 11):

1. Autonomy, the right of individuals to make decisions for themselves, which others must respect (12).
2. Nonmaleficence, the concept "do no harm."

3. Beneficence, the duty to promote good, and the dictum *summum bonum*—
   "Human happiness and well-being is the highest good" (13).

Since autonomy is a cardinal principal, it is the health professional's duty to
respect the patient's right to refuse treatment or to have treatment withdrawn.
Many cases and statutory laws support the ethical concept that an adult person
can choose to accept or refuse treatments, even if the latter decision could lead
to death.

The right to refuse treatment is not an absolute right, and at times it may be
outweighed by compelling state interests. These include the following (14):

1. The state's interest in the preservation of life.
2. The state's interest in protecting third parties.
3. The state's interest in preventing suicide.
4. The state's interest in maintaining the ethical integrity of the medical profession.

However, since virtually all states have viewed respirators, artificial nutrition,
and hydration as a form of treatment that a competent individual with a disease
as debilitating as ALS may refuse, there has never been a case in which removal
of an ALS patient from a ventilator has been negated by a court due to "compelling state's interest" (15).

Health care professionals are increasingly faced with the ALS patient who is
ventilator-bound and requests extubation (16). Such patients are almost invariably
competent. Physicians who are faced with this situation have several obligations:
to ascertain that the patient is competent; to fully inform the patient about the
prognosis with and without the ventilator; and to reassure the patient that whatever
treatment plan is chosen, the physician will not abandon him and that comfort
care will be provided (8). Physicians should take particular care not to coerce
the patient into more aggressive treatment than he wishes by exaggerating the
suffering he will undergo in the absence of treatment. Although it is psychologically difficult to extubate respirator-dependent patients, knowing they will die as
a direct result, this action is the ethically correct one when the competent patient
has chosen it. Physicians have the ethical duty to follow the rational health care
wishes of their competent patients. This premise has been tested and validated
in several high court judicial rulings, and courts have invariably granted patients
dying of ALS the right to have their ventilators discontinued (17).

Physicians must be aware themselves how much easier it is to withhold than
to withdraw treatment, although this is not ethically justified. Treatment was
begun based on potential benefit and the patient's informed consent. If benefits
are less or risks are much greater and discomfort is much more than anticipated,
treatment should be discontinued. The difference between withholding and withdrawing treatment is much more a psychological issue than an ethical one.

If unhappiness and pain predominate despite all efforts, and it is the patient's wish to die, it is our obligation to let him. However, in spite of that being very easy to say, and a straightforward ethical principle to go by, there are indeed paradoxes involved in its actual application. Society expects the physician to be a healer, not a taker of life. On the other hand, they do applaud compassionate doctors who end the suffering of patients. There is the "slippery-slope" principle, which has expressed marked reservations about aiding patients in relieving suffering, using treatment that might shorten their lives. Also, once begun, physician-assisted suicide may well be prone to be used more and more. On the other hand, patients expect the right to die with dignity and clearly want physicians to carry out their expectations.

Advance Directives

Most states now having "living will" statutes, often called "natural death" acts. As of October 1991, forty-five states (Massachusetts, New York, Michigan, Nebraska, and Pennsylvania excluded) had living will legislation. The living will is a document given by a competent person to direct extended form of care in case of subsequent incompetency or to give advance direction of the level of care desired when the individual's condition is terminal (18). Under such statues, patients may state their views about the medical treatment they would want at some future time if they are too ill to do so. An alternative form of advance directive is a Durable Power of Attorney for Health Care, with which an individual appoints another person to speak for him if he becomes incapable of expressing his preference as to his medical treatment (19). A single document may encompass both approaches. It may appoint another to speak on the individual's behalf, but may also include specific directions as to the individual's desires (20). Durable power of attorney is legal in forty-three states as of October 1991 (excluded are Alabama, Alaska, Arizona, Maryland, Hawaii, Nebraska, and Oklahoma).

The enactment of living will statutes in many states has been a direct response to popular pressures. Nonetheless, these statutes often contain enough restrictive provisions to rob them of much usefulness. The statutes typically limit living wills to the withdrawal of "life-sustaining treatment" from patients who are "terminally" ill. In California, for example, a living will may only authorize the withdrawal of a procedure that "would serve only to artificially prolong the moment of death . . . where death is imminent whether or not such procedures are utilized" (21). Theoretically, an ALS patient could not be removed from a ventilator on the basis of that interpretation of a living will, since death would not be imminent if he were on a ventilator. Comas or persistent vegetative states are not terminal conditions, and patients in such states may live for many years without ever regaining consciousness if supportive treatment is provided. Fortunately, that is a very rare occurrence in ALS. A dilemma would arise if a patient in a chronic vegetative state developed cancer. Then no living will adopted under a statute like that of California's could authorize withholding the life-saving surgery, since neither the coma nor the cancer would be a terminal condition, as defined under the statute.

The California Act contains other restrictions that weaken the living will. It allows the execution of living wills only by patients who have been diagnosed as terminally ill at least fourteen days before they execute the document. Obviously, many patients diagnosed as terminal will be too ill to maintain decision-making capacity for two more weeks. Also, this does not leave any advance decision-making capacities for someone whose illness has a sudden onset causing incapacitation, such as a stroke or hypoxic encephalopathy.

Regardless of the wording of a living will, its wishes might still not be carried out. A family member might say "I don't care what my father says. I want him treated," and the physician would often follow the family member's wishes. The written directives are useful but, in their ordinary level of detail, they are often vague and may be potentially misleading. Physicians may be thrust into the unenviable role of having to make interpretations from vague directives. For example, a typically written directive may state that the patient "refuses life-prolonging therapy" and "extraordinary measures" if he is in a "hopeless, terminal state." Is an ALS patient on a ventilator in a hopeless, terminal state? From a logical standpoint, one would say of course; on the other hand, one could argue that death would not be imminent as long as he is on the ventilator. Fortunately, this dilemma has been resolved with ample court precedents allowing ALS patients to be removed from a ventilator.

I always advise patients to be as specific as possible in the wording of a living will. For example, rather than a blanket statement indicating that no life support systems are wanted, I recommend that patients state specifically what they do and do not desire regarding feeding tubes or ventilators. In regard to the latter, I also recommend that patients state something like "although not wanting long-term ventilatory support, if I am unable to breathe on my own, I might opt to have ventilatory support for a short period of time, if necessary, during pneumonia or subsequent to aspiration." Also, if patients are started on ventilatory support and the quality of life eventually becomes so poor that they no longer desire to continue on the ventilator, it should be stated specifically in the living will that they have the option to be removed from the ventilator. Use of precise language should aid in adherence to their wishes.

In general, the Durable Power of Attorney for Health Care may be more useful as an advance directive because it provides greater flexibility for responding to specific clinical situations. With knowledge of the patient's values and preference, as well as with the patient's living will, a proxy can make appropriate judgments for a given situation. However, since ALS patients almost always maintain their mental capacities, the Durable Power of Attorney for Health Care rarely comes into play.

It is imperative for hospitals to develop policies asking all adult patients at the time of admission if they have prepared an advance directive or would like information on how to do so, since the patient's self-determination act is part of a federal law that went into effect in November 1991. The law is quite inclusive since hospitals, HMOs, nursing homes, and other health care facilities that received Medicare or Medicaid funds must follow this guideline and inform patients of their right to make treatment decisions, utilizing advance directives such as living wills and durable power of attorney.

In the situation where no specific advance directives exist, a proxy decision maker (next of kin or official guardian) should be appointed (22). The proxy decision maker, just as the proxy who has the Durable Power of Attorney for Health Care, should be instructed to attempt to reproduce the decision that the patient would have made in this particular situation if he were able to do so. If the proxy has no knowledge of the patient's preference and values, he should attempt to balance the goals of beneficence and nonmaleficence in order to choose the proper level of treatment.

Orders To Limit Treatment

Cranford has classified aggressiveness of treatment into four descriptive categories that may be continued or discontinued, depending on the prognosis, the patient's prior wishes, or the proxy's decision:

1. Technology—those interventions that are often expensive, invasive, sometimes burdensome, and may invoke an allocation of scarce resources such as respirators, pacemakers, heart/lung machines, and dialysis;
2. Medications such as antibiotics, vasopressors, digitalis, and insulin;
3. Hydration and nutrition;
4. Basic care related to maintenance, comfort, hygiene, and dignity (23).

"Do not resuscitate" orders exclude only a portion of level 1 care, usually the use of defibrillators, intubation, and respirators in the case of a cardiac or respiratory arrest for an ALS patient. However, it is common practice for physicians who want to reduce level of care in hopelessly ill patients to exclude the entire level 1 care as well as level 2. Whether or not to withdraw level 3 care in a patient who maintains consciousness is often problematical.

Legal Aspects of Terminating Treatment

From the legal standpoint, the case of an ALS patient who desires to be removed from a ventilator is quite straightforward. The courts dealing with these types of cases have uniformly supported the patient's right to decide. Unfortunately, many times physicians and others involved are not as aware of the legal rights of the ALS patients, and difficult situations may occur.

The Cruzan case, which was decided by the U.S. Supreme Court in 1990, was quite supportive of the individual's right to determine her fate regarding medical care. The Cruzan decision stated ''we assume that for purpose of this case, that a competent patient has the constitutional right to decide their own fate in health care circumstances.'' Therefore, although the Cruzan decision did not go as far as some people would have liked in regard to incompetent patients, the statement regarding competent patients is quite straightforward (17).

Only two years after the 1976 landmark Karen M. Quinlan decision, which was the groundbreaking case on death and dying, a case of an ALS patient became the first decision attesting the right of a competent individual to be removed from life support.

Abe Perlmutter was a 73-year-old taxi driver who developed ALS and subsequently became ventilator-dependent (24). He remained in command of his mental facilities and could speak, although with great effort. He eventually desired to be removed from the ventilator, realizing that he would die. Actually, he had attempted to disconnect the ventilator himself and had succeeded on one occasion; hospital personnel, alerted by the alarm on the respirator, reattached it. His family supported his decision to be removed from the ventilator; however, the hospital declined to honor his request, largely out of fear of both criminal and civil liability, which the court conceded ''cannot be discounted.'' The patient, therefore, petitioned the court for an order restraining hospital personnel from interfering with his decision to have the respirator removed. The state intervened in opposition to the petition, arguing that it had an overriding duty to preserve life and that the termination of this supportive care would constitute an unlawful killing under state law. The case then went to court. The judge said that the constitutional right of privacy and the common law right of self-determination needed to be adhered to and the patient had the right to be removed from the ventilator. Therefore, this case established the precedent that the countervailing state's interest, i.e., preservation of life, did not supersede an individual's right of autonomy when the illness is as severe as that of an ALS patient on a ventilator.

Catherine Farrell was 37 years old and respirator-dependent from ALS for three years. By the time she reached the point when she wanted the respirator stopped, she had lost sixty pounds and most of her muscle function; however, she could blink her eyes and could talk with some difficulty. Her husband took the case to court, saying that his wife wanted the respirator to be discontinued because her quality of life had declined and she was tired of suffering. The case was decided in 1987 by the New Jersey Supreme Court (25).

In all such cases, there must always be a careful examination of the patient:

1. Why does the patient want the ventilator removed?
2. What is the psychological state of the patient?

The issue of depression almost always comes into play. Is there a reactive depression to a severe chronic illness, or does the patient have a major psychotic depression that renders him unable to make competent decisions? There is no one definition of competency. The main definition that is utilized is that the patient understands the proposed treatment, its risks and benefits, and understands the risks and benefits of any alternative to the proposed treatment such as the absence of treatment. Regarding depression, as long as there is nothing that seems out of the ordinary and the patient can still make a competent decision, it is considered a typical reactive depression. No one wants a patient to make a decision such as to be removed from a ventilator because they feel isolated or abandoned. However, a law states that once a reasonable evaluation is made and, if indicated, there has been an attempt to treat depression, then one can go in a short time to the next step.

Catherine had two young sons, which brought up the point of the state's interest of dependent third parties. Is this a reason that the state would tell a patient that she has to stay alive, since there are children who need her? In this case, they were teenagers who were capable of doing alright on their own and were being cared for by their father. The court made a very strong statement that the state's interest is in preserving life, but that here the quality of life is so poor, so minimal, and so racked with pain that it would be unfair to force its continuation against the patient's interest (25). This is a common remark that courts make in these cases, with judges usually being very supportive of patient's rights.

The last example, which is also especially interesting, is a 1986 case (26) involving a woman named Beverly Requena, who could only blink her eyes in response to questions and communicated by using a computer. She had been on a ventilator and tube feeding since her admission to the hospital over a year before the case came to court. She was fully competent. However, she wanted the feeding tube withdrawn rather than the ventilator. That is where she drew the line. Individual patients draw the line in different areas. Some want everything done, some want everything but a ventilator, and some do not want a feeding tube. However, if it is the individual's decision, then we should respect it. The hospital was a Roman Catholic hospital, and the position of the church in terminating nutrition and hydration has not been completely clarified. There are some spokespeople who always say it is wrong to terminate this treatment, while there are others who say that tube feedings can become extraordinary care that patients need not accept. In this case, the staff said that removal of the feeding tube and hydration violated their own moral and ethical principles and they did not want to participate in it, while another hospital seventeen miles away said that it would take the patient. The patient said she did not want to move since she had been at that one hospital for over a year and, aside from that one problem, she was quite happy there. The conflict was whether she had to move seventeen miles away to a second hospital to have her feeding tube removed, or have it done at the original facility. The judge ruled in her favor and stated that in view of her devastating illness and extremely poor physical condition, her interests were the predominant ones, and health care professionals had to adhere to her wishes.

In the issue of legal liability, there are no cases regarding nontreatment at the end of life in which physicians have been held criminally or civilly liable for participating in decisions to forego treatment. They must be careful, be sure the patient is competent, and assure family agreement. Once they do, there is no risk involved. On the other hand, there is risk in going ahead with treatment that patients do not want. There have been successful law suits in which there were clear grounds to stop treatment, and the physician or hospital refused. Usually it is the hospital, and the hospital has been held responsible for the cost of care. There is also the question of whether the hospital or physicians could be held responsible for battery. Therefore, it is more of a risk to say that I will not go along with what the patient wants, than to go along with what the patient desires. This has clearly been a shift in attitude over the last few years.

Physician-Assisted Suicide and Euthanasia

The taboo against doctors discussing how they have helped patients commit suicide has certainly ended. Last year a Rochester, New York, physician described in the *New England Journal of Medicine* how he had prescribed barbiturates to help a patient kill herself (27). Since that time, other physicians have revealed their roles in responding to requests from mentally competent patients to help them die. In addition to physician-assisted suicide, physicians have raised the dose of a drug, knowing that it was far beyond what was needed to control a patient's pain and would be considered a lethal overdose. Others have prescribed enough sedative or hypnotic medication for the patients to take themselves to cause death.

Dr. Jack Kevorkian, a Michigan pathologist, has devised a "suicide machine," in which patients turn on an intravenous system that provides a lethal overdose. The key is that the patient himself has to turn on the switch, so it does fit the definition of suicide. Two years ago, Dr. Kevorkian connected a woman suffering from Alzheimer's disease to the suicide device and watched as she pushed the button and died. He was severely criticized because he had known the woman, Janet Atkins, for only a few days. Although she clearly had Alzheimer's disease, she was still functioning at a reasonable level and had been playing tennis only a few weeks previously. Last year he was subjected to even more criticism by providing the "suicide machine" for one patient with pain secondary to multiple sclerosis and another one who probably had a fibrositis syndrome. In none of the cases has the State of Michigan prosecuted Dr. Kevorkian for either manslaughter or homicide; charges were pressed by the district attorney and subsequently dismissed by the court.

The debate on euthanasia has become quite heated over the last few years.

Initiative 119 on euthanasia in the state of Washington was defeated by a very small margin (56–44 percent) last year. If it had passed, Initiative 119 would have made Washington the first place in the world to pass a law authorizing doctors to assist in suicides or to give lethal injections to patients who have asked to die. Therefore, euthanasia is still illegal in the United States.

In the Netherlands, euthanasia officially remains a crime, punishable by up to twelve years in prison, but it is practiced fairly commonly and openly there, protected by a body of case law and by strong public support (28). Estimates are that 5,000–8,000 Dutch lives are ended by euthanasia each year (9). In 1985, a Government Clinic Commission on euthanasia issued a report recommending a change in a criminal code to permit euthanasia; however, this has not yet been passed. In 1984 the Dutch Medical Association suggested stringent guidelines for performing euthanasia. Four essential conditions must be met:

1. The patient must be competent. This excludes many groups of patients in whom the question of withholding life-sustaining treatment has been most prevalent in the United States, such as advanced Alzheimer's disease, retarded individuals, and persistent vegetative state.
2. The patient must request euthanasia voluntarily, consistently, and repeatedly over a reasonable time, and the request must be well documented.
3. The patient must be suffering intolerably with no prospect of relief, although there need not be a terminal disease. Therefore, depression for which there is treatment would not be a reason for euthanasia, whereas ALS might be.
4. Euthanasia must be performed by a physician in consultation with another physician not involved in the case. The usual method is to introduce sleep with a barbiturate, followed by a lethal injection of curare (9).

There are a few vigorous advocates of euthanasia, including medical ethicists, who say that afflicted patients have a right to medical help in committing suicide or to a peaceful death by lethal injection. However, the vast majority of ethicists and physicians are still opposed to such measures; they do defend the patient's right to choose or refuse treatment and criticize physicians for aggressively prolonging the lives of dying or comatose patients with modern technology.

The nation's major religious faiths have adhered to traditional patterns in being opposed to euthanasia. Protestants, Catholics, and Jews hold life as "a gift from God over which humans only have stewardship" (17). Leaders of the country's two largest Christian groups, the Roman Catholic Church and the Southern Baptist Convention, reiterate their opposition to all forms of euthanasia or suicide. A similar view is expressed by leaders of both Orthodox and Conservative Judaism. However, Initiative 119 in Washington has also found religious advocates, mostly from liberal and mainline Protestant churches where euthanasia and assisted suicide appear to become increasingly accepted. One year ago, the General Synod of the 1.6-million-member United Church of Christ passed a resolution referring

Amyotrophic Lateral Sclerosis

to euthanasia and suicide and affirming "individual freedom and responsibility to make a choice in these matters." The Pacific Northwest College of the United Methodist Church endorsed Initiative 119.

Medical ethicists, although obviously concerned about the choices facing dying patients and their families, also give far more attention to the consequences of legalizing euthanasia for the medical profession, the health care system, and public policy in general than just its effects on individuals and their families (28). Many ethicists, including some who do not oppose assisted suicide in all circumstances, question whether doctors should ever be involved in such practices or in aiding the death of suffering patients who ask to die. An important principle of medical ethics is that doctors have an exceptionally intimate, private, and powerful relationship with their patients, who are extremely dependent and vulnerable. To inject into this relationship a legal power to cause death would alter the role of medicine drastically and ominously. Another aspect of the debate surrounding euthanasia focuses on whether such measures place society on a "slippery slope" that could lead to the elimination of unwanted individuals or whole categories of people, such as the retarded, seriously disabled, or senile. Supporters of Washington Initiative 119 emphasize that to be eligible for "aid in dying" (the term used in the measure), a person must be conscious and mentally competent, must be certified by two doctors within six months of death, and must sign a voluntary written request witnessed by two unrelated and impartial adults. Opponents said that these requests were not specific enough and that, for example, the determination could be made by a dermatologist and a pathologist.

The public seems to be of two minds about doctor-assisted suicide. People expect physicians to be healers, not takers of lives, but they applaud compassionate doctors who help patients end their suffering. They also express reservations about being treated by doctors who admit that they would help patients commit suicide. In expressing fear that approval of doctor-assisted suicide could create a "slippery slope," one woman said, "I'm worried because it just becomes a little easier the second time and each time thereafter until it becomes routine." Yet patients often assume the right to die and expect the physician's help in carrying out their wishes. Physicians thus receive a contradictory message from some of those they serve: "Have the utmost respect for life, but do otherwise when we tell you."

References

1. Gillon R. Telling the truth and medical ethics. *Brit Med J* 1985, 291:1556–1557.
2. Culver CM, Gert B. Basic ethical concepts in neurologic practice. *Semin Neurol* 1984, 4:1–8.
3. Bernat JL. Ethical and legal duties of the contemporary physician. *Pharos* 1989, 52(2): 29.
4. Peabody FW. The care of the patient. *JAMA* 1927, 88:877.

5. Brett AS, McCullough LB. When patients request specific interventions: Defining the limits of the physician's obligation. *New Eng J Med* 1986, 315:1347–1351.
6. Paris JJ, Crone RK, Reardon F. Physicians' refusal of requested treatment: The case of Baby L. *New Eng J Med* 1990, 322:1012–1015.
7. Prinz LA. Is withholding hydration a valid comfort measure in the terminally ill? *Geriatrics* 1988, 43:84–88.
8. Nelson WA, Bernat JL. Decisions to withhold or terminate treatment. *Neurol Clin* 1989, 7:759–773.
9. Angell M. Euthanasia. *N Eng J Med* 1988, 319:1348–1350.
10. Beauchamp TL, Childress JF. *Principles of Biomedical Ethics,* 2nd ed. New York: Oxford University Press, 1983.
11. Gert B. *Morality: A New Justification of the Moral Rules.* Oxford: Oxford University Press, 1988.
12. Beauchamp TL, Childress JF. *Principles of Biomedical Ethics,* 3rd ed. New York: Oxford University Press, 1989.
13. Gillon R. Beneficence: Doing good for others. *Brit Med J* 1985, 291:44–45.
14. Superintendent of Belchertown State School v. Saikewicz, 370 N.E. 2d 417 (Mass. 1977).
15. Healy JM. Legal issues. In: Smith RA, ed. *Handbook of Amyotrophic Lateral Sclerosis.* New York: Marcel Decker, 1992.
16. Goldblatt D, Greenlaw J. Starting and stopping the ventilator for patients with amyotrophic lateral sclerosis. *Neuro Clin* 1989, 7:789–806.
17. Bernat JL. Ethical issues in neurology. In: Baker AB, Baker LH, eds. *Clinical Neurology,* Vol. 1. Philadelphia: J.B. Lippincott, 1991.
18. Areen J. The legal status of consent obtained from families of adult patients to withhold or withdraw treatment. *JAMA* 1987, 258:229–235.
19. Eisendrath SJ, Jonsen AR. The living will: Help or hindrance? *JAMA* 1983, 249:2054–2058.
20. Schneiderman LJ, Arras JD. Counseling patients to counsel physicians on future care in the event of patient incompetence. *Ann Intern Med* 1985, 102:693–698.
21. Hall MA, Ellmann IM. *Health Care Law and the Ethics.* St. Paul: West Publishing Co., 1989.
22. President's Commission for the Study of Ethical Problems in Medicine and Biomedical and Behavioral Research. *Making Health Care Decisions: The Ethical and Legal Implications of Informed Consent in the Patient-Practitioner Relationship.* Washington D.C.: US Government Printing Office, 1982.
23. Cranford RE. Termination of treatment in the persistent vegetative state. *Semin Neurol* 1984, 4:36.
24. Satz v. Perlmutter, 362 So.2d 160 (Fla. App.) Aff'd, 379 So.2d 359, 1978.
25. In the Matter of Kathleen Farrell, 108 N.J. 335 (Supreme Court of New Jersey), 1987.
26. In the Matter of Beverly Requena, 213 N.J. Super 475 (Superior Court of New Jersey), 1986.
27. Quill TE. Death and Dignity. *N Eng J Med* 1991, 324:691–694.
28. Council on Ethical and Judicial Affairs, American Medical Association. Decision near the end of life. *JAMA* 1992, 1267:2229–2233.

19

Hospice: A Family Approach to Amyotrophic Lateral Sclerosis

N. Michael Murphy, M.D., and Barbara Thompson, O.T.R.

The hospice is dedicated to providing care and comfort to all who are involved with far-advanced illness when the pursuit of a cure is contributing little or nothing to the quantity or quality of life. ALS creates pain, unrest, and mourning in everyone it touches. Since these are major concerns of hospices and curative treatment is not available for ALS, it is appropriate that the hospice become involved as early as possible to temper the stresses and strains in the family and so improve the quality of life for all.

The modern hospice evolved within the last half century mainly as a response to rampant technology that engulfed medicine, paid little attention to the feelings of all involved, and usually promoted treatment of one sort or another right up to the bitter end. It was becoming difficult to die in peace and rare to die at home. Most individuals with far-advanced illnesses died in hospitals which, in their anxiety-producing clinical sterility, are the antithesis of a quiet, comfortable, loving, and familiar environment in which we would wish to die.

The hospice is still considered by some as a death sentence and a place of doom and gloom, and it is feared that if a patient becomes involved she will give up or lose hope. Our experience is much more optimistic; with enhanced communication and connectedness in the family, the ever-present tension related to the fear of dying lessens, and it becomes more possible to focus on the possibilities for each day as it arises, and eventually to die in peace.

The first part of this chapter is concerned with a short history of the hospice movement together with organizational details. There follows some consideration of ALS as it affects the whole family with an outline of the family meeting, which we consider to be a necessary and powerful catalyst to more tolerable management of the last weeks and months of life. The chapter ends with a review of the care of some of the more common symptoms with which hospice staff are likely to be involved.

The Hospice

In the literature, hospice refers to both a place or environment and the nature of the relationship between guest and host (1).

Records of ancient hospices date to the fourth century A.D. As way stations for travelers and pilgrims, hospices proliferated in the Middle Ages. Often based in monasteries, these early hospices provided refuge for those in need. Hospices subsequently disappeared and did not reappear until the seventeenth century, when the Sisters of Charity in Paris opened several houses to care for people who were ill, indigent, or dying. During the next two centuries, the work of these nuns and their successors inspired the formation of hospices in Germany and Ireland (2).

In 1900, five Irish Sisters of Charity founded St. Joseph's Convent in London and began visiting the sick in their homes. Two years later, they opened St. Joseph's Hospice with thirty beds for the dying poor. Simultaneously in the United States, Rose Hawthorne Lathrop established a domiciliary facility for seriously ill people, which was funded through community support. The term *hospice* became synonymous with care for the dying (3).

The hospice movement of the twentieth century developed in response to the unmet needs of patients dying in traditional medical environments. Through her work as a nurse and social worker in England, Dame Cicely Saunders recognized the necessity of developing an alternative program of care for persons with advanced illness for whom there was no hope of a cure. With this intention, Saunders became a physician and subsequently opened St. Christopher's Hospice in 1969. Based in a London suburb, St. Christopher's gained an international reputation and became the model for hospice programs in the Western world (4).

In 1971, St. Luke's Hospice opened in Sheffield, England, under the direction of Professor Eric Wilkes. Whereas St. Christopher's Hospice offered only inpatient care, St. Luke's offered inpatient care, home care, and day treatment services. The first Canadian hospice opened in 1973 at the Royal Victoria Hospital in Montreal under the medical direction of Dr. Balfour Mount. The Connecticut Hospice in New Haven became the first hospice in the United States, opening a home care program in 1974 and an inpatient facility in 1980.

By the late 1970s there were over two hundred hospice programs in the United States, with many variations in the scope of services and organizational models. Explosive growth in the type and number of hospices led concerned providers to recognize the need for principles of hospice care and standards for developing programs. This crucial consensus was achieved by the National Hospice Organization (NHO) soon after its first annual conference in 1978 (5). Basic tenets and characteristics of a hospice program were identified, and the National Hospice Organization Standards (1979) provided the following statement on the philosophy of hospice:

"Dying is a normal process, whether or not resulting from disease. Hospice exists neither to hasten nor to postpone death. Rather, hospice exists to affirm life by providing support and care for those in the last phases of incurable disease so that they can live as fully and comfortably as possible. Hospice promotes the formation of caring communities that are sensitive to the needs of patients and families at this time in their lives so that they may be free to obtain the degree of mental and spiritual preparation for death that is satisfactory to them" (6).

With the surge in the hospice movement during the 1970s, Congress mandated the Health Care Financing Administration (HCFA) to study hospice and its potential impact on the Medicare and Medicaid programs. This study ultimately showed that hospice was a cost-effective means of caring for the terminally ill, and 1982 legislation provided hospice benefits to Medicare beneficiaries. These regulations established beneficiary requirements, reimbursement standards and procedures, the required scope of services, and the conditions for a program to become Medicare certified. Additional legislation, approved in 1986, allocated federal funds for an optional state Medicaid hospice benefit. Individual states could thereby choose to amend their Medicaid plans to provide beneficiaries with coverage for hospice care. In 1990 Congress passed legislation extending coverage to eligible beneficiaries. As a result, residents in nursing homes are now eligible for Medicare hospice benefits when their stay is reimbursed through Medicaid or private pay.

Under the Medicare hospice benefit, care must be provided by a Medicare certified hospice program. According to a 1990 NHO census, there were 1,123 Medicare certified hospice programs in the United States, and 140 more had certification pending (7).

To receive hospice care under Medicare, an individual must be entitled to Part A of Medicare and have a physician certify a prognosis of approximately six months or less. Eligible beneficiaries then transfer their coverage from traditional Medicare to the Medicare hospice benefit. In electing the hospice benefit, which is more comprehensive than regular Medicare, the individual waives the right to regular Medicare benefits except for payment to their attending physician and treatment for medical conditions unrelated to the terminal illness. The individual may revoke the hospice benefit at any time and resume regular Medicare benefits. If revoked in the middle of an election period, the remaining days in that election period are forfeited.

Medicare hospice beneficiaries are entitled to receive hospice care for two election periods of ninety days each and one election period of thirty days. Legislation approved in 1990 provides for an additional unlimited fourth benefit period when there is evidence of disease progression and certification by the hospice medical director that the person remains terminally ill (8). Private insurance coverage for hospice care varies from one policy to the next but usually covers hospice care.

Along with the eligibility requirements defined by the Medicare hospice benefit, participating hospices usually develop additional criteria for admission to their programs. For instance, eligibility requirements can vary with respect to the presence or absence of a primary caregiver in the home. Certain types of care, such as intravenous antibiotic or fluid replacement therapy, may not be available through the hospice, and most hospices do not admit the ventilator-dependent.

Regardless of whether a hospice is an offspring of a hospital, freestanding, or community based, it must meet criteria established by HCFA in order to be Medicare certified and eligible for reimbursement through Medicare and Medicaid. The hospice must provide a full complement of services in both home and inpatient settings. Core services that must be provided directly by the hospice include:

- Nursing care by or under the supervision of a registered nurse
- 24-hour on-call availability of nursing services
- Physician services: the hospice medical director assumes overall responsibility for the medical component of the hospice program. Usually, the hospice medical director serves as a consultant to the attending physician and does not assume the role of the primary care physician
- Social work services
- Pastoral care services
- Volunteer services: the hospice must utilize volunteers in defined administrative or direct care roles and provide ongoing training to volunteers
- Bereavement follow-up.

The following services can be provided directly by the hospice program or indirectly through contractual arrangement:

- Home health aide and homemaker services
- Occupational, physical, respiratory, and speech therapy
- Medical supplies and appliances, including drugs and biologicals, deemed necessary by the interdisciplinary team for palliation and symptom management
- Durable medical equipment (4).

Although the primary thrust of hospice care is in the home setting, inpatient care must be available as needed for symptom control, respite care, or terminal care in the last days of life if it becomes impossible at home. Some hospices operate freestanding facilities or hospice units within hospitals; others utilize designated hospice beds within affiliated hospitals or nursing homes when inpatient care is needed.

The Hospice and ALS

The hospice philosophy and structure are ideally suited to assist people with ALS and their families to live as fully and comfortably as possible in the final stages of illness. Meticulous attention to symptom control, experience in providing care to people who are approaching death, and resources to support families through this process can ease the anxiety, fear, and worry that invariably accompany the progression of ALS. Increasingly, people with advanced ALS are benefiting from support available through hospice programs.

Hospice programs in the United Kingdom have the longest history of caring for those with ALS. In particular, St. Christopher's Hospice (1967) opened with at least ten percent of its ward beds for people with advanced neurological illnesses (9). St. Christopher's Hospice continues to serve people with ALS and has contributed to an increased awareness of hospice and ALS through publication of retrospective studies on this subject.

In the United States, the relationship between ALS patients and hospices is younger and less developed than in the United Kingdom. This is due in part to the relative newness of hospice in the United States, and as a result of differences between the structure of hospice in the United States and the United Kingdom. Some hospices are unfamiliar with the disease and its management and hesitate to admit patients because of concerns regarding prognosis and possible lengths of stay. Increased collaboration between hospices and individuals or institutions experienced in the care of people with ALS can enhance the willingness of hospices to become involved and promote effective management of problems associated with the disease. This form of collaboration among health care providers not only improves the quality and continuity of care from diagnosis to death, but also can help to sustain the caregiving abilities of involved health care professionals through pooling of resources, experience, and support (10).

Hospice Referral

It is essential that the emotional needs of the patient and family be addressed from the earliest stages of the disease. This chapter is designed to demonstrate the value of the comprehensive services offered through hospice. Although it would be ideal to utilize the full range of hospice services throughout the course of the illness, the decision on the part of a health care provider to introduce hospice into discussions needs to be informed by an appreciation of the constraints on hospice programs as well as an understanding of the patient's and family's psychological and medical needs. The following list outlines criteria that can be used by a Medicare certified hospice to determine eligibility for admission:

1. Approximate prognosis of six months or less, bearing in mind that the longer the family is on the program the closer will be the interpersonal relationships that improve the effectiveness of hospice care.
2. DNR status.
3. Progressive dysphagia, decreased oral intake, progressive weight loss, and a decision not to use a feeding tube. Persons with supplemental feeding support may be appropriate for hospice care if they are experiencing a progressive decline in pulmonary function.
4. Progressive respiratory compromise.
   A. Early symptoms
      • shortness of breath, with or without exertion
      • shortness of breath while eating
      • inability to blow one's nose, raise secretions, cough, and sigh
      • shallow breathing
      • inability to sleep in a supine position due to diaphragmatic weakness that is relieved when the person returns to an upright position
      • pulmonary function testing demonstrates that respiratory capacity is less than fifty percent and is deteriorating. (Respiratory fatigue is generally experienced when vital capacity (VC) is less than 1.5 liters (11))
      • increased anxiety and/or restlessness especially during the night hours
   B. Later symptoms
      • visible use of accessory muscles for breathing
      • continued decline in respiratory function. At a VC less than 1 liter, people are usually without any respiratory reserve (11). Respiratory ability is further compromised by an ineffective cough and an inability to manage saliva.
      • abnormal blood gases
      • morning headaches due to increased CO_2 levels
      • confusion or hallucinations resulting from hypoxia and/or hypercarbia

The Family and ALS: The Family Meeting

At St. Peter's Hospice, we invite every family to meet with us within a few days of our initial contact. We affirm that life-threatening illness affects everyone in the family and that if we come together and share experiences, concerns, and worries, the additional stress of hiding fears and feelings will be lessened and connectedness will be enhanced, and this will make each family member feel less isolated in the ordeal of ALS.

This sounds simple and reasonable, and the most cohesive of families are usually very eager for the gathering. But for most families, despite loud protestations of their closeness, the idea of the whole family coming together is terrifying. Usually, feelings of love and rage have rarely been expressed completely and openly, especially in front of strangers, even when felt intensely. If the family has had little experience in sharing these powerful everyday feelings, they will be terrified at the thought of sharing the avalanche of emotions set off by loss: fear, rage, grief, and a sense of unreality and being out of control, to name but a few.

Patients and families often ask us, at a time when death is in the offing, what possible use it would be to talk, since they fear that it will only make the situation more painful. If it is simply talking the way we usually talk in families, this would be so. Usually, one person talks and the others argue and interrupt. Thoughts and feelings are not permitted to unfold. It is a daily experience of interrupted intercourse that rarely bears fruit and seldom leads to enhanced connectedness and understanding of all concerned. We are not usually lovingly heard and witnessed by one another in families, but when it does happen, there is the magic of soul-to-soul connectedness. This helps to transcend the aches and pains of everyday life, even the frightening manifestations of ALS, which seem so much more powerful when we feel alone, unheard, and unwitnessed.

Most hospices do not arrange family meetings routinely but will do so at the request of family or if there is extreme chaos. It is our belief that one or more gatherings should be held for all families because life-threatening illness always brings with it a greater or lesser degree of chaos, and there is always much to say even though we might be afraid to say it.

Looking back at having guided several thousand family meetings over more than a decade, it still seems impossible that anything will be accomplished during the hour or two of the family meeting. There is often a thick atmosphere of tension and distrust. We may have been regaled beforehand with stories of who does not talk to whom and tales of black sheep, disputes, hurts, and a list of family members who have died who were never fully grieved and whose mourning is reawakened by the ALS. We are warned not to upset Mother and not to say anything to Father because he "doesn't know." Skeptical, frightened, or hostile family members, who would ask us what we could possibly hope to accomplish and why we would want to upset people at this time, were enough to send us into a frenzy of apology and doubt in the early years of facilitating these family gatherings. But gradually, as we felt less pressure to rescue and fix and became less judgmental and analytical and more the fully attentive witness, we began to notice that miracles were happening. Feelings were shared, hurts relinquished, old losses mourned. Not completely, and occasionally it seemed as though there was hardly any movement, but quite often we were left with the feeling of peace and lightness that follows all being said and done.

Since the objective of hospice care is for patients to live and die at home and more than four out of five are able to do so, most of our family meetings are held at home. As guides or facilitators of the meeting, we suggest that we meet around the patient's bed or chair or perhaps around the kitchen table or on the patio. There may be up to thirty family members and friends, or there may be no family, but we still hold a family meeting because we believe that our lives and continuity depend on the telling of tales to anyone who will listen and be witness.

A man who was born in Turkey and was being cared for in the Hospice Inn had no family, so in a literal sense there was no family meeting, but for an hour or so two hospice staff became family and listened to a whole series of poignant tales of his life. The murder of his father in Turkey, the family's flight to Persia and then Lebanon, and his eventual move to Boston. Stories about his mother and siblings and the magic of the paradise that was Lebanon. Then his loneliness and fears as cancer advanced, and his relief to be safe in the Hospice Inn with two people to listen to his story. That is what he needed: witnesses to his life and his linkages.

The Story of the Illness

The facilitator usually begins the meeting by asking the patient to tell the story of the illness. The accuracy of dates and facts is of little importance. It is the images and feelings that need expression. If it is Father who has the illness, he will often turn to Mother to ask her to tell the story. She has always been custodian of wounds as well as the life and soul of the family in the transitions of birth, marriage, and death, and she is often the designated family storyteller. She has always talked to the doctors and relayed news to the family, and she is the one who has dispensed love and comfort to an emotionally paralyzed and inarticulate husband. But it is a family myth that the feminine and the nurturing only resides in Mother and that it is her role to run interference for death. Father needs to acknowledge his own wounds and face his own shadow, so Mother is gently encouraged to listen for now and tell her version later so that all can hear what he has to say. Perhaps this is the first time they have heard the story from him, and often their fears and worries now unshielded by Mother are almost palpable. Telling the story removes it from the realm of the shadowy unspeakable into the light of day in ordinary consciousness. Usually, he regains some confidence as he tells the tale and seems more connected to both family and facilitator, ready now to move into the underworld of his fears about living and dying.

The Story of His Worries and Fears

Dad will probably say that his principle concerns are for his wife and children. The facilitator asks him how he met his wife, what she is like, how he feels about her, and how he evaluates their marriage. These powerful questions evoke jokes or nervous laughter sometimes verging on uproar in the family, but gentle persistence often leads to words he had never uttered. The surprise is that the disappointments, disillusionments, and resentments can be let go when voiced, and room is made for the expression of vulnerability, tenderness, and love that has seldom if ever been heard from Father and is often so difficult to express for men who hide behind their unemotional and strong facade like the Wizard of Oz.

Dark secrets can be aired. For example, his own alcoholism, which created immense pain within the family without any resolution other than the frequent expression of explosive rage from all involved. The tragedy was that his drinking produced torrents of anger and guilt, which are still just below the surface. When Dad tells the story in the context of his own parents' alcoholism and how he missed out on his children and they on him, and they listen with no interruption and a minimum of judgment, compassion, forgiveness, and intimacy are possible, and this would never occur without the story being told.

When he tells of the children, he usually starts with facts and figures; their grades, degrees, and successes. It is much more difficult for him to express feelings of love and the heartbreaking sadness of having to leave them. He will say that they know he loves them without his having to say it, but the story of his love needs to be spoken, and, as with any other good story, the children never tire of hearing it. It is most important that grandchildren be involved in the family meetings. This may be very difficult for the adults who want to shield them, and they will frequently say the children are too young to understand. Although three-year-olds may not understand the words, they are very much in touch with the feeling tone of those they love, and excluding them conveys a message that death is something to be hidden.

In the early days of the hospice, one of us (N.M.M.) was facilitating a family meeting presided over by Mr. Ryan, whose wife, eight children and their spouses, together with several grandchildren, were present. It was a love fest! He told stories of a wonderful marriage with many struggles and had something loving and supportive to say about everyone in the room and they about him. There was much laughter and many tears. After about two hours, he was exhausted, as we all were, and I was winding up proceedings by asking whether he had any questions or anything more to say. He sat up on the couch and said that he wanted to speak to his five youngest grandchildren, who had been wandering in and out of the room but had not been directly addressed. Ranging in age from about six to nine years old, they sat on the floor in a semicircle by his feet, and the following is my recollection of what he said: "Children, I have cancer and it is nobody's fault. It just happens. I am going to die and won't be there to see you grow up, but I want you to know that you have each been a joy in my life, and you will always have my blessing and my love." There was not a dry eye in the room for any of the witnesses to this most sacred event. I have repeated this story many times to grandparents and others because Mr. Ryan reminded us how important it is for grandparents to take leave of their grandchildren face-to-face if at all possible. They are best friends, so often, and unconditional lovers, and it is an act of betrayal if the grandparent leaves without saying goodbye, delegating the heartbreaking task to the parents. An interesting sequel to this glorious family meeting took place about six years later when

I was stopped by one of Mr. Ryan's sons-in-law, who told me how powerful that event was for him and that it gave him the courage to be intimately present for his twenty-two-year-old daughter by his first marriage, who died of cancer two years after Mr. Ryan's death.

We continue the story of Dad's fears and worries, and he is asked about concerns for himself. He dismisses the question initially but when pressed will say that he does not wish to suffer. Then, if he permits himself to give it voice, he will say that he is fearful about choking to death and wonders how he will die. At that point, it is possible to tell him a story of how it will probably be, having been with many people who have died from ALS, most of whom died at home. We tell him that people become progressively weaker and probably less able to move. Swallowing may become difficult, but we can always keep his mouth moist to relieve distress from thirst. If breathing becomes more shallow, he will retain carbon dioxide and become progressively more drowsy. No struggle. No gasping, and a respirator is not necessary. Drugs can relieve discomfort, but they are frequently not necessary. At some point, often in his sleep, he will simply breathe out—expire—and not have the strength to breathe in again. Simple, quiet, and if in the company of prepared and loving family who are present and unpanicked, there is the peacefulness of being fully connected. It is not so much the words that are said, but the openness, clarity, and caring, and we have heard many times a relieved sigh with some variant of "Oh! Is that all it is?"

Stories of Roots

This is a chance for Father to tell of his connections with his ancestors. It is surprising how little many people know of parents, grandparents, and beyond. A few facts but not many stories, and it is stories that give a sense of connectedness and solidarity with the past. It is the stories that define us. Many will say that their parents came from abroad and would never speak to them about their painful past. This leaves subsequent generations without any tales to tell and pass along. We need to tell and hear the sad stories along with the happier ones; otherwise the picture of our roots is incomplete. Reflections about parents, siblings, and growing up often reveal continuing pain from deaths unmourned and loving words unspoken. Bringing these memories and images from the shadowy past into the present allows some mourning to take place and lessens the deep pain that resulted from holding on to the story rather than mourning and letting it go. This in turn makes it possible to die in peace, unattached to the rage or grief of preceding losses and deaths. If this is not done, Father will expect that the mode of his death will be like that of his mother or father with its physical pain and terrors of long ago repeated for him; in his fantasy, he redies their deaths along with his own.

The Family Tells of Him

Mother starts by telling her story. How they met and her view of the ups and downs of the marriage. She is always asked how the illness has affected her, and this usually evokes tears and worries about present and future, together with stories of other losses and disconnections in her life. Her worries are for his comfort and for the relief of his suffering, and she may voice some of the fears she has concerning future unknowns and what life will be like without him.

Some secrets may emerge; a very common example already alluded to is alcoholism. Dad may have resurrected this trouble when he told his story, but more commonly it is Mother or one of the children who speaks of it. She recalls that the twenty years of his drinking were awful for both her and the children, and there was a repetitive sequence of drunkenness, abuse, financial problems, and absence, but she usually adds that he was wonderful when he was sober. The children are invited to say what it was like for them. Embarrassment, shame, anger, fear, a sense of never having known Dad and constantly worrying for Mom. The object is not to be judge and jury for Father or to inflame his guilt. That is already present in overabundance. It is to acknowledge and speak of a piece of family history that actually happened but had been banished into the underworld to ferment and almost always reappear in subsequent generations if not aired. The fact that they can all speak of this, feel feelings, listen to one another, and not dash out of the room is a source of wonder to all of them. The story is out. It no longer needs to be hidden, and there is now less of a barrier in dealing with the facts and fantasies of Father's advanced illness. Additionally, this airing may be the opportunity for other family members to take responsibility for their own alcoholism or other difficulties, and there have been many instances of the family meeting being the catalyst for change in individuals within the family.

Some family secrets are harder to let go of than others, so the suffering is likely to be handed on. There was a family meeting around the bedside of a middle-aged woman who was dying of breast cancer. Her husband was by her side and had been extremely attentive and almost over-solicitous during her few days in the Hospice Inn. Her daughter sat at the end of the bed with her husband. There was an impenetrable stiffness and superficiality at the beginning of the meeting. Mother lay with her eyes closed, said she had no worries, and did not have much to say about husband or daughter. Father held her hand and rhapsodized about his wife and their marriage and how heartbreaking her illness had been for him. The daughter was initially quiet and said a few things about her mother but suddenly stood up and delivered a startling and heartrending story. She said that she had been immersed in an incestuous relationship with her father for ten years and talked of the pain, shame, and nightmares of her childhood, from which she was only now emerging with the help of both a therapist and a loving husband. Her father made a variety of interjections of denial, but her mother listened with eyes open, and it was to her mother that she was talking. This dialogue continued off and on for the several days before she died. The daughter forgave her mother's lifelong closed eyes, and they struggled with their new intimacy. Father remained denial-coated and disconnected.

Most children are not plagued by such painful memories, and the family meeting is an opportunity for them to remind and remember, laugh, cry, hug, thank, and take their leave. Even if Dad appears to be unconscious, the children are encouraged both in the family meeting and when they have time alone with him to hold his hand and tell him anything they would like to say. Even in the most wanting of relationships, we can always express our sadness that we missed out on one another and thank our parent for giving us life.

Reflections on the Family Meeting

The family meeting is reminiscent of the story told about the first of four tasks set by Venus for Psyche that had to be completed if she was to be reunited with Eros. Venus set before her a huge pile of mixed dark and light seeds with the instruction that she was to separate them before nightfall. She started the task but quickly realized that it would never be accomplished in time. At that moment, an army of ants arrived and separated the seeds in short order, well before sunset.

When the family meeting starts, it seems impossible that anything will be accomplished; there is too much pain and too much rage. Children have not lived up to parents' expectations and parents have not fulfilled the real and imagined needs and wishes of their children. Oddly enough, in this sacred setting of the family meeting, presided over by impending loss that facilitates the letting go of trivial resentments and bickering, some sorting out does happen.

Common Symptoms and Signs of ALS in the Hospice

We close this chapter with a few notes in response to questions often asked about ALS symptom management in the hospice setting.

Constipation results from immobility, paralysis of abdominal muscles, and decreased fluid intake. Caregivers need to be instructed in a bowel management program.

Pain or discomfort can result from muscle spasms or as a consequence of prolonged immobility. Medications, physical therapy, and occupational therapy may be useful, depending on the specific nature of the problem. Massage is particularly valuable.

Decreased mobility changes one's ability to engage in daily activities and perform role functions within the family and community. Additionally, it results in greater demands on caregivers. Occupational and physical therapy can address areas of dysfunction, assist people in adapting to role changes, recommend appropriate assistive devices and equipment, and teach caregivers how to assist with self-care and daily activities. Loss of physical control and the ability to "do" may be helped by meditation, visualization and counseling.

Salivation becomes difficult to manage as the oral musculature weakens and dysphagia worsens. Drooling can be annoying and embarrassing for people with ALS. Management can include use of a suction machine, proper positioning, avoidance of certain foods, and the use of medications to reduce secretions.

Fatigue commonly accompanies ALS and reports increase as the disease progresses, particularly as the respiratory muscles weaken. Occupational therapy for instruction in energy conservation techniques and relaxation therapy can be useful.

Difficulty with communication is usually progressive, and people with ALS frequently express fear of being unable to communicate. It is imperative that they have access to equipment and training in alternative methods of communication if speech and writing become impossible to perform. Various devices ranging from simple communication boards to sophisticated augmentative communication devices are available. As covered providers under hospice, the speech-language pathologist and occupational therapist can be called on to assess areas of communication difficulty. ALS clinics and knowledgeable practitioners can provide invaluable help to hospices in meeting the communication needs of people with advanced ALS. Some hospices have arranged contractual agreements with speech-language pathologists and occupational therapists who have experience in managing ALS. This type of arrangement can help to maintain the continuity of care as people with ALS transition onto hospice programs.

Insomnia may result from an inability to change one's position in bed and from discomfort associated with immobility. Insomnia frequently accompanies changes in respiratory status coupled with a fear of dying during the night, which is common to many people with far-advanced illness. Various management approaches should be considered: alternative positioning, assistance with position changes, bed pads that improve weight distribution, relaxation training, and use of medications. It is most important to give voice to the fact that many persons with ALS worry that they may die in the night. Bringing this fear into the open frequently lightens it, making it easier to let go into sleep.

Anxiety may be expressed as restlessness, agitation, or insomnia. Feelings of loss of control and fears or worries related to the progression of the disease and eventual manner of death need to be addressed in the family meeting.

Dysphagia is a distressing problem in ALS. One study involving the review of 124 people who died of ALS showed that none "choked to death" (12). Nevertheless, people with ALS commonly articulate a fear of "choking to death" and it is helpful to provide reassurance that, although they may experience "choking episodes," "choking to death" is not the manner of death from ALS. Additionally, it is helpful to counsel family members on how to assist someone who is experiencing a "choking episode," as these can be anxiety-producing for everyone. The speech-language pathologist can provide instruction on how to decrease the likelihood of problems associated with dysphagia. The option of using a feeding tube has usually been discussed well in advance of admission to hospice. Although it is possible to have a feeding tube inserted after hospice admission, it is not common. People with ALS, family members, caregivers, and health care professionals may express concerns about "starving to death" as oral intake decreases. Use of this emotionally charged phrase in discussions with people with ALS and families should be abandoned because it can conjure fearful images that do not accurately portray the process. Typically, people with advanced ALS do not complain of a gnawing hunger or pain resulting from decreased ability to take food by mouth. The process is usually gradual and accommodated to in stages. Appetite wanes and fatigue increases, along with visible weight loss. Likewise, fear of dehydration need not be a motivating factor for having a feeding tube. Even for those who elect to use a feeding tube, the amount of fluids given is often decreased in the advanced stages of the disease so that the body is not burdened by excess fluids. It is very important to maintain scrupulous attention to mouth care as fluid intake decreases. Dehydration toward the end of life does not cause discomforting symptoms other than dry mouth. The zeal of physician and family to promote intravenous fluids at this stage may delay death for a short time, which may in turn add to the agony rather than relieve discomfort.

Occasionally, a hospice patient may elect to discontinue use of a feeding tube for nutritional support. It is important for this type of decision to be discussed openly with the family, as caregivers can sometimes interpret the decision as a failure on their part to provide adequate support or care.

Respiratory problems usually prompt discussion of hospice as one alternative response. If, after a series of discussions with physician and family, an individual with ALS decides that he or she does not wish to utilize ventilatory support in the event of respiratory failure, it is appropriate to consider hospice. Clearly, it is important that this area of discussion occur well in advance of serious respiratory difficulties and within the context of the family system so that a consensus can be reached on how to respond as changes in respiration occur. Once a person with ALS has been admitted to hospice, various forms of palliative treatment can be utilized to ameliorate the effects of respiratory compromise. These can include: noninvasive ventilatory support, nasal oxygen, percussive treatments, proper positioning, relaxation training, and medication. A fear of "suffocating to death" commonly produces anxiety for both the person with ALS and family members. Gentle yet open discussion surrounding the likely progression of the disease and manner of death can soften fear. Reiterating the 24-hour on-call availability of support through hospice and the option of hospice inpatient admission for terminal care can also be reassuring. Providing people with ALS and their families with knowledge of what to expect helps to prepare them for death and can enhance their ability to make the most of their remaining time together. Even in the final hours of life, people can connect with loved ones in ways that can help ultimately to sustain family members during the bereavement process. An essential vehicle for helping people with ALS and families throughout the course of the disease is the family meeting, which has been discussed earlier.

Drugs and ALS

There is still some reluctance to use morphine sulfate in far-advanced illnesses, especially when there is any hint of respiratory compromise. Hospices have demonstrated its efficacy in the pain control of cancer, and such issues as addiction and ever-escalating doses are theoretical rather than real problems. In ALS, toward the end of life, there may be a mixture of restlessness, agitation, aching discomfort, fear, anxiety, and sleeplessness that responds extremely well to the use of low dose morphine in a dose of 5–10 mg oral elixir every four hours. Lorazepam is usually tried first, and occasionally is used along with morphine in a dose of 1–2 mg. daily.

A Caveat

While meticulous attention to signs and symptoms is basic to hospice care, it must be remembered that it is much easier for patient, family, and staff to focus on tangible symptoms than to express something of the shadowy fears of the unknown and the pain of the relentless and progressive losses in ALS. The next chapter, in which mourning is discussed, is essential reading, since mourning colors every sign and symptom to a greater or lesser extent. For example, narcotics are often prescribed without much question when sleeplessness is reported. If the insomnia is induced by mourning that creates tension over falling asleep for fear that there will be no awakening, a narcotic may compound the anxiety as the patient strives to fight off the effects.

A provocative quatrain by the psychiatrist R.D. Laing is a caveat for caregivers:

Take this pill.
It helps you not to shout
It takes away the life
You're better off without.

Pills and potions are all too often given to deaden life rather than to enhance its quality.

When faced with the relentless decline of ALS, coupled with family distress and a personal feeling of inadequacy and helplessness, we are eager to prescribe something to take it all away. Fight and flight have been ingrained into us; we fight disease and then back away when our doings are no longer helpful. We are not taught that we have a vital place in mourning with our patients. Antidepressants are no substitute for presence and are rarely needed. When we are dying of ALS or anything else, we need someone to mourn along with us; we need someone to listen, witness, and be thoroughly present, and we can be a powerful force in this role.

References

1. Saunders C. The modern hospice. In: Wald FS, eds. *In Quest of the Spiritual Component of Care for the Terminally Ill: Proceedings of a Colloquium.* New Haven: Yale University School of Nursing, 1986.
2. Hadlock D, Physician roles in hospice care. In: Corr CA, Corr DM, eds. *Hospice Care: Principles and Practice.* New York: Springer, 1983.
3. Corless I. The hospice movement in North America. In: Corr CA, Corr DM, eds. *Hospice Care: Principles and Practice.* New York: Springer, 1983.
4. Thompson B, Wurth MA. The hospice movement. In: Tigges KN, Marcil WM, eds. *Terminal and Life-Threatening Illness: An Occupational Behavior Perspective.* Thorofare, NJ: Slack, 1988.
5. Thompson B. Occupational therapy with the terminally ill. In: Kiernat JM, ed. *Occupational Therapy and the Older Adult: A Clinical Manual.* Gaithersburg, Md.: Aspen, 1991.
6. National Hospice Organization. *Standards of a Hospice Program of Care.* Alexandria, Va.: Author, 1981.
7. Hospice News Service. It's now official: the medicare hospice benefit is "here to stay." *New York State Hospice Association Newsletter.* February 1991.
8. Selinske C. The fourth hospice benefit period. *New York State Hospice Association Newsletter.* March 1991.
9. Saunders C. Walsh TC, Smith M. Hospice care in motor neuron disease. In: Saunders C. Summers DH, Teller N, eds. *Hospice: The Living Idea.* London: Edward Arnold, 1981.
10. Thompson B. Amyotrophic lateral sclerosis: integrating care for patients and their families. *Am J Hospice* 1990, 7:27–32.
11. Hillel A, Miller R. Bulbar amyotrophic lateral sclerosis: patterns of progression and clinical management. *Head Neck* 1989, 11:51–59.
12. O'Brien T, Kelly M. Saunders C. Motor neurone disease: a hospice perspective. *Brit Med J* 1992, 304:471–472.

20

Mourning and Amyotrophic Lateral Sclerosis

N. Michael Murphy, M.D.

Introduction

With reasonable physical health, or even in the face of considerable sickness, we seldom contemplate or allow into full consciousness the possibility that we can die at any time. Denial of death is everyday fare for most of us, but that inner innocence or naivete which maintains the myth of our physical immortality becomes sorely tried or even shattered by the diagnosis of any life-threatening illness. The implications of ALS are particularly hard to ignore since all the literature speaks of a fatal outcome, and the muscular decline is an ever-present reminder of finitude and death. This loss of health and innocence in ALS evokes the expression of a whole range of feelings that may be frozen by denial or given full exposure, which is the prelude to acceptance of what is happening. These responses, induced to varying degrees in patient, family, and caregivers are the subject of the first part of this chapter. The second part focuses on some aspects of care for those who are suffering or have suffered from loss, be they the ones with ALS, their families, or their caregivers.

Mourning and the Response to Loss

Loss transports us into a journey that ranges back and forth along a path that ends with integration and acceptance. In ALS or any other terminal illness, death may intervene at any time with the trials and tribulations imposed by the loss still unresolved. We will retain some degree of denial, but most of the time will move beyond it. Most will not continue to rage incessantly against the coming of the night, but may become stuck in a state of bereavement and need a kindly nudge in order to leave it behind. Grief is a prelude to letting go or dying and will be shunned as long as death is denied or avoided or while we are consumed by our response to bereavement.

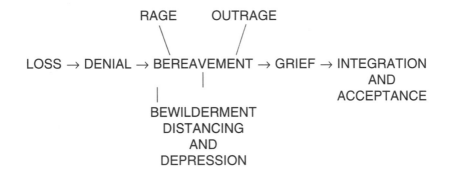

Denial is a natural, self-protective response to any event that disconnects us from that which provides nurture or self-esteem. In the event of sudden death of someone close, or the sudden, unexpected diagnosis of an illness such as ALS, the immediate response is usually some variant of "Oh, no!" Taken literally, this is an exclamation denying the truth of what has just been told in an attempt to obliterate the fear and chaos inspired by the life-threatening diagnosis and to restore equilibrium. Usually the individual does not maintain the stance that the incident never happened, and asks a series of questions that help to confirm the new reality. With a life-threatening illness, most will breach their denial to some degree but will often shore it up again with the aid of family members who are terrified at the prospect of loss and hide behind the possibility of doing something—anything at all—to dissipate the helplessness and fear.

Some physicians are models of sensitivity as they speak of that which is difficult to hear and still remain fully present and available. Others protect themselves by disgorging unpalatable facts over the phone or even in hospital corridors. Medical schools give scant attention to teaching students how to digest painful information and reframe it for their patients simply, clearly, and compassionately. We need to give only as many of the facts as the one with ALS needs at the moment, all within a framework of compassion and gentle hopefulness, not the false hope of the blusterer who dangles insubstantial half-truths with the justification that he does not want to take away all hope. He does not understand that real hope and optimism are always appropriate in life-threatening illness; not that the condition will be cured, but that in a loving atmosphere, with truthful communication and connectedness, we will experience the hope and preciousness of each day, and the peace that comes from having settled our technical and emotional affairs.

Bereavement is defined in the Oxford English dictionary as the state of being deprived, robbed, or stripped, usually of immaterial possessions. Thus, if we feel that we own someone or something that is then lost, we will believe that we have been robbed. The feelings that accompany this robbery usually include all manner of rage and outrage.

If we believe that we have a birthright to good health, and that muscular power, control, and integrity which have been painstakingly promoted and learned from our earliest days are "ours," we will experience bereavement with rage, outrage, and bewilderment when it is taken away by ALS. If we believe that a loved one belongs to us, then the death threat and gradual taking away of that person will cause us to go through all the pain of the bereaved. Since we are human and have been brought up to believe in ownership, we will feel bereaved many times in our lives. Those who are able to love without attachment and are not tied to goods, chattels, or the inalienable right to good health are less apt to become engulfed by anger and more ready to accept whatever comes their way.

Rage is a word associated with being mad, going berserk, running amok, and losing control. When we say that we are mad, we do not usually imagine that we mean it literally, that we are really insane or are out our minds. But the fact is that if we maintain rage, we are insane and incapable of responding in a healthy manner to the realities of the moment.

A well-respected physician, who had authored several books and was a wonderful teacher and observer of others, was wheeled into my office by his wife. I had no idea he was physically sick until that moment, but one look at his intense jaundice and emaciated state and it was clear that he was close to death. He said that he had asked to see me because he was afraid that he was going out of his mind and wanted my opinion. His story was that carcinoma of the pancreas had been diagnosed several months earlier, and since then he had been involved in a continual technological nightmare of surgery, chemotherapy, and tests. In his words, he barely had time to catch his breath. It was as if he had been holding his breath and suspending his feelings for the past months, aided and abetted in this denial by his intellect, his family, and a horde of physicians. Now he was beginning to experience feelings of rage, translated by this cultured man into feelings of loss of control and fear of losing his mind or going mad. With a little gentle nudging and a couple of family meetings the following week, he was able to acknowledge his rage and leave it behind. At that point, he was ready to grieve with his family, share stories, and express tender feelings, all of which had been a lifelong difficulty for this logical, controlling man. He died a few hours after the second family gathering, peacefully, with all said and done.

Charles was a fear-filled man who raged against the diagnosis and manifestations of ALS. His rage and fear were such that he developed unremitting angina that was uncontrollable with medical treatment. This created a dilemma between the risk of surgery in one whose respiration was already affected by ALS and the prospect of pain for the rest of his life. He elected to undergo surgery, which completely relieved the angina, but then he was compelled to face his bereavement and address the rage over the perceived rape of his physical integrity. The rage and madness over his state and the outrage that this happened to him abated as he gave it voice. Years before, his teenaged son had died in a climbing accident, and at that time and subsequently he avoided his grief and dealt with bereavement by banning all thought and talk of his son. With his own life-threatening illness, he initially avoided having to deal with his feelings by almost killing himself with angina, breaking his heart rather than allowing himself to feel broken-hearted. The next year provided him with the time to experience his bereavement and grief over the loss of his son, and this in turn gave him the courage to mourn his own losses and impending death. Six weeks before he died, his younger sister was killed in a motor vehicle accident. He attended her funeral in a wheelchair and appeared to be fully present to his outrage and sadness over her death. It seemed as though her death gave him permission to let go and die, and the last few weeks of his life were relatively comfortable and peaceful.

Outrage at being the subject of life-threatening illness is rage that is more focused and controlled. The one outraged screams "Why me?" or the relative cries out against this happening to a good person like mother when there are so many worse people out there who are perfectly free of illness. Outrage blames an unjust God or sees the illness as a punishment. It storms against a missed diagnosis or fastens blame for what is happening on anyone or anything. It is like paranoia as it projects the insanity of the situation on to an outside source, unwilling or unable to understand or accept the randomness and impersonal nature of terminal illness. It is an attempt to avoid the impotence of medicine and its regular inability to control outcomes. Rage and outrage disconnect us from each other and our world just at the time we most need connectedness and love. Its main purpose is to stave off grief, which is the necessary prelude to connectedness, acceptance, and integration.

Betty was in her early sixties when she came to see me following surgery for what proved to be metastatic colon cancer. She said that she had foregone chances to live independently or get married in order to take care of her chronically ill mother, who eventually died twelve years before the diagnosis of her colon cancer. Her mother never said a word in gratitude and seemed to be in a perpetual state of rage, outrage, or their internalized associate, depression. The thirty years of caregiving produced little joy and a constant stewpot of anger, and mother's death offered little emotional relief since they had never shared anything but rage and had not allowed themselves to connect through grief, which in turn leads to integration, permitting the exchange of love. The stewpot continued to simmer for the next decade, during which she looked after her meek and mild father until his death. The long awaited peace and happiness, expected as a birthright, especially with the departure of her parents, never happened. Two years after her father's death, she was diagnosed with colon cancer, and I remember the spirit of her words, if not their actual form, as she raged and bubbled in my office: "It is not fair. After all I did for my parents. Now I expected to enjoy myself and travel, and look what has happened. If there is a just God in heaven, He will take this cancer away, and I am going to sit here until He does!"

That is exactly what she did. She sat on her stewpot of rage with her spiritual arms folded and did little else for the nine months until she died. No softness, no grief, no letting go. No kindness to herself for her service to her parents even though it was reluctantly given. No tears for the little girl within her who never felt loved. She died as she lived; a stony monument to self-righteousness and outrage, fending off the comfort and love that was within her reach.

Bewilderment is the state of losing one's way or being unable to grasp what is happening. It is beyond denial in that there is an understanding that all is not well. But there is a numbness or apathy that does not admit to feelings, especially rage, outrage, or grief.

Distancing results from not wishing to become too emotionally involved. Some family members and friends keep their distance from the one with ALS, and so never accompany the dying person though grief to acceptance and a place of new intimacy born of having gone through the emotional refiner's fire together. If we keep our distance, we protect ourselves from grief but do not experience intimacy. We will not have to say goodbye, which many of us believe too painful, but this ensures that we will be forever nagged by the wish that we had made some expression of love; that we had told our loved one that she was important to us and would be sorely missed. It is paradoxical that such an expression is a necessary prelude to letting go, and it is only after we let go that we are free to be nourished by the everlasting images and stories that are the real essence or soul of the one who has died.

Physicians, nurses, and other caregivers frequently distance themselves from their patients. We have been taught by words or example that it is not good to become too involved. How much is too much has never been clearly defined other than the proscription related to sexual behavior with patients. Are we permitted or do we permit ourselves to love a patient or mourn her loss? If we grieved for each of our patients who died, there is the fear that we would burnout or go mad. Oddly enough, it is our resistance to mourning and our stubborn maintenance of distance that is a frequent cause of chronic anger and burnout among caregivers. If emotionally we will go the whole distance with patients and their families and be prepared—or unprepared—to weep and also to attend the wake or funeral, we will have done everything possible so that we can then let go and move on. Those who distance emotionally and feel that their work is done, as soon as they run out of technical tricks, never experience completion and peacefulness with their patients who die. This, like any form of interrupted intercourse, is, by definition, incomplete and unsatisfying. It is the failure to accompany the family to the end that creates in caregivers a continuous sense of bereavement.

Burnout means being consumed by the fire of rage, and this in turn precipitates fight or flight. We will fight by becoming even more angry and distanced, and we will fly by changing specialties, leaving medicine, or committing suicide.

Grief: We will go to any extreme in our attempts to avoid grief. We have been admonished to hold back tears and be brave. Little John Kennedy saluting the coffin of his Dad. The show must go on. Keep the stiff upper lip, and be "strong."

We are uncomfortable with feelings, and being emotional in a male-ordered world is considered little short of sinful, and most certainly weak. In the face of grief, many physicians, especially the pseudo-masculine, macho ones, will provide and encourage tranquilizers and sleeping pills so that its expression is muted. Others will prescribe antidepressants rather than listen to the rage and outrage and assist their patients in the delivery of their grief. There is the fear that being very emotional in grief will lead to breakdown and this inspires the fear of madness and even the fantasy of incarceration in a mental hospital. It is not always accepted that grief is the normal final expression of loss and being out of control.

The story of Dante's Inferno is a vivid reminder that the pain of grief cannot be avoided if we wish to emerge from mourning. The Inferno was imagined as a round pit with steep sides, and almost all of the sufferers tried to escape the flames by scrambling toward the periphery and attempting to get out by clawing their way up the steep sides. Just a few realized that the only way out was through an opening in the middle of the pit. The flames of grief will end only if we travel into their midst.

We are uncomfortable with grief because it is both the harbinger of death and the beginning of its acceptance, and in our society death is hopeless, a failure, and the greatest of all possible negatives. We may never say die. So it is common in families for each of the members to experience grief but to do their crying alone. Over and over again I have heard variations on the theme of a daughter who was heartbroken over her mother who had advanced ALS. When I asked if she had shared her fears with mother, she was shocked, saying that she did not want to upset her and that she needed to remain strong for her. What a sad dissipation of soulful feelings. I will always remember a daughter who was the devoted caregiver for her much-loved mother: "When I am down, she holds me while I cry, and when she is sad and tearful, I am able to hold and comfort her. We are each there for the other." If we share grief and be witnesses for one another, we experience the connectedness that we crave, and it becomes the prelude to acceptance and peace. Mourning does not end while grief is in the closet.

We often wonder whether children should witness our grief and we attempt to protect them from feelings, both ours and their own. It is a real gift to share our tears and sadness with children. We are telling them by example that the loss of grandmother to ALS is painfully heartbreaking, and that these feelings are both appropriate and very much worth sharing. Children who are "protected" from feelings are fundamentally deprived, and are being taught that the feelings induced by loss are dangerous and not to be expressed. When feelings of loss are pushed underground, they do not disappear and may be transformed into chronic fear and anxiety to emerge in full force at the next appearance of life-threatening illness.

Integration and acceptance may be at hand when we have ceased fighting and raging against the coming of the night. Tears have been shed for the child within, and she is at peace. We have grieved with our family and have ceased to hide behind endless procedures and other doings. We have let go of family and friends and are now able to be a human being rather than a human doing, simply being with ourselves and our family for whatever time remains.

I remember Melba, a marvelous, energetic, humorous woman I had the privilege of knowing at different stages of ALS. In the early days she raged, but in listening to herself and being listened to, the anger seemed to evaporate in a mist of wit and wisdom. She grieved for her husband and children, and she wept for herself, and there was a wealth of healing and love between them all as they laughed, cried, and told stories. As her breathing became very shallow, talking was almost impossible, but at that point, all had been said and done. There was nothing more to say. She died quietly and peacefully, simply breathing out—expiring.

I had several taped interviews with Joan, a most remarkable woman who had lost the ability to speak and swallow a few months before my last interview. She had been living independently, but profound muscular weakness had made it necessary for her to leave the area and move in with family. She was able to type with one finger on a word processor and her words conjure up images of acceptance and letting go that move me beyond words:

" . . . it is not easy to part from each other. That is why we should make the most of our time and be open and trusting I'm not saying anything new. I want to say that it seems to me since I am no longer verbal, I talk a lot! It is ironic and a little sad. I don't feel sick. I keep thinking it's a big mistake and I'm waiting for someone to correct it. At least God has big shoulders, but I still think or rather I wish he had overlooked me! It is amazing. I am still struggling to hold on to life, and at the same time there are those who throw theirs away. How sad for them who have never known joy of life.

"Do not feel sorry for me; I have peace and love. At times I get a sense of life slipping away and it is frightening, but at the same time I know I will be fine.

"What is important is never to let ALS be a person instead of seeing your loved one as the person with ALS. I have seen time and time again when family members become isolated from one another. It is a gift of love that we remain connected. It is an obligation for both the person with ALS and the caregiver. It is not ALS that cuts us off. It is our fear and lack of love for one another.

"Finally, I want to thank you all for your generosity, friendship, and love. For being there with me, sometimes in silence, sometimes with soft suggestions, but always dealing with me as a person, as an individual. I wish I had the ability to tell you all how much you have given me. I'm not alone, traveling in uncharted waters. You have kept me safe, close to shore, and when I've drifted too far, you have gently guided me back to safety. I thank you, all my friends. You are my heroes.''

Caring for Those Who Mourn

Caring for the Patient: The prerequisite for caregiving is that the caregivers understand the process of mourning for the one with ALS and are also able to articulate how this process is affecting themselves. If we are frightened of rage, we will discourage its expression in the families to whom we are giving care. If the expression of sadness rocks our need for self control, and we have been raised to worship the stiff upper lip and the belief that any public expression of grief is not positive or is an admission of defeat, then we will be routed by the tears of our patient and so be of little help.

Openness and connectedness among all involved are essential to good care. Family connectedness is enhanced and encouraged by the family meeting, which should be held soon after the diagnosis and repeated at the request of the family or whenever they appear to be stuck in the journey of mourning. It is important to address technical questions and any symptoms that may arise, but it is tempting to remain focused on these practical issues and not give voice to the responses to loss. Anticipation of the losses of ability to talk, swallow, and breathe, and skillful discussion of these issues over time will usually avert a crisis response, born of widespread denial, which may well lead to the patient being impelled into a course of action which, on greater reflection, he would not want. A peaceful death, when all has been said and done, is much more likely when all involved have given their full attention to both body and soul.

Caring for the Family: Isadora Duncan (1), reflecting on her own grief following the death of her two small children:

"The next morning I drove out to see Duse, who was living in a rose colored villa behind a vineyard. She came down a vine covered walk to meet me, like a glorious angel. She took me in her arms and her wonderful eyes beamed upon me such love and tenderness that I felt just as Dante must have felt when, in the 'Paradiso,' he encounters the Divine Beatrice.

"From then on I lived at Viareggio, finding courage from the radiance of Eleanora's eyes. She used to rock me in her arms, consoling my pain, but not only consoling, for she seemed to take my sorrow to her own breast, and I realized that if I had not been able to bear the society of other people, it was because they all played the comedy of trying to cheer me with forgetfulness. Whereas Eleanora said: 'Tell me about Deidre and Patrick,' and made me repeat to her all their little sayings and ways, and show her their photos, which she kissed and cried over. She never said, 'Cease to grieve,' but she grieved with me, and, for the first time since their death, I felt I was not alone.''

Isadora might have said: ''Don't cheer me with forgetfulness nor keep me in denial nor drug me into apathy and distance. I need to grieve. I need to be held, so that my anger and hurt flows out of me, and I need love to help me cry. Don't tell me to get on with my life and cease to grieve because at that moment we become disconnected and I am plunged deeper into loneliness.''

The family will have mourned to a greater or lesser extent while the patient was alive. Few will still be in denial or ''in shock'' at the time of death. Most will have left their rage and anger behind, but some will experience bereavement after the death of their loved one even though they were the most meticulous and loving of caregivers. Mrs. B told me that the eighteen months after the death of her husband from ALS were quite awful. Their marriage was intimate and unusually exciting, but the year of his illness was filled with losses that seemed to follow one another without respite. He coped with each crisis with dignity, humor, and compassion for all right up to the moment of his death, which followed removal from a respirator at his request. But Mrs. B, caught up in her husband's crises especially toward the end, never allowed herself to feel the rage and anger while he was alive, and after he died she was engulfed by overwhelming resentment at the disease and the turmoil it created in her life. She had worked alongside her husband, and that ceased. Recreationally, physically, emotionally, sexually, her life was turned upside down, and after his death some of her rage was vented toward her image of him and toward the ''selfish'' decision he made to disconnect the respirator. After his death, when the hubbub of family and friends quieted down, she became almost paralyzed by anger and depression. Gradually, through talking about her feelings over and over again with a handful of nonjudgmental friends, she was able to move from rage to grief. She stressed to me how important it was for her to solicit these few friends to come and share their feelings about her husband and invite them to listen to her. Without her encouragement, they would not have come and shared painful feelings, which was the necessary prelude to moving on.

Self-help groups are very good for some of those whose loved ones have died. The death can be a precious opportunity to mourn many other losses that have gone unmourned. If this happens, the individual's life may take on a new zest, freed from a dark pall of unremitting bereavement and grief from the past. I frequently advise and encourage counseling for those who have been involved with a death since many are ripe for change at that moment.

Caring for the Caregiver: We look for and are expected to provide answers even when there are none. There is great uncertainty in medicine, and yet we are not taught how to deal with it, emotionally and interpersonally. ALS offers caregivers the perfect opportunity to confront helplessness and to go beyond it and realize we are only helpless in doing but never in being. Because of our illusions of professionalism we will be bereaved by ALS. We will be angry at

the disease, the patient, or the family, or else distance ourselves behind a procla-
mation that there is nothing to be done. It is not a waste of valuable professional
time for a physician to be with someone afflicted with ALS, although it may be
one of our most difficult challenges because of our own discomfort, not the
patient's. Our grief and sadness will be evoked, and we may wish to flee, especially if there have been significant others in our lives who have died and for
whom we never mourned.

I believe that all caregivers who provide care for the dying, including all physicians and nurses as well as many others, need to participate in a workshop that
focuses on their mourning, past, present, and future, and the workshop needs
repeating at least once or twice during a career. The "soul searching" workshops
I have given for several years last two or three days and include time for visualiz-
ing or imagining our own death so that we can experience some of our fears and
apprehensions about death, and so be more in touch with what our patients are
experiencing. Workshop participants also experience a simulated family meeting
when they are the ones who are dying and are finishing up their business with
those they love by saying what needs to be said. There is also time in the workshop
to mourn other losses, and there are many opportunities to experience the art of
being an impeccable listener and witness. Being a nonjudgmental, fully present
witness is difficult and unfamiliar. We are so practiced in half-listening, interrupt-
ing, and dispensing advice. Experiencing the power of witnessing and being
witnessed is one of the great surprises for workshop participants. They also learn
a few techniques on how to nudge and encourage others to move along the
route of mourning. The workshop is extremely personal, and in experiencing and
processing the personal we become more empathic caregivers who are less prone
to fight and flight.

Since death is still considered as failure and technology is becoming ever more
insistent in medicine, it is doubtful that medical and nursing schools will give
the lead by having this kind of workshop experience as an essential part of the
curriculum. This should not deter smaller groups from introducing such workshops, and the collaboration, interpersonal connectedness, and skills of individuals who are members of caregiving groups for ALS and cancer will be much
enhanced as a result.

Another suggestion for ALS caregiving groups is that there be an hour, every
week or two, when caregivers gather together to discuss the process of their own
mourning and that of the patients and families with whom they work. This is a
time when personal reactions to caregiving, families, helplessness, the anger of
others, and a box full of other feelings may be aired and witnessed. If we work
with the dying for long, we will certainly be reminded of the past or future deaths
of our own mothers, fathers, brothers, lovers, and of ourselves. We will have the
opportunity to rehearse a little what it might be like when someone close to us
dies, and we need a safe place where we can discuss this. Having been part of
such a "process group" in St. Peter's Hospice for the past fourteen years, I know

of its usefulness. But I also know that these meetings can be filled with feelings, and that many caregiving groups abandon them because of discomfort with exposing their vulnerability before colleagues with whom they have to work every day. I believe the intention behind any process or support group is the key to failure or success. If the intention is confrontation and analysis, then sooner or later the group will self-destruct. If the intention is to encourage the expression of feelings that will be lovingly witnessed without judgment and without being pulled apart, the group may become a vital force in the care of the caregiver.

Reference

Duncan I. *My Life*. New York: Liveright Pub, 1927.

21

Long-Term Care: The Financial Realities

Brian S. Gould, M.D.

Historical Overview

Although health insurance can trace its origins back to the 1850s, insurance policies have consistently emphasized protection from certain major costs of acute illness such as hospital confinement, surgery, and anesthetics. It was not until World War II that health care coverage broadened to provide additional benefits for general medical services such as physician fees. Even then the general pattern of little or no coverage for extended illnesses and lengthy hospital confinements was maintained. It was not until the 1950s that commercial insurance carriers initially and Blue Cross and Blue Shield plans later mitigated some of these limitations by popularizing major medical coverage, in which the extraordinary costs of catastrophic illnesses were matched with higher benefit levels, but only after the satisfaction of significant deductible costs. In general, the health insurance system has offered excellent protection for the health care costs associated with acute, highly technical medical care—particularly hospitalization—but is far less adequate for low-tech services and chronic conditions, even when they are disabling.

Consequently, despite many innovations in health care financing during the last twenty years, such as employer self-insurance, the growth of health maintenance organizations, and other managed care delivery systems, it can still be said that virtually all private health insurance plans continue to emphasize the same three basic coverage categories: hospital care, surgical fees, and physician services.

Health care that falls outside of these areas—for example, preventive services, convalescent and long-term care, or specialized non-physician services such as physical therapy, chiropractic, or psychological treatment—exists either as specifically defined benefits subject to narrowly qualified coverage and limits, or they are not covered at all. Therefore, those in need of long-term care usually ''drop out'' of the health insurance system at some point into dependence on other insurance, private funds, or public sector programs.

The most common type of supplemental insurance is disability coverage. Although it is often thought of as a type of health insurance, this is a misconception. Disability insurance must be obtained separately from different sources than health insurance, is built around a significantly different benefit design, and carries unique qualifying conditions.

In general, disability insurance is designed to pay benefits only when and if the beneficiary is rendered totally disabled by the definitions of the policy (although policies now frequently contain additional provisions for partial disability as well). Health-related functional disability is defined for insurance purposes in terms of occupational capacity—either fitness to meet the demands of one's regular occupation or, using the language of many current plans, any occupation for which the beneficiary is ''reasonably qualified by training, education, and experience.'' Policies offering coverage for partial disability usually augment this with additional benefits based on the loss of income resulting from disability rather then degree of functional incapacity.

Sources for disability insurance include individual or group policies that are purchased separately from health insurance and require the payment of an additional premium either by working individuals or their employers; workers compensation, which only provides benefits for disabling injuries occurring on the job or caused by occupational circumstances; veterans disability benefits, which offer limited benefits to those who served in the armed services; and Social Security. Under the provisions of the Social Security program, most working people qualify for a monthly income benefit once they reach retirement age, have been disabled to the point that they have been unable to work for an extended period, or have a certain illness. (Although a seemingly broad program, the reality of actually navigating successfully the necessary qualifying procedures for Social Security coverage, especially as a disabled beneficiary, can be daunting.)

Medicare

Since its passage in the United States in 1965, Medicare has been the national federally funded health insurance program for the elderly and, since 1973, the disabled. Although originally intended to finance hospital, physician, and other acute care services, Medicare has been broadened to include coverages that are still uncommon in private health insurance. It is a two-part program: Part A now covers hospital, nursing home, and home health services; Part B extends coverage to physician services, outpatient hospital services, and limited ambulatory care. Enrollment in Part A is automatic for individuals age 65 or older who receive Social Security benefits, and can also be qualified for by end-stage renal disease, or twenty-four months of total and permanent disability. Part A recipients may voluntarily elect to participate in Part B, which requires the payment of a small monthly premium ($29.90 in 1991).

Part A hospital insurance covers 90 days of confinement per benefit period, which renews whenever the beneficiary has been out of the hospital for at least 60 days. This coverage pays for all hospital services but currently required coinsurance payments are substantial: $628 per benefit period, plus for the 61st to the 90th hospital day, the beneficiary is required to pay $157 per day. Medicare also contains a benefit referred to as "lifetime reserve days." This is coverage for an additional 60 days of hospital care, but is not renewable and carries an additional hefty coinsurance requirement of $314 per day. These hospital benefits can be used only once during the beneficiary's life.

Of particular interest to the ALS patient is the Medicare skilled nursing facility (SNF) benefit. The Medicare beneficiary is entitled to 100 days of skilled nursing per benefit period, renewable following 60 days outside of the institutional setting. Previously, this benefit was contingent on the qualification that there is a medical necessity for skilled nursing and/or skilled rehabilitative services present. However, in the last few years this qualification has been broadened to include the concept of needed skilled supervision or skilled management by a registered nurse for what Medicare refers to as "an aggregate of unskilled services." This reinterpretation is intended to apply to the type of situation in which technical procedures, such as ventilator care or infusion therapy, are not required, but the volume and complexity of the unskilled services necessitated by the underlying medical condition are such that overall supervision by a nurse is necessary and appropriate. Such situations are not uncommon with the types of disability caused by ALS.

For approval, SNF confinements must follow a qualifying acute hospital stay of a minimum of three days and must obtain a certification of medical necessity from the treating physician. The initial 20 days of SNF stay have no coinsurance liability, while the 21st to the 100th day require coinsurance of up to $78.50 per day.

It is appropriate to note at this point that although Medicare attempts to achieve the uniformity of a national health financing program, it is administered under contract by a number of private insurance companies across the United States acting as regional fiscal intermediaries for the federal government. Consequently, one encounters a certain amount of unfortunate but inescapable variation in the interpretation of the guidelines governing the application of Medicare benefits. Those of us who speak and write on this topic never fail to encounter specific cases with experiences that contradict any generalizations made regarding the proper administration of benefits in the program. The sophisticated beneficiary learns to read the guidelines and is not inhibited about challenging the local F.I. when their actions appear to be in error.

By congressional intent, the most ample benefit in the Medicare program is home health care. It is designed to encourage as much home treatment for the chronically ill as possible. Therefore, in the Medicare program the home health benefit is unique in being essentially unlimited without any coinsurance requirement. The qualifying requirements for home health care are relatively simple: physician certification of medical necessity for intermittent skilled care administered under the physician's plan of care by a certified home health agency. It is important to note that this benefit does call for a primary service to be delivered which would be either skilled nursing, physical therapy, or speech pathology. However, once the primary service is delivered, then secondary services such as nurse's aide, occupational therapy, social services, and miscellaneous supplies and durable medical equipment may also be paid, even though neither Medicare skilled nursing nor home health care benefits cover custodial care per se.

Perhaps not surprisingly, the previously described variability in the interpretations of the various regional fiscal intermediaries are often encountered in the medical reviews of this type of care. While we are not aware of a single case of a ventilator-dependent patient being denied skilled nursing care or home care, gaining coverage approval for less dire situations, such as extended visits by a nurse's aide or a particularly expensive piece of adaptive equipment, can require the utmost assertiveness by the beneficiary. This problem is particularly difficult for the disabled ALS patient who cannot afford to purchase assistive technology and is dependent on the Medicare benefit to restore communication capability. Expensive but effective assistive technology has a high potential for noncoverage, but a successful appeal may be all but impossible without it.

Medicaid

Medicaid is a joint federal-state program that has come to play a key role in financing medical care for the poor as well as those impoverished by their illnesses. As such, unlike the other insurance programs discussed previously, Medicaid is a means-tested program. That is, its benefits are restricted to only low-income individuals who meet categorical qualifying criteria, as well as maximum income and assets requirements. For example, the categorical criteria for welfare assistance opens the Medicaid program to the elderly, children from single parent families, recipients of AFDC, the disabled, and recipients of financial assistance under the Supplemental Security Income program (SSI).

Although states have considerable discretion in setting their own benefit levels and eligibility criteria, qualifying for the aged, blind, and disabled has become more consistent nationally as it has keyed off the SSI assistance program. Similarly, as federal contributions for the Medicaid program were progressively reduced during the early 1980s, the various state asset standards governing Medicaid eligibility were also made more uniform. Currently families are allowed to possess a home, a single automobile worth up to $1,500, and other personal property up to $1,000.

Even more than Medicare, Medicaid has had a goal of attempting to provide comprehensive health care coverage to the eligible poor. When, in the early 1970s, the exploding cost of the program nationally made this goal appear unrealistic and resulted in a cutback in general medical benefits, coverage for specific classes of individuals and services to the disabled were still being expanded, until today the Medicaid program contains the most extended long-term care coverage of all.

As the health insurer of last resort and the only source of coverage for true long-term care services for the most severely and permanently disabled individuals, Medicaid has been severely impacted by the reductions in funding of the last decade. Medicaid is the primary source of funding for 40 percent of all nursing home residents, at an average cost per resident in excess of $22,000 per year. Typically, long-term nursing home residents consume their life savings until they qualify for poverty assistance, because they lack the ability to cope with this level of expenditure over a sustained period. From 1978 to 1984, total Medicaid nursing home expenditures increased from $6.2 billion to $10.9 billion at a rate of almost 10 percent a year. Despite every cutback of acute care benefits and provider fee levels, aggregate Medicaid expenditures continue to increase without any sign of letup.

For this reason, an entirely new area of health law has developed, intended to assist the chronically disabled individual plan for the long-term legal and financial consequences of the disease. Planning tools for such circumstances include the Durable Power of Attorney, authorizing someone else to act on behalf of the patient to handle the patient's financial (and, in some situations, medical) affairs, and the establishment of an irrevocable trust in which all assets are placed into the trust and managed for the individual's long-term benefit. Both approaches are serious and binding steps, so they must be approached with careful consideration and knowledgeable consultation. An experienced health law attorney familiar with the specific laws of the state in which one resides would be essential to this process.

The Future

It seems all but certain that long-term care will be one of the early beneficiaries of the rise of health care on the national policy agenda. Changes in tax law, insurance regulation, and liberalization of Medicaid eligibility, all designed to expand the insurance support for health care services, are likely to extend to long-term care as well. In recent tests, the American electorate has been consistent in voting a consensus that the financial barriers to needed medical care should be lowered (and removed if possible) for more people.

Additionally, the apparent market ''failure'' of private long-term care insurance now seems to have been a premature conclusion. Several health insurance companies are finding that better informed consumers are in fact willing to purchase these supplemental benefits while they are still young and healthy, and several other life insurance carriers are enjoying the market popularity of life insurance plans that provide for accelerated death benefits as a means of nursing home and home care financing. All in all, this is a hopeful situation that promises more balanced private/public support for long-term care in the near future.

Acknowledgment

This chapter is a compilation of remarks presented during a panel discussion, ''Financial Realities of Long-Term Care,'' at the symposium ''Toward Effective Advanced Management of ALS'' held in Cleveland in June 1991. I gratefully acknowledge the discussion by our panelists: Mary Foto, OTR, FAOTA, Blue Cross of California, Woodland Hills, California; Barbara J. Smith, JD, MBA, Squire, Sanders, & Dempsey, Cleveland, Ohio; and Dolores Holden, RN, ALS and Neuromuscular Research Foundation, San Francisco, California.

22

ALS: The Experiences of Health Care Professionals

Marlene A. Ciechoski, M.S., R.N.

The challenge to health care professionals working with patients with amyotrophic lateral sclerosis and their families is unique in its nature and scope. A vast armamentarium of ideas, interventions, and energies is required. To impart some of the breadth and depth of working with ALS patients/families is to speak through the pages of this chapter in a way quite different from reading pages in a text. A careful exploration of the literature reveals a paucity of information about the effects of the ALS experience on health care professionals. The literature about working with patients with cancer, AIDS, or other potentially fatal illnesses refers to this "strain and drain syndrome" on the health care professional, but little of this is evident in the ALS literature. Each illness demands its own specific considerations. The paltry attention to the responses of health care professionals working with ALS patients/families suggests a need to focus on this particular situation.

The terms *therapist*, *health care professional*, and *professional caregiver* are used synonymously throughout this chapter. The idea is to be inclusive in looking at the experiences of these professionals. Additionally, each reader may feel more comfortable with a certain role title with which he identifies. The importance of this inclusive concept with regard to the dynamic relationships within the interdisciplinary ALS team is discussed later. The initial emphasis is on the nature of the illness and its psychological manifestations in the patient/family. The profound multidimensional effects of the illness on patient and family serve to set the stage for the next two sections. The third section discerns the experience of the professional caregiver, how he responds to the changes in patient and family relationships and to the progressively worsening condition of the patient. The ALS journey, no matter how brief or lengthy, exacts a particular stress on the therapist. The final section addresses the importance of the therapist's cognizance of his responses within the settings in which the health care professional practices. Critical examples capture a sense of the ideas and attitudes of the health care professional and how his reactions may indeed be a reflection of the experiences of the patient and family.

ALS—The Illness

To appreciate the magnitude of ALS and its impact on patient, family, and health care professional, it is important to review salient points about the illness. Physically, ALS is a progressive neuromuscular disease. The deterioration it effects is manifest in a multitude of ways. The individual has overwhelming weakness (1). There is precious little energy. The simplest task becomes a major project. Difficulty in speaking and eventual loss of speech emphasize the patient's inability to communicate wants and needs. Loss of speech is accompanied by significant loss of self-esteem. The patient may experience a great sense of isolation and withdraw into a very private world. Problems with choking, swallowing, and copious secretions further impair comfort and function. Drinking fluids may become frightening and dangerous. Eating, which heretofore may have been pleasurable, is difficult and exhausting. Despite hours invested in eating small quantities of food, inadequate nutrition and then malnutrition result in remarkable dehydration and weight loss (2).

Immobility is another major component of the progression of the disease. The inability to walk even with assistance causes important changes in daily lifestyle. Reliance on a wheelchair may promote safety and save energy, but it also represents another terrible milestone in the course of the illness. When no longer able to use his hands, the patient moves into another area of disappointment and dysfunction. He can neither feed himself nor drink without assistance. He cannot bathe or dress himself. He is not able to adjust his glasses. He cannot grasp a hand outstretched in greeting. Progressive respiratory problems enhance anxiety and vice versa. The acute fear associated with dyspnea magnifies the fatal nature of the disease to the patient. In summary, ALS makes the hundreds of tasks of daily living laborious, if not impossible (3,4).

The Patient, The Family, The Illness

When the spectrum of ALS surrounds the patient and family, everyone and everything are forever changed. The arrival of a diagnosis is frequently preceded by months or years of confusion and uncertainty. Numerous clinicians, diagnoses, and treatments are not unusual. In fact, careful history taking may reveal that the patient has seen many physicians, has had multiple diagnoses, and very often has endured a wide variety of medical, surgical, pharmaceutical, and physiatric therapies (5). A thirty-eight-year-old man, for example, had five different diagnoses ranging from carpal tunnel syndrome to a herniated lumbar disk. He also had as many surgical procedures. The quest to find out just what is wrong is both frustrating and frightening to the patient and family.

Patients whose ALS has not yet been diagnosed react strongly to news that they have some musculoskeletal problem, mood disorder, or stroke. When medical-surgical interventions are tried with no positive outcome, the patient is even more discouraged and perplexed. One woman was adamant in her pursuit of a diagnosis after being told by a physician that she had early arthritis. Later she was told that many of her complaints were related to menopause. Another patient with speech problems underwent thousands of dollars of dental surgery only to find out that her slurred speech was still present. An elderly woman had been treated for three years as having had a stroke.

Establishment of a diagnosis is a two-edged sword. On the one hand, the months or years of pursuing an answer may result in a short-lived sense of relief. On the other hand, the diagnosis of ALS cannot help but bring a tremendous onslaught of anxiety, fear, and denial. Many patients and family members have only heard of ALS in a fleeting note or commentary. Others know that Lou Gehrig died from it. When the diagnosis is communicated, some people want to know more about the disease. Others want only limited information or no knowledge of the illness at all (6).

In the early phases of the illness, patient and family alike often reflect attitudes of hope and a will to conquer. They are interested in finding treatments and achieving a cure. Often much of the factual information given about the disease process is met with denial. In the majority of situations, this is frequently a time when there is strengthening of ties between patient and family members. A solidarity of will and purpose that is directed toward changing the diagnosis or reversing the disease process is unconsciously begun and later consciously acknowledged. One family voiced that "there was nothing that together they could not change." Others frequently remarked that they would be the ones to help find the right treatment resulting in cure.

As the disease progresses, despair replaces hope, and the patient and family are angry, anxious, and depressed. Both are faced with significant changes in roles and life-styles (7). If the patient's work had been the major source of income, this will eventually not be possible. If the family caregiver produced the major earnings, this can also mean a dramatic change. If both patient and caregiver work outside the home, a significant, if not complete, loss of income can result.

Role changes, however, are not limited to the earning of wages. The part that each individual patient and family member plays within the design of the family system may be altered forever. In one family, the wife-mother-patient who routinely planned family activities, especially those including extended family members, was no longer able to accomplish this. She expected that the husband-father-caregiver would set aside time to do these things. He, in turn, was overwhelmed with the expectations of wage earner, social planner, and caregiver. Similarly, the children in the family may be expected to participate in the care of the patient and the maintenance of the household. Siblings of the patient or perhaps elderly parents may be called upon to expand their role in the day-to-day care of the patient. Families who previously had been working toward the accomplishment of particular goals, such as buying a home or providing school tuition, may need to downsize or even eliminate their plans. The effect of ALS on the patient and the family system is profound. Individuals who heretofore related lovingly and respectfully to each other may find that their interactions are marked by arguments and dissension. The pressures that are brought to bear by the illness take a great toll on the individual and collective psyche of the family system. For some people, the presence of ALS can be a unifying factor. Family members who previously were loosely connected to each other may now feel more bonded and share mutual hopes. This, however, appears to be an exceptional response.

The progress of ALS continues as a physically and psychologically enveloping experience. The patient must cope with increasing difficulties in daily life. Emotionally, fears of helplessness and dependency abound (8). In fact, ALS, as described by one family, pervades every ''nook and cranny'' of human existence.

There is an inverse relationship between the increasing dependency of the patient and the family caregiver's responsibility to provide for the patient's needs. As the patient experiences greater inability to care for himself, the family has more doubt about its ability to care for the patient. Not only do the physical needs of the patient require more time and energy of family caregivers, but numerous psychological issues continue to emerge.

New relationship difficulties form because of the acute stress on the family system. Patient and family members may now have unrealistic expectations of each other. One individual may believe that the other person need only give more time and energy in order to accomplish a task. Another member may think that responsibilities are unfairly distributed or that people are not sharing the work equitably. Old problems are also resurrected to complicate the situation. Unsettled differences among family members and rivalries between the patient and his relatives create more friction. In one family, the husband-patient had always insisted on being the sole decision maker. His wife-caregiver had been struggling to create a reciprocal framework for decision making. As the patient's illness progressed and his dependence on his wife increased, he insisted on absolute authority to make decisions that affected all family members. His wife, angry and ambivalent about her tremendous responsibilities and negligible authority, openly challenged the husband's demands, resulting in repeated disagreements and escalating arguments.

Throughout the course of illness, decisions of significance may have to be made. Paramount among these are gastrostomy tube, ventilator support, and caregiving resources. Particularly difficult are decisions related to whether the patient can continue to be cared for at home. The multiple decisions that must be made exact an unusually difficult toll on both patient and family. Each is affected by the decisions reached. Therefore, decision making as a conjoint process between patient and family members is of critical importance. Minor and major decisions affect the quality of life of the entire family. One family had enjoyed leisurely dinner hours together. The patient wanted to continue this practice and delay his evening care needs until much later than usual. His family caregiver initially attempted to comply but later registered anger and annoyance when it interfered with the caregiver's opportunity for a few hours of rest before working an 11 P.M. to 7 A.M. job. Patient and family reached agreement by restructuring the time allocated for dinner. Some of the patient's physical care was better distributed throughout the day and evening hours. In another family, a patient who previously decided to refuse ventilator support changed his mind and opted for a ventilator when needed. The family caregiver was astounded at the change because of the decision previously agreed on with her husband. She believed she could care for him up to the point of his needing ventilation, but was overwhelmed by the prospect of assuming this additional responsibility.

The demands of decision making by patients and families are great and complex. Accordingly, they must live in light of the decisions they have made. Because of this, it is crucial that health care professionals respect and adhere to decisions made by the patient and family members. We can offer our best assistance and guidance while recognizing and accepting the ultimate right of the family unit to determine its own direction (9).

The Impact of ALS on Health Care Professionals

Along with the dearth of material in the literature on the effects of ALS on patients and families, there is insufficient focus on the response of health care professionals to the ALS experience. Selecting to work with ALS patients and families is especially difficult because the therapist is continuously faced with limited solutions to urgent and ever-changing problems.

Despite the highest level of compassion for the patient and family, the health care professional is confronted with feelings of inadequacy and ambivalence. He experiences a sense of defeat by the illness and is overcome by the multitude of problems associated with it. There is not a sphere of the therapist's physical, emotional, intellectual, or behavioral self that is not touched, to a greater or lesser degree, by the illness. Physically he may complain of headaches, GI distress, or generalized malaise. Emotionally he may be amazed at the intensity of his anger and depression. He may feel overwhelmed by the constant drain on his feelings.

He may lose self-confidence and feel incompetent in his role. Often he may show unrealistic optimism or intense pessimism about the patient's condition (10).

Similar to the feelings of patients and families, the ALS therapist is devastated by the illness. The nature of the responsibility for others serves as a catalyst for the development of stress in the health care professional (11). If the ALS therapist is to work successfully with the patient and family, he must be aware of his own level of stress. In every health care system there are two central individuals, one in need of skilled sensitive care and the other seeking to fill that need (12). A delicate balance occurs between offering professional closeness and maintaining emotional distance. This balance prevents unmanageable stress and possible burn-out (13).

A phenomenon that often manifests itself throughout the course of illness is the "mirroring effect" between patient and therapist. Stress in the patient may rise or fall depending on his perceived and actual state of illness. In a similar manner, the stress experienced by the health care professional may also increase and decrease in direct proportion to that of the patient. For example, a patient verbalized his anger at his family, who he viewed as unresponsive to his needs. The therapist, in turn, empathized with the patient because he perceived his colleagues as being unsupportive to him in his role. One health care professional, in another situation, verbalized how patients sometimes get to him. Within a short period of time he encountered several patients with significant progression of symptoms. The therapist expressed doubts about his abilities to work with these patients. He felt doomed to failure in dealing with the tremendous difficulties the patients experienced.

Unrecognized and unresolved stress may lead to acting-out behaviors that impede the patient-family-therapist relationship (14). The therapist with a high level of stress that is not dealt with risks feeling negatively toward the patient and family. He may project blame on the patient and family and perceive the patient as self-centered and narcissistic. He may believe that he is working longer and more diligently than his colleagues. He may see the patient as selfish and demanding. Despite the professional caregiver's need for relief, he may feel guilty about his wishes to be free of responsibility for the patient and family.

In response to stress faced by ALS professionals, the therapist develops his own patterns of defense. One unproductive pattern is to avoid involvement with the patient. In this way, he may minimize his sense of personal loss and pain. This behavior tends to lead to a fixed style of dealing with patients. The therapist may find himself utilizing a standardized, nonstop talking approach. Further manifestations of stress and discomfort in the professional are seen in criticism about the internal structure of the practice site. The therapist may express unhappiness about his working conditions. He feels anger and frustration toward other professionals with whom he is working (15). One professional, exhausted by the difficult nature of his work with patients, approached each encounter with great reluctance. He asked his colleagues to time his visits and to interrupt his appointment with the patient within five minutes of its beginning. Another therapist voiced his frustration with the work schedule; he believed fewer patients should be seen in the clinic on any given day.

These behaviors are means by which the therapist relieves his own discomfort. He is confronting the terminal nature of the illness in the face of his own sense of loss and despair. Health care professionals working with ALS patients and families are in a heartbreaking situation from the initial contact with the patient and family, to listening to the diverse accounts of how and when a diagnosis was reached, to the course of illness, to the eventual death of the patient, and to the need for continued support of the family survivors. The behaviors are representative of the levels of stress experienced by the therapist rather than any expression of inhumanity. Regardless of the emotions evoked by the illness, professional caregivers, in electing to work with patients and families, identify and utilize numerous mechanisms in coping with their own feelings and attitudes.

Coping with the stress inherent in his role requires a keen sense of self and the ability to identify and implement various stress reduction strategies. One therapist routinely goes for a walk during his lunch hour to relax and focus on pleasant thoughts. Several members of the ALS team meet three times a week for an aerobics class to promote release of tension.

Although some stress is thought to be challenging and growth-producing, excessive levels of stress are potentially counterproductive (16). Particularly in the work situation, stress may be minimized through the help of colleagues (17). For example, in an environment of cohesiveness, open and free communication, mutual respect, and esprit de corps, the individual may be quite comfortable discussing his tension with other colleagues. One therapist identified a surge in his stress level whenever families talked about moving the ALS patient to a nursing home. The therapist felt secure in speaking with several team members about his responses. When his associates accepted these concerns without criticism, the health care professional was able to understand why nursing home placement provoked a stressful reaction. In another situation, the professional caregiver spoke about difficulty in communicating clearly when he felt a significant level of stress. His expression of humor in a self-deprecating way was met with delight by his colleagues, and the stress abated.

Other ways to facilitate reduction of stress may take place outside the work setting. Extracurricular activities such as participation in sports, attending the theater, or visiting friends promote mental and physical well-being (18). In a more formal manner, the therapist may seek out another colleague external to the work area with whom to discuss his experiences with patients and families. This avenue provides an excellent conduit for the therapist to understand and relieve stress. The reduction of unmanageable stress is crucial to the therapist's ability to function productively and effectively with ALS patients and families.

Central to the therapist's role in working with the ALS patient and family is the basic philosophy and goal of assisting the patient to live as fully as possible in whatever span of time he may have. The core of the professional caregiver's work lies in a sense of caring for and about the patient and family. The therapist concentrates on the challenges of the numerous factors with which he is confronted. He is a constant and purposeful observer of the physical deterioration of the patient, witnesses the overwhelming emotional torment in the patient and family, sees the patient's loss of productivity, the ebbing away from participation in the world, and eventual death. The ALS therapist is privy to the disintegration of the family unit. He sees the economic pressures on the family, is moved by the family's social isolation and, often, the disappearance of human support from friends and community.

In offering his skills, compassion, and caring to patients and families, the therapist adopts a framework in which to approach his work. This enables him to remain goal-oriented with clearly delineated objectives. Although the professional caregiver accepts the terminal nature of the illness and acknowledges the eventual reality of the loss of the patient, he also retains a sense of optimism about the achievement of specific objectives. To do otherwise invites over- or underaction in response to the needs of patient and family.

The devastating impact of ALS on patients and families requires an enormous amount of creativity, energy, commitment, compassion, and resourcefulness on the part of health care professionals. The needs for care of an ALS patient, especially in the latter stages of the illness, are impossible for one primary caregiver to fulfill. The physiological and psychosocial effects of this illness on patients and families can be comprehensively addressed by a team of ALS professionals. This group is generally comprised of nurse, mental health specialist, social worker, neurologist, physical therapist, occupational therapist, nutritionist, specialized equipment technician, speech pathologist, and pulmonary therapist. This array of professional talent, educational background, and expertise is vital in response to the complexity of problems that both patient and family experience.

The professional ALS team typically practices in an outpatient clinic setting where patients and families are seen in initial visits and follow-up appointments. The team, however, is not simply a group of people who work together in the same geographical place. Rather, it is a dynamic group of highly skilled professionals who are goal-directed and passionate about serving this population. The ALS team collaboratively defines and fulfills its philosophy and mission of promoting the best quality of life for patients and families living with ALS. The care provided is tailored to meet the individualized needs of patients and families. The team members offer the knowledge and competencies of their respective professional disciplines to patients and families. The collective talent provides even greater resources to patients and families.

This cadre of professional caregivers function, with skill and experience, in an atmosphere that is nontraditional and nonhierarchical. Each team member presents evaluations and recommendations to the team. These, in turn, are incorporated into the overall plan of care by mutual agreement among team members.

Decision making is shared by the team and is not the domain of any one discipline. Leadership among team members emerges as a result of the needs of patients and families (19). For example, one family (patient, wife, and daughter) expressed confusion, frustration, anger, and ambivalence with the mounting needs of the patient and the lack of time for social relationships. It was apparent to the team that the emotional needs of the family as a whole were of primary importance at this time. Although the physical needs of the patient were addressed, it was readily understood and accepted by the team that the mental health specialist would have the major portion of time to work with the family. Assessment and implementation of plans of action are often done spontaneously and occur smoothly in the interdisciplinary setting.

On the ALS team, the typical medical model of providing care gives way to a structure based on the needs and concerns of the patient and family. The team of health professionals is characterized by several special attributes. At its core, the team has a shared commitment to the people it serves. It is a cohesive group that functions interdependently and collaboratively in fostering open communication among its members (20). Individual opinions, ideas, and information are encouraged and welcomed without fear of criticism. Basic to a team approach is an atmosphere that is both nonjudgmental and supportive. The team is cognizant of a genuine and honest style of relating to each other. It is sensitively aware of acknowledging and respecting each member's views (21). Perceptive and compassionate awareness of the needs of patients and families also requires professional caregivers to be in touch with their own and their colleague's sensitivities.

The ALS team that strives to support its members individually and collectively enhances its opportunities to be of major assistance to the people it serves. Health care professionals working with ALS patients and families render services to persons in one of the most profoundly difficult circumstances of life. The ALS team most effectively meets this challenge when its members honor, respect, and sustain each other in their endeavors to accomplish their goals. The professional caregivers who choose to work with ALS patients and families accept enormous responsibility for people experiencing an overwhelming calamity in their lives.

In conclusion, much has been spoken of and written about the heroic character of the individual with ALS and his family. Without doubt the strivings of both to persevere in coping with the illness is indeed both noble and courageous. To include the health care professionals in this characterization is also fitting and appropriate. The professional caregiver, challenged in the face of this confounding illness, is undaunted in his pursuit to care. The mind of the ALS team is the collective ingenuity of its members. The heart of the team is its uncompromising compassion and gallant efforts on the behalf of the patient and family.

Acknowledgments

I thank Marguerite Termini, M.A., R.N., and Steven M. Bende, Ph.D., for their outstanding support and critical review of the manuscript.

References

1. Caroscio JT (ed). *Amyotrophic Lateral Sclerosis.* New York: Thieme Medical Publishers, Inc., 1986.
2. Montgomery GK, Erickson LM. Neuropsychological perspectives in amyotrophic lateral sclerosis. *Neurol Clin* 1987, 5:61–81.
3. Rose FC, The management of motor neuron disease. In: Cosi V, Kato AC, Parlette W, Pinelli P, Poloni M, eds. *Amyotrophic Lateral Sclerosis.* New York: Plenum Press, 1987.
4. Norris FH, Smith RA, Denys EH, The treatment of amyotrophic lateral sclerosis. In: Cosi V, Kato AC, Parlette W, Pinelli P, Poloni M, eds. *Amyotrophic Lateral Sclerosis.* New York: Plenum Press, 1987.
5. Ginsberg N. Living and coping with amyotrophic lateral sclerosis: the psychological impact. In: Caroscio JT, ed. *Amyotrophic Lateral Sclerosis.* New York: Thieme Medical Publishers, Inc., 1986.
6. Horta E. Emotional response to amyotrophic lateral sclerosis and its impact on mangement of patient care. In: Caroscio JT, ed. *Amyotrophic Lateral Sclerosis.* New York: Thieme Medical Publishers,1986.
7. Luloff PB. Reactions of patients, family, and staff in dealing with amyotrophic lateral sclerosis. In: Caroscio JT, ed. *Amyotrophic Lateral Sclerosis.* New York: Thieme Medical Publishers, Inc., 1986.
8. Sebring DL, Moglia P. Amyotrophic lateral sclerosis: psychosocial interventions for patients and their families. *Health and Soc Work* Spring 1987, 113–120.
9. Baumann A. ALS—decision making under uncertainty: a positive approach. *Axon* December 1991, 41–43.
10. Bond M. *Stress and Self Awareness: A Guide for Nurses.* Rockville, MD: Aspen, 1986.
11. Sutherland VJ, Cooper CL. *Understanding Stress: Psychological Perspectives for Health Professionals.* London: Chapman and Hall, 1990.
12. Francoeur RT. *Biomedical Ethics: A Guide to Decision Making.* New York: John Wiley, 1983.
13. Scott CD, Hawk J, eds. *Heal Thyself: The Health of Health Care Professionals.* New York: Brunner/Mazel, 1986.
14. Doyle D. Staff stress: prevention and management. In: Turnbull R, ed. *Terminal Care.* New York: Hemisphere Publishing, 1986.
15. Bailey R, Clarke M. *Stress and Coping in Nursing.* London: Chapman and Hall, 1989.
16. Milsum JH. *Health, Stress, and Illness. A Systems Approach.* New York: Praeger, 1984.
17. Frude N. *Understanding Family Problems: A Psychological Approach.* New York: John Wiley, 1991.
18. Rhodes C. Staff stress: the nurse. In: Turnbull R, ed. *Terminal Care.* New York: Hemisphere Publishing, 1986.
19. Dunlop RJ, Hockley JM. *Terminal Care Support Teams: The Hospital-Hospice Interface.* New York: Oxford University Press, 1990.
20. Shaw ME. *Group Dynamics: The Psychology of Small Group Behavior.* New York: McGraw-Hill, 1981.
21. Doyle D. Staff stress: prevention and management. In: Turnbull R, ed. *Terminal Care.* New York: Hemisphere Publishing, 1986.

23

Patient and Family Support Groups in ALS

Helen Ann Bower, M.S.W., L.C.S.W.

The value of a support group for ALS patients, their families, and caregivers is its effectiveness in helping this population cope with the emotional distress and changes in daily living occasioned by the illness and disability. Although the needs of the ALS patient and the needs of the family/caregiver differ in some fundamental ways, it has been our experience that support groups are most effective when they include both the patient and the family/caregiver.

A diagnosis of ALS presents a unique combination of threats and demands difficult decisions from the patient and family within a relatively short period of time. Under ideal circumstances, the patient and family will have a close relationship with a physician who is familiar with ALS and a network of extended family and friends who can provide the support that the patient and family will need to survive emotionally and psychologically. The ALS support group can be an integral part of this network.

Theoretical Benefits of Support Groups

There are many therapeutic forces in support groups that are particularly useful in helping individuals mobilize coping strategies for dealing with crisis and damaged self-esteem. Support groups can also be effective in diminishing somatization, increasing patients' awareness of the connection between their psychosocial problems and their physical symptoms, and decreasing unnecessary patient visits to primary care providers.

Sharing information, that is, both didactic instruction from neurologists, pulmonologists, physical therapists, nutritionists, occupational therapists, communicative disorders experts, and so on, as well as shared experiences and knowledge among members, facilitates mastery and allows members to make informed decisions.

Universalization, or the understanding that one's feelings and experiences are not unique, often diminishes the feelings of being isolated and alone.

Support groups provide the opportunity for *modeling*, in which both the successes and failures of others provide a yardstick for measuring one's own performance.

Group norms and group support for *communicating* without condemning and for listening can improve the quality of interpersonal interaction and enrich the quality of family relationships.

Peer support, in which providing advice and understanding to someone else helps one enhance self-esteem by permitting one to be in a giving as well as a receiving role, is another therapeutic aspect of support groups.

Emotional catharsis. Shared painful or "unacceptable" experiences and feelings that are accepted by others can be liberating and growth-producing; this is especially important for the family member or caregiver who is close to burnout.

Reality testing, in which feedback from others and the opportunity to observe how others cope provides a more accurate perception of ones own strengths and liabilities.

Although not all patients or family members/caregivers wish to participate in support groups, our studies have shown that the need for bereavement counseling in survivors is lessened for those who have participated in support groups.

Goals of the ALS Support Group

The goals of our ALS support group were determined by the patients, the family members and caregivers, and the clinical social work facilitator. These goals are to provide information, hope, and a feeling of power and control. The support group belongs to its members; it provides a place where both patients and families can feel safe talking about their concerns and where they find the reassurance that they are not alone.

The functional and visible deterioration caused by ALS is progressive and inevitable; cognition is very rarely affected. Therefore it is important to allow the ALS patient to make decisions rather than infantalizing him by expecting the family/caregiver to do this for him. Knowledge about adaptive equipment, communication devices, and life support equipment can help the patient maintain some degree of personal autonomy as he becomes increasingly physically dependent. Family and patient training by an interdisciplinary rehabilitation team can maximize the patient's abilities and enable the patient and family to find ways to actively enjoy life, rather than giving in to ALS before it is necessary.

It is important to recognize that we will not always be successful in reaching these goals, despite our best efforts. This was best exemplified for our group by the attitudes of two of our member couples. One couple enjoyed traveling and continued to do so. As the patient became progressively weaker, they found nicknames for each piece of adaptive equipment that he needed: his soft collar became "Horace"; his electric wheelchair became the "Hup-mobile." His last act, shortly before going on a ventilator, was to walk his daughter down the aisle at her wedding. "I'll do it even if she has to let me sit on her train and pull me," he said. That was not necessary: leaning on each other, they walked the long aisle together. The other couple, both active professionals, retired within a month of the patient's diagnosis and stayed at home with each other, terrified that each new ache or pain was further exacerbation of ALS. Eventually they cut themselves off from all their friends and, five years later, they still rarely leave their home even though the patient is physically capable of participation in many activities. The patient's spouse has become increasingly depressed, angry, and resentful by this forced "intimacy" and isolation and is unable to provide any meaningful emotional support to the patient. Their home has become a house of silence.

Focus of Our ALS Support Group

We have found it important to include both patients and family members/caregivers in our support group. Sometimes the group meets as a whole; more often, they divide into a group of patients and a group of family members/caregivers. Often the group meets as a whole to hear a speaker and ask questions before dividing into separate groups. Since information is one of our major goals, we believe it is important to allow the patient and family members to hear the same information at the same time. This increases trust within the patient/family constellation, and it increases the patient's ability to make informed choices for himself.

Topics for discussion in the patient group and in the family group often share a similar theme, although not necessarily on the same evening. Issues for patients include:

- The fear of being a burden, which can be restated as a goal of maintaining a feeling of self-worth and a hope of feeling like a whole person who continues to be a contributing member of the family.
- The fear of expressing feelings—anger, sorrow, despair—which can be restated as a goal of feeling connected to significant others, having someone in whom to confide one's deepest feelings without having to fear abandonment. Feeling connected allows the patient to continue to be involved in family activities and decisions, to be treated like a person and not a patient, an adult and not a child.

- The fear of becoming hopelessly dependent with the loss of all personal dignity. This can be restated as a goal of maintaining control and autonomy, making decisions regarding treatment, taking the responsibility for being an active participant in managing major symptoms.
- The conflict of despair versus acceptance as one struggles with having to relinquish lifelong hopes and dreams and experiences grief over the loss of function and the ultimate loss of life.

Defense mechanisms commonly seen in patients include denial, projection ("I should go to a nursing home so I won't be a burden"), displacement, regression, and overcompensation.

Issues for Family Members/Caregivers

- The need to learn how to manage stress. Sessions for family members often become sessions in caring for the caregiver. Family members need permission to take care of themselves so that they can continue to provide care for the patient. They are encouraged to get respite as often as possible; to set aside time for exercise and recreation; to get adequate sleep and nutrition; and to learn relaxation techniques. Guided imagery for both patients and caregivers is offered.
- How to maintain emotional health. Caregivers often need permission to get their own needs met. They express fear of letting the patient know what their needs are—something we call "Why can't you read my mind?" Family members often struggle with feelings of resentment, guilt about resentment, anger, despair, helplessness, and hopelessness.
- The fear of being unable to provide hands-on care when the time comes. This can be restated as a goal to learn how to provide care within one's own comfort level and to feel good about what one is able to do.
- The fear of expressing feelings, which can be restated as a goal of establishing open communication with the patient. This is often a frightening concept for both patients and caregivers: they report that their lives together have consisted of talking about things and events, not about feelings. The effort is worthwhile according to several family members: "It was like peeling an onion; when we finally got to the core of who we really are and how we feel, it was like falling in love all over again"; "We are closer now than at any other time in our lives—in a strange way ALS has been a blessing."

Family members are encouraged to partialize, to break down the problem into manageable parts, to ask others for help. They remind each other to take things one day at a time, to make each day count. Some of our family members keep journals. Others work with the patient to record a memory book for their children and grandchildren.

Conclusion

ALS is a unique disease. The stresses and the challenges it creates for patients and families/caregivers can be alleviated by participation in support groups. Supportive relationships with others who share similar problems diminish feelings of isolation, encourage healthy styles of communication, enhance self-esteem, and build the confidence that comes from knowing at the end that one has done all that was possible. By offering information and hope and encouraging autonomy, the support group enables the patient and the family/caregiver to maintain dignity, alleviates feelings of anxiety and suffering, and assists both in reaching a state of acceptance over how they have managed ALS.

Suggested Reading

Berkman B, Bonander E, Kemler B, et al. *Social Work in Health Care: A Review of the Literature.* Chicago: American Hospital Association, 1988.

Carlton TO. Group process and group work in health social work practice. *Social Work with Groups*, 1986, 9, 5–20.

Galinsky MJ, Schopler JH. Practioners' views of assets and liabilities of open-ended groups. In: J. Lassner, K. Powell, and E. Finnegan (eds.) *Social Group Work: Competence and Values in Practice.* New York: Haworth Press, 1987.

Garland JA, Jones HA, Kolodny R. A model for stages of development in social work groups. In: S. Bernstein (ed.) *Explorations in Group Work: Essays in Theory and Practice.* Boston: Milford House, 1965.

Gitterman A. The use of groups in health settings. In: A. Lurie, G. Rosenberg, and S. Pinsky (eds.) *Social Work with Groups in Health Settings.* New York: Prodist, 1982.

Lieberman MA. Group properties and outcomes: A study of group norms on self help groups for widows and widowers. *Internat J Group Psychother* 1989, 39:191–208.

Lieberman MA, Borman LD. *Self-Help Groups for Coping with Crisis.* San Francisco: Jossey-Bass, 1979.

Lonergan EC. Group intervention for medical patients—a treatment for damaged self-esteem. *Group* 1980a, 4:36–45.

Lonergan EC. Humanizing the hospital experience: Report of a group program for medical patients. *Health Soc Work* 1980b 5:53–63.

Lubin B, Lubin AW. *Comprehensive Index of Group Psychotherapy Writings.* Madison: Internat Univ Press, Inc., 1987.

Northen H. Social work with groups in health settings: Promises and problems. *Soc Work Health Care* 1983, 8:107–121.

Roback HB (ed.). *Helping Patients and Their Families Cope with Medical Problems.* San Francisco: Jossey-Bass, Inc., 1984.

Toseland RW, Siporin M. When to recommend group treatment: A review of the clinical and the research literature. *Internat J Group Psychother* 1986, 36: 171–202.

Walls N, Meyers AW. Outcome in group treatments for bereavement: Experimental results and recommendations for clinical practice. *Internat J Ment Health* 1984–85, 13: 126–127.

Yalom ID. *The Theory and Practice of Group Psychotherapy*. New York: Basic Books, 1975.

24

The Role of the National Voluntary Agency in ALS

Lynn M. Klein

The role of the voluntary agency in dealing with ALS is multifaceted. Representing 30,000 people in the United States living with ALS, the mission of the organization is well-defined: to raise funds to support cutting-edge research, to increase public and governmental awareness, and to assist patients and families in coping with the day-to-day challenges they face living with ALS. The ALS Association (ALSA) is the only not-for-profit voluntary health agency in the United States dedicated solely to amyotrophic lateral sclerosis.

Research

Research into the cause, prevention, and ultimately the cure of this devastating disease is the driving force behind The ALS Association. Research on ALS is very complex, spanning a broad field—from what makes cells die to definition of the disease processes. Seemingly no single researcher can comprehend it. And it has been difficult to attract investigators to take on the challenge of a puzzle no one else has been able to solve since it was first identified by Charcot in 1869! The organization actively recruits and provides stimulus for young neuroscientists to develop an interest in ALS research. Attendance at major neurological conferences provides the Association an opportunity to interact with the scientific community, providing information on its expanding grant programs and patient services. Developing credibility and strong partnerships within this prestigious constituency has increased both the quality and quantity of ALS grant proposals received in the past few years.

ALSA has a well-respected grant program that attracts new researchers from prestigious institutions every year. Part of this program includes awards for "starter" or short-term grants, designed to allow scientists to develop preliminary data on a new or promising hypothesis and then apply later for a larger, long-term award from ALSA, the National Institutes of Health (NIH), or other private sources.

The Association receives over one hundred abstracts each year. They are screened by the chairman of ALSA's Research Committee of the Board of Trustees and the co-chair of the Scientific Review Committee for merit, innovativeness, relevance, and whether ALSA has funded earlier or similar work by the principal investigator. Approximately forty researchers are then invited to submit full applications.

Why not invite all to submit full applications? Two reasons: to save the principal investigators whose projects stand little chance of funding the work of preparing a full application; and to enable ALSA's Scientific Review Committee to review in-depth a manageable number of applications in one day.

Grant proposals received are peer-reviewed by the Scientific Review Committee comprised of prominent neurologists and scientists with expertise in neurology, epidemiology, genetics, immunology, virology, pathology, chemistry, and molecular biology. The proposals are graded in two areas—scientific merit and relevancy to ALS. Only the highest-scored projects are recommended for funding by the committee. These recommendations are presented to ALSA's Board of Trustees, who determine the grants to fund, dependent on research dollars available. About 30 percent of the applications submitted are funded each year. Since origination of the grant program, The ALS Association has awarded over 180 grants, with grant expenditures nearing $13 million in ALS-specific research.

Recently, there is a new ripple in ALSA's ever-widening research program—the "think tank" workshop. Outstanding young neuroscientists, highly respected in their fields, gather for two days in a workshop environment designed both to stimulate new ideas and to interest the participants in doing research on ALS.

ALSA is committed to do all it can to support the greatest number of the best research projects and is committed to a leadership role in the ALS arena.

Patient Services

The current status of the organization of health and human services does not provide a method within the necessary bureaucratic structure to coordinate services in the community. It becomes difficult to meet the special comprehensive needs of individuals afflicted with chronic disabilities like ALS. Government programs are designed to support institutional activities such as medical research and certain forms of qualified reimbursement, but experience to date reflects that the quality of personal-care programs and the coordination of special services required are much better achieved by the efforts of citizens working cooperatively at the community level. To meet this need for linkages among services in order to assure a continuity of care, we have voluntary groups. They have a long social history and are thoroughly embedded in the social structure for the purpose of coordinating help to solve problems of various types. Making professional and voluntary services available in a compassionate and humane manner can greatly improve the quality of life for patients and families (1).

On a national level, The ALS Association is an information, resource, and referral service for persons with ALS (PALS®), their families, and the health care community. Through the personalized attention of a patient services coordinator, information is provided on management of the symptoms (managing ALS or MALS manuals), answers to specific problems, current research trends (including clinical trials), available national resources, and referrals to health care professionals with an interest and expertise in ALS. The toll-free patient hotline is the link for thousands of PALS®.

Few diseases create as great a sense of hopelessness and despair on the part of both patients and medical professionals as ALS. Historically, people diagnosed with ALS have been told there is nothing that can be done, to go home and wait to die. PALS® provide a clear example of the problems of management in many types of neurological diseases. Of critical importance to the person with ALS is the ongoing need for adaptation to unique problems and a changing range of special services as the unpredictable course of the disease unfolds.(1)

Recognizing the need to address this long-standing problem, ALSA developed the ALSA center program. Certification of these ALS clinics establishes a national standard of care for the multidisciplinary team approach in management of ALS.

Applications for center status are received from across the country. They are then reviewed by the the ALSA center certification committee, an ad hoc committee of the Association. Recommendations for certification are made on the basis of criteria including having an ALS-specific clinic with a multidisciplinary team of professionals dedicated to providing quality care for PALS; appropriate diagnostic facilities; availability of services irrespective of race, color, creed, or financial status; affiliation with a local ALS Association chapter; and a willingness to exchange information with other ALSA centers. Certification is for a period of two years. Recertification is considered after on-site visit by select members of the Certification Committee. There are currently seven ALSA centers objectively chosen by strict criteria.

The centers are a team effort for patient care and clinical management providing maximum utilization of resources. For ALSA centers, the program provides increased prestige, the advantage of collaborative work with other centers, improvement in patient care and potential research, and increased patient referrals through ALSA's patient information bank.

For The ALS Association, the centers are one more step forward in fulfilling its mission. They provide increased visibility, an enhanced patient network and even greater use of its resources, and help in facilitating fund raising for patient support and research.

Most important, the centers provide ALS patients and referring physicians easy access to the highest standard of outpatient care on a regional basis, easier availability of up-to-date research and medical information as well as easy access to diagnostic and therapeutic referral centers.

Of primary importance to ALSA is the education of the health care community. The Association co-sponsors accredited professional educational conferences with prestigious institutions such as UCLA (University of California at Los Angeles) and the Cleveland Clinic Foundation, addressing the physical, psychosocial, and financial problems facing ALS patients. In-service training programs at skilled care facilities, home health agencies, and hospitals are also held throughout the year.

Public Awareness

Although ALS has been with us for over 120 years and its incidence is greater than Huntington's disease and equal to that of multiple sclerosis, a major challenge of the voluntary organization has been to establish the identity of ALS in this country. Unless the general public knows about ALS and its devastating effects on life, how can we expect them to help? Without the ongoing support of generous donors, the funding of research grants, patient services programs, and chapter development become impossible.

In a similar manner, because of the nature of the disease and lack of understanding, there is a need for a basic education program for the general public. In a more targeted fashion, the awareness program for ALS patients and family members is to let them know there is an available resource for information and assistance; a resource for basic information about the disease, treatment of symptoms, and direction to national and local medical and social/human resources.

From a professional standpoint, it is again necessary to publicize the existence of the association as a resource for the health care community, which may not be well informed about the disease. Also for the scientific community, to let it know about current research trends and grant programs and to encourage it to take up the challenge of ALS research.

Advocacy for patient support and increased government research dollars should be a priority for the voluntary agency. As the state of the economy declines, so do contributions and research support by National Institutes of Health. The voluntary agency, often as members of a coalition of other not-for-profit agencies, has to take a leadership role on behalf of the patients for increased or even continued support to find the cause and cure of this disease.

A successful public awareness program requires commitment— commitment of the Board of Trustees who govern the organization, commitment of the grass roots constituency, and a commitment of resources, both people and financial, a commitment that involves allocation of necessary funds to carry out the job correctly. Sometimes public awareness programs are perceived as rather unimportant—as an unnecessary expense, rather than an investment. Also, a public awareness program is separate from direct mail, donor marketing, and so on, although the basic messages are consistent. The success of a voluntary agency can be affected by the success of its public awareness programs and ability.

The ALS Association conducts an ongoing effort to create an ALS awareness among the public, including the placement of articles, features, and public services ads in major newspapers and magazines and on radio and television. The association's quarterly newspaper, *LINK*, has a circulation that includes ALS patients, families, physicians, scientists, donors, government officials, the media, institutions, foundations, corporations, and individuals interested in ALS. It includes current information on research, disease management techniques, assistive technology, and information of interest to all these groups.

The Association is constantly striving to expand its public and professional education programs so that an ALS identity is firmly established. Only an aware public will insure that full resources are brought to bear on solving this serious problem.

The Role of the Chapter

In order to be successful in the battle against ALS, work must be done on all fronts, national and local. There are specific aspects of The ALS Association's goals as an organization that cannot be fully realized without a presence in every community in the country. The association must reach out to every locale with information about ALS.

Chapters of the voluntary agency are the grass roots units committed to carrying out the mission of the national organization at the community level. While receiving tax-exempt status as part of a national organization, chapters are incorporated in their own state as a not-for-profit organization and are governed by a volunteer Board of Trustees.

The success of The ALS Association is determined in part by the strength and effectiveness of its chapters and their committment to the association's goals. These goals are pursued through fund raising to support the Association's national research program and local patient programs, patient services to aid present and future patients and families, and education of the public and professional community.

The Association is supported by voluntary gifts and voluntary efforts, all of which are to be used for the programs of The ALS Association, whether at the national or local level.

On a local level, ALSA chapters provide more of the direct hands-on patient services. All chapters have at least one support group that meets on a regular basis. Many chapters have extensive patient services programs including equipment loan pools, a home care consultant, van transportation, an ALSA center, augmentative communication equipment loan pools, and respite programs. The level of services provided by the chapter is directly related to the financial abilities of the chapter and the number of volunteers available to direct the programs.

ALS patients and their families must learn how to survive, cope, and *live* with a chronic disability. Chronic illness—illness that will not get better—demands tremendous intellectual and emotional energy to cope and function. ALS, a chronic neuromuscular disease, demands extraordinary energy of individuals and their families. The reality is that most learn to live with their chronic disability by exchanging information on "how to do it." By being active in an ALS support group, the patients and their caregivers will learn not only more about this disease that has invaded their lives, but also more about themselves and how they can *live* with ALS. The Association's chapters are in a unique position to help through support group meetings. Support groups have many benefits for individuals, the greatest of which is learning that they are not alone.

In areas of the country where a need for support has been identified but lacks the leadership support necessary for a chapter, Freestanding Support Groups are developed. These groups meet on a regular basis. They do not conduct fund raising or public awareness programs, although their very presence in the community creates awareness and often raises money.

A complete association network is an essential key to meet the needs of the ALS population in this country and to generate the funds necessary to solve the mystery of ALS, the challenge of our time.

Reference

1. Slater RJ. A model of care: matching human services to patient's needs. *Neurology* 1980, 30:39–43.

25

Resources for ALS Patients and Their Families

Kristen L. O'Donovan, L.S.W.

ALS Resources

ALSA Centers

An ALSA Center is certified by ALS Association. These centers are certified on the basis that they have a clinic for ALS patients with a multidisciplinary approach and service availability is offered irrespective of race, color, creed or financial status. The ALSA Centers also have an affiliation with a local ALS Association Chapter and a willingness to exchange information with other ALSA Centers.

The following is a list of ALSA Centers located nationally:

ALS & Neuromuscular Research
  Foundation
California Pacific Medical Center
Pan Med Building, Room 110
2100 Webster Street
San Francisco, CA 94115
415/923-3055
Forbes H. Norris, Jr., MD

University of Chicago
Motor Neuron Disease Clinic

University of Chicago Medical
  School
5841 S. Maryland Avenue
Box 425
Chicago, IL 60637
312/702-6221
Raymond P. Roos, MD

Motor Neuron Disease Clinic
University of Michigan Medical
  Center

Dept. of Neurology
1914-0316 Taubman Center
1500 E. Medical Center Drive
Ann Arbor, MI 48109
313/936-7165
Mark B. Bromberg, MD, Ph.D.

Harry J. Hoenselaar ALS Clinic
Henry Ford Hospital
2799 W. Grand Blvd.
Detroit, MI 48202
313/876-2594
Daniel S. Newman, MD

ALSA Center
Cleveland Clinic Foundation
Dept. of Neurology—S90
9500 Euclid Avenue
Cleveland, OH 44195

216/444-5418
Hiroshi Mitsumoto, MD

ALS Clinical Services Center of
    Hahnemann University
Hahnemann University Hospital
Broad & Vine Streets
Mail Stop 423
Philadelphia, PA 19102
215/448-8090
Howard Natter, MD

ALS Clinic Dept. of Neurology
College of Medicine of the University
    of Vermont
Dept. of Neurology
1 South Prospect Street
Burlington, VT 05401
802/656-4588
Rup Tandan, MD, MRCP

ALS Clinics

California

University of Southern California
School of Medicine
Dept. of Neurology
Hospital of the Good Samaritan
Neuromuscular Center
637 S. Lucas Avenue
Los Angeles, CA 90017
213/975-1270
W. King Engel, MD

Children's Hospital of San Francisco
Neuromuscular Disease Research
    Program
3700 California Street
San Francisco, CA 94119
415/387-8700
Robert G. Miller, MD

ALS Referral Center
Center of Neurological Study
11211 Sorrento Valley Road

Suite H
San Diego, CA 92121
619/455-5463
Richard Smith, MD

Florida

University of Miami
School of Medicine
ALS Clinic
Dept. of Neurology D4-5
P.O. Box 01690
1501 N.W. 9th Avenue
Miami, Florida 33136
305/547-6732
Robert Shebert, MD
Walter Bradley, MD

Illinois

Les Turner Foundation
Northwestern University Medical
    School

303 E. Chicago Avenue
312/908-5886: Lois Insolia Center
Teepu Siddique, MD
Scott Heller, MD, Co-Director

Massachusetts

Tufts-New England Medical Center
Dept. of Neurology
171 Harrison Avenue
Boston, MA 0211
617/956-5000
Theodore L. Munsat, MD

Minnesota

Mayo Clinic
Dept. of Neurology
200 S.W. First Street
Rochester, MN 55905
507/284-2675
Anthony J. Windebank, MD
William J. Litchy, MD
Jasper Daube, MD

Missouri

Regional Neuromuscular Disease
    Center (127-C)
Veterans Administration Medical
    Center
4801 Linwood Blvd.
Kansas City, MO 64128
816/861-4700
Barry Festoff, MD
Joseph Schulte, MD

Washington University
School of Medicine
Neuromuscular Research Center
Dept. of Neurology
660 S. Euclid

Box 8111
St. Louis, MO 63110
314/362-7170
Alan Pestronk, MD

New York

University of Rochester
ALS Clinic
P.O. Box 673
Rochester, NY 14641
716/275-2542
David Goldblatt, MD

Mt. Sinai Medical Center
1 Gustave Levy Place
New York, NY 10029
212/241-8323: Administrative
    Secretary
Mark Sivak, MD
ALS Clinic: 212/241-8168
                 Telephone Mail System
(Please be patient. Leave a message and
    someone will call you back
    promptly.)

St. Vincent's Hospital & Medical
    Center
ALS Clinic
152 W. 11th Street
New York, NY 10011
212/790-8314
Harry Bartfeld, MD

Pennsylvania

University of Pittsburgh
School of Medicine
ALS Clinic
322 Sciafe Hall
Pittsburgh, PA 15261
412/648-9200
Robin Conwit, MD

Wisconsin

ALS Clinical Research Center
University Hospital & Clinics

600 Highland Avenue, J6-504
Madison, WI 53792
602/263-9057
Benjamin R. Brooks, MD

Worldwide Associations for MND/ALS

Africa

South Africa

Diane Husband
Motor Neurone Disease/ALS Support
  Group
Swiss Farm
Upper Hillcrest Road
Somerset West 7130
Cape
South Africa
Tel: International (   )
  +27 24 514252

Tunisia

Professor M Ben Hamida
ALS Society of Tunisia
Institut de Neurologie
La Rabta 1007
Tunisia

Uganda

The Biruduma Students Muscular
  Dystrophy Association
P.O. Box 596
Mbarara
Uganda

North America

Canada

Joanne M. Brown, National
  Executive Director
ALS Society of Canada
90 Adelaide Street East
Suite B101
Toronto, Ontario
M5C 2RA
Canada
Tel: International (   )
  +1 416 362 0269

United States of America

Robert V. Abendroth, Acting Director
The ALS Association
21021 Ventura Blvd.

Suite 321
Woodland Hills, CA 91364
USA
Tel: International (   )
  +1 818 340 7500

Forbes H. Norris, Clinical Director
Dee Holden Norris, Executive
  Director
ALS & Neuromuscular Research
  Foundation
2351 Clay Street
Suite 416
San Francisco, CA 94115
USA
Tel: International (   )
  +1 415 923 3604

Wendy Fisher, Executive Director
The Les Turner ALS Foundation Ltd.
3325 West Main Street
Skokie, IL 60076
USA
Tel: International (   )
   +1 708 679 3311

Evelyn McDonald
The ALS/Patient Profile Research
   Project
P.O. Box 15981
Seattle, WA 98115
USA
Tel: International (   )
   +1 206 527 5114

Latin & South America

Agentina

Dr. Alberto Dobrovsky
Hospital Frances—La Rioja 951
Seccion de Enfermedades
   Neuromuscular
Centro Neurologico
Buenos Aires 1211
Argentina

Brazil

Associacao Brasileira de Distrofia
   Muscular
Edificio da Biologia
Sala 348
Cidade Universitaria
San Paulo—S.P.
Brazil

Colombia

Ivan Dario Arteaga
Fundacion Omega
Carrera 30 No. 89-79 (La Castellana)
Bogota

Colombia

Tel: International (   )
   +57 1 2365004

Mexico

Fydenmac
Paseo de la Reforma No., 6900
Edificio Nayarit
Entredad, Dep. 7
Tlatelolco, 06900 D.F.
Mexico
Tel: International (   )
   +52 583 73 71

Uruguay

Dr. O. Vincent, Assistant Neurologist
ALS/MND Group in Uruguay
Instituto de Investigaciones
   Biologicas Clemente Estable
Av. Italia 3318
Montevideo
Uruguay 11600
Tel: International (   )
   +598 2 47 16 16

Asia

India

R. Janardana Rao, President
Indian Muscular Dystrophy
   Association (IMDA)

21-136, Batchupet
Malchilipatnam—521 001 (A.P.)
India
Tel: International (   )
   +91 8672 2817

Japan

Yukio Matsuoka, Secretary General
Japan ALS Association
9-10-701, Shin-ogawa-Cho
Shinjuku
Tokyo 162
Japan
Tel: International ( )
  +81 3 3267 6942

Pakistan

Mrs. Shahida Abdullah,
  Administrator
Ma Ayesha Memorial Center for Care
  and Control of Neuromuscular
  Diseases
SNPA-22 Block 7/8 (near
  commercial area)
FMCHS
Karachi
Pakistan

Philippines

Joel Pelayo
Group Leader
The ALS Association Philippines
  Support Group
78 Misikap Extension
Central District
Diliman
Quezon City 1100
Metro Manila
Philippines
Tel: International ( )
  +63 2 922 8274

Australia

Mavis Gallienne
Motor Neurone Disease Association
  of Australia
P.O. Box 262
South Caulfield
Victoria 5162

Australia

Tel: International ( )
  +61 3 596 4761

Hon Secretary
ALS—Motor Neurone Disease
  Research Institute Inc.
20 Mons Road
Westmead
NSW 2145
Australia
Tel: International ( )
  +61 2 891 2073

Norman Minton, President
Newcastle & Hunter Region Motor
  Neurone Society
P.O. Box 75
Warners Bay
NSW 2232
Australia

John Wearne, President
Motor Neurone Society of
  Queensland
P.O. Box 380
Morningside
Queensland 4170
Australia
Tel: International ( )
  +61 7 396 8360

Alison Kinson, Chairperson
Motor Neurone Society of South
  Australia
P.O. Box 27
Hackham West
South Australia 5163
Australia

Marie MacDonald, President
Motor Neurone Society of Western
  Australia
320 Rokeby Drive
Subiaco

Western Australia 6008
Australia
Tel: International (   )
   +61 9 382 1159

John Hughes, Chairperson
Motor Neurone Society of Tasmania
P.O. Box 769
Devonport
Tasmania 7310
Australia

Guam

Madeleine V. Bordallo
Guam Lytico & Bodig Association

P.O. Box 1458
Agana
Guam 96910
Tel: International (   )
   +671 472 3581

New Zealand

Pat Jones, Secretary
Motor Neurone Disease Association
   of New Zealand
P.O. Box 1613
Auckland
New Zealand
Tel: International (   )
   +64 9 410 4034

Europe

Croatia

Miralem Mehmedovic, President
Savez Drustava Distroficara Hrvatske
(Union of Muscular Dystrophy of
   Croatia)
Zagreb, Nova Ves 44
Croatia
Tel: International (   )
   +38 41 271 849

Denmark

Jette Moller
Muskelsvindfonden
Vestervang 41
DK-8000 Arhus C
Denmark
Tel: International (   )
   +435 86 13 97 77

France

Gerard Beneteau, President
ARS Association pour la Recherche

sur la Sclerose Laterale
   Amyotrophique
Forum Saint-Eustache
1 rue Montmartre
75001 Paris
Tel: International (   )
   +33 1 45 08 04 00

Association de Lutte Sclerose
   Laterale Amyotrophique
Centre Regional de Gerontologie
   Sociale
2 Place de la Major
13002 Marselille
France

Irish Republic

Eithne Frost, Administrator
Irish Motor Neurone Disease
   Association
Carmichael House
North Brunswick Street
Dublin 7

Irish Republic
Tel: International (   )
 · +353 1 730230

Italy

Mauro Codini
Associazione Sclerosi Lateral
  Amiotrofia
c/o Centro Medico di Riabilitazione
Via per Revislate
Veruno 28010 (NO)
Italy
Tel: International (   )
  +39 322 830101

Netherlands

VSN, ALS-diagnosewerkgroep
Lt. Gen. van Heutszlaan 6
3743 JN Baarn
Netherlands
Tel: International (   )
  +31 2154 18400/20500

Eric Trietsch, Secretary
ALS Research Fund
Joos van Clevelaan 8
3723 PG Bilthoven
Netherlands
Tel Evenings:
  International (   ) +31 30 280346
Tel Days:
  International (   ) +31 30 533591

Portugal

Fernando Moragdo, President
Associacao Portuguesa de Duencas
  Neuomsculares
Servico de Neurologica
Hospital de Santa Maria
7600 Lisboa
Portugal

Tel: International (   )
  +351 1 797 8821

Romania

C. Vasilescu, President
Neuromuscular Diseases Association
  of Romania
Institute of Neurology
C.P. 61-42
RO-75622 Bucharest
Romania
Tel: International (   )
  +40 0 756273

Spain

Dr. Jesus Mora
ADELA (Asociacion Espanola de
  ELA)
Apartado Correos 108
28912 Alcorcon
Madrid

Sweden

Mia Lundstrom
NHR (Neurologiskt Handikappades
  Riksforbund
Box 3284
S-103 65 Stockholm
Sweden
Tel: International (   )
  +46 8 14 03 20

Switzerland

Mr. W. Parlette
International ALS/MND Research
  Foundation
Tiradelza di Monteggio
Termine
CH-6998
Switzerland
Fax: International (   )
  +41 91 732232

Turkey

Prof Coskun Osdemir
Association of Muscle Disorders
Yesilkoy
Hotboyu No 12
Istanbul
Tel: International (   )
  +90 1 5331374/5242535

United Kingdom

Peter Cardy, Director
Motor Neurone Disease Association
P.O. Box 246

Northhampton
NN1 2PR
UK
Tel: International (   )
  +44 604 250505/22269

Anne Jarvis, Projects Director
Scottish Motor Neurone Disease
  Association
50 Parnie Street
Glasgow Scotland G1 5LS
UK
Tel: International (   )
  +44 41 552 0507

Voluntary Agencies Providing Services to ALS Patients

THE ALS ASSOCIATION
21021 Ventura Blvd., Suite 321
Woodland Hills, California 91364
(818) 340-7500
(800) 782-4747

The ALS Association is a not-for-profit voluntary health agency that provides research, patient services, public and professional education and volunteer programs for ALS patients and their families.

MUSCULAR DYSTROPHY ASSOCIATION
3561 E. Sunrise Drive
Tucson, Arizona 85718
(602) 529-2000

Provides services to patients with muscular dystrophy and related neuromuscular disorders, including ALS.

NATIONAL MULTIPLE SCLEROSIS SOCIETY
205 E. 42nd Street
New York, New York 10017
(800) 624-8236

MS Society has been known to provide equipment to ALS patients depending on budget and MS patient population needs.

SHARE FOUNDATION
Southeastern Massachussetts Univ.
North Dartmouth, Massachussetts 02747
(508) 999-8214

Non-profit organization that assists people who need augmentative communication equipment. Will assist with developing program or device and will assist with funding.

I.V.U.N. NEWS
International Ventilator Users Network
4502 Maryland Avenue
St. Louis, Missouri 63108
(314) 361-0475

Links ventilator users with each other and with health care professionals interested in home mechanical ventilation.

NATIONAL LIBRARY SERVICE FOR THE BLIND AND HANDICAPPED
Library of Congress
Washington, DC 20542

A free national library service providing recorded and braille materials to blind and handicapped persons. Fifty six regional and ninety two subregional libraries are currently part of the network servicing U.S., Puerto Rico, Guam, and the Virgin Islands.

Suggested Reading and Resources

Suggested Reading	Where to Order
Managing ALS (MALS) Manuals I Finding Help II Managing Muscular Problems III Managing Breathing Problems IV Managing Swallowing Problems V Solving Communication Problems	The ALS Association 21021 Ventura Blvd. #321 Woodland Hills, CA 91364 (818) 340-7500 (800) 782-4747
In Sunshine And In Shadow Edited by Judy Oliver	The ALS Association Keith Worthington Chapter 340 Mission Road Suite B-10 Prairie Village, KS 62206 (913) 648-2062
This Far And No More Andrew Malcolm	Time Books New York, New York 10022 1987 Random House

Amyotrophic Lateral Sclerosis
   Edited by:
      James T. Caroscio, M.D.

Thieme Medical Publishers
81 Park Avenue South
New York, New York 10016

We Are Not Alone
   Learning to Live with Chronic Illness
   By Sefra Kobrin Pitzele

Thompson & Company
Minneapolis, MN

Amyotrophic Lateral Sclerosis
   Therapeutic, Psychologic, and
   Research Aspects
   Edited by:
      V. Cosi
      Ann C. Cato
      William Parlette
      P. Pinelli
      M. Poloni

Plenum Press
Plenum Publishing Corporation
233 Spring Street
New York, New York 10013

Realities in Coping with Progressive
   Neuromuscular Disease
   Edited by:
      Leon I. Charash
      Robert E. Lovelace
      Stewart G. Wolf
      Austin H. Kutscher
      David Price Roye
      Clare F. Leach

The Charles Press
P.O. Box 15715
Philadelphia, PA 19103

Family Caregiver's Guide
   By Joan Ellen Foyder

The Futuro Company
5801 Marimont Avenue
Cincinnati, Ohio 45227

Amyotrophic Lateral Sclerosis
   A Teaching Manual for Health
   Professionals

Publisher:
ALS Health Support Services
12815 N.E. 124th Street
Kirkland, WA 98034

Beyond Rage—How to Cope With
   Emotional Problems of Chronic
   Physical Illness
   By Joann LeMaistre, Ph.D.

Alpine Guild
P.O. Box 183
Oak Park, Illinois 60303

Express Yourself
   By Peg L. Johnson

Pegijohn
6432 Fifth Avenue So.
Richfield, MN 55423

Home Health Care
   By Joann Friedman

W.W. Norton & Co. Ltd.
500 Fifth Avenue
New York, New York 10110

Neuromuscular Disorders
  A Guide for Patient and Family
    By Steven P. Ringel

Raven Press
1185 Avenue of the Americas
New York, New York 10036

Non-Chew Cookbook
  by J. Randy Wilson

Wilson Publishing, Inc.
P.O. Box 2190

Glenwood Springs, CO 81602

Meals For Easy Swallowing
  By Vicki Appel
    Sandy Calvin
    Gena Smith
    Donna Woehr

Muscular Dystrophy Association
3561 E. Sunrise Drive
Tucson, Arizona 85718
(605) 529-2000

Handbook of Living Will Laws
  1992 Edition

Society for the Right to Die
250 West 57th Street
New York, New York 10107

Catalogs for Daily Living

Enrichments
Bissell Healthcare Company
P.O. Box 579
Hinsdale, Illinois
(800) 323-5547

Catalog of every day aids for daily
  living.

Fred Sammons
Box 32
Brookfield, Illinois
(800) 323-5547

Catalog for health care professionals
  equipment, orthotics, ADL's, etc.

Video Tapes

It's Your Choice
  An education video presenting
    information to people who need to
    make an informed decision about
    whether to use a ventilator.

The ALS Association
21021 Ventura Blvd.
#321
Woodland Hills, CA 91364
(818) 340-7500

(800) 782-4747

A Thief in the Night
  Narrated by Michael Gross
    11 minute information video on
      ALS and The ALS Association

The ALS Association
21021 Ventura Blvd.
#321
Woodland Hills, CA 91364
(818) 340-7500
(800) 782-4747

Right to Die True story of one woman's fight with ALS	Loan The ALS Association 21021 Ventura Blvd. #321 Woodland Hills, CA 91364 (818) 340-7500 (800) 782-4747
One More Season Charlie Wedemeyer Story	Loan The ALS Association 21021 Ventura Blvd. #321 Woodland Hills, CA 91364 (818) 340-7500 (800) 782-4747
Ask the Experts 11 leading ALS experts Philadelphia ALS Chapter	Loan The ALS Association 21021 Ventura Blvd. #321 Woodland Hills, CA 91364 (818) 340-7500 (800) 782-4747

Audio Tapes

State-of-the-Art Management of ALS Series of audio tapes of Managing ALS Conference, 1988 Long Beach, California	Loan The ALS Association 21021 Ventura Blvd. #321 Woodland Hills, CA 91364 (818) 340-7500 (800) 782-4747
Toward More Effective Management in ALS Series of audio tapes of Managing ALS Conference, 1991 Cleveland, Ohio	Loan The ALS Association 21021 Ventura Blvd. #321 Woodland Hills, CA 91364 (818) 340-7500 (800) 782-4747

Communication

AT & T National Special Needs Center 2001 Route 46 Parsippany, New Jersey 07045 (800) 233-1222	Special communication products for people with hearing, vision, motion, and speech impairments.

Index

337